Marc Sindou
Yves Keravel
Aage R. Møller (eds.)

Hemifacial Spasm

A Multidisciplinary Approach

SpringerWienNewYork

Prof. Dr. Marc Sindou
Hôpital Neurologique, Lyon, France

Prof. Dr. Yves Keravel
Hôpital Henri Mondor, Creteil, France

Prof. Dr. Aage R. Møller
Department of Neurological Surgery, University of Pittsburgh, Pittsburgh, U.S.A.

Printed in Austria

Typesetting: Thomson Press (India) Ltd., New Delhi 110001

Printing: DAN, Ljubljana, Slovenia

Graphic design: Ecke Bonk

Cover illustration: Posterior operative view of the left cerebello-pontine angle in a patient operated on for a left Hemifacial spasm due to a neuro-vascular conflict between the facial nerve and the PICA. [**7**: facial nerve, **8**: cochleo-vestibular nerve, **9**: glosso-pharyngeal nerve, **10**: vagal nerve; **floc.**: flocculus; **V**: vertebral artery, **pica**: postero-inferior cerebellar artery, **L**: labyrinthine artery] Left: A pica loop is cross-compressing infero-laterally (arrow-heads) the Root Exit Zone (REZ) of the facial nerve, hidden by the cochleo-vestibular nerve. Right: The offending PICA loop has been pushed away (downward) from the facial REZ (7) with a microsucker.

Printed on acid-free and chlorine free bleached paper

With 95 partly coloured Figures

Library of Congress Cataloging-in-Publication Data

A hemifacial spasm : a multidisciplinary approach / M. Sindou, Y. Keravel. A.R. Møller (eds.).
p. cm.
Includes bibliographical references.
ISBN 3-211-82792-7 (alk. paper).
1. Face—Movement disorders. 2. Spasms. I. Sindou, Marc, 1943– II. Keravel, Yves, 1944– . III. Møller, Aage R.
[DNLM: 1. Facial Muscles—physiopathology. 2. Facial Muscles—innervation. 3. Spasm. 4. Facial Nerve—physiopathology. WE 705 H488 1997]
RC418.H46 1997
617.5′2—dc21

ISBN 3-211-82792-7 Springer-Verlag Wien New York

Preface

Hemifacial spasm constitutes a severe disability, not only aesthetic because of the visible involuntary contractions affecting the muscles on one side of the face, but also functionally for daily life. This chronic disease has no curative medical treatment and is almost never, even slightly, favourably influenced by sedative medication. Its psychological consequences are really devastating, isolating the patient from his environment and destroying his social life.

Until recently, this peculiar syndrome had remained enigmatic. But during the last two decades, important advances have been made in the comprehension of its mechanisms and the efficacy of its treatment. A neurovascular conflict has been recognized as the almost constant cause of the disease. Microsurgical vascular decompression by liberating the nerve from the cross-compression exerted by an elongated neighbouring artery at the root exit zone of the facial nerve from the brain stem is the curative treatment. Botulinic toxin injected in the facial muscles turned out to be helpful to alleviate the facial contractions, even though its effects are generally transient. Taken as a palliative treatment, botulinic toxin injections can be indicated in those patients who do not want or would not tolerate an open surgery.

A wide range of specialists are involved in the diagnosis and the management of this disease: neurologists, ophthalmologists, neurophysiologists, electromyographists, neuroradiologists and, of course, neurosurgeons. For these specialists, this multidisciplinary review of the topic will be of interest.

Marc Sindou
Yves Keravel
Aage Møller

Contents

Introduction

Hemifacial spasm (HFS) is a rare disorder (its incidence is less than 1 in 100,000 in the U.S.A.) that is *characterized* by involuntary contractions of muscles on one side of the face. As defined by Wilkins (Wilkins, R. H. Hemifacial spasm: A review. Surg. Neurol. 36: 251–277, 1991), HFS is a syndrome of spontaneous and gradual onset that has as its hallmark the intermittent twitching of the muscles of facial expression on one side of the face. Typical HFS – which is the most common form of this disorder – begins in the orbicularis oculi muscle and subsequently spreads to involve other muscles that are innervated by the ipsilateral facial nerve. Voluntary facial movements often trigger the involuntary contractions of the face. Characteristically, the frequency and intensity of the spasms increase over a period of 1–10 years, and they may be followed by a sustained spasm. The spasms may fluctuate in severity and they are often affected by stress, but generally the spasm becomes more pronounced and truly disabling over time. HFS has *great cosmetic and psychological effects*, and in its advanced forms the patient's vision can be affected. HFS occurs almost exclusively in *adults*; the average age of patients in HFS studies is in the mid-fifties. The *sex ratio is slightly higher in females* than in males (incidence of 0.81 versus 0.74 per 100,000) (Auger, R. G. and Whisnant, J. P. Hemifacial spasm in Rochester and Olmsted County, Minnesota, 1960 to 1984. Arch Neurol 47: 1233–1234, 1990). The *left side of the face is affected twice* as often as the right side. The objective *electromyographic signs* of HFS are rhythmically-occurring discharges at high frequencies (20 to 200 Hz), with almost complete synchronization of the discharges within the ipsilateral facial muscles (i.e., *synkinesis*). There is a characteristic abnormal muscle contraction in patients with HFS that can be demonstrated by electrically stimulating one branch of the facial nerve while recording EMG responses from a muscle that is innervated by a different branch of the facial nerve.

Previous to the last two decades this peculiar disease had remained an enigma and was *resistant to all kinds of treatments*. But *within these two last decades important advances* in ascertaining the pathophysiology of HFS have been made which has led to an increase in the efficacy of treatment.

There have been two main *hypotheses* regarding the mechanisms involved in HFS. Gardner (Gardner, W. J. Crosstalk – the paradoxical transmission of a nerve impulse. Arch. Neurol. 14:149–156, 1966) proposed that an abnormal cross-transmission between individual fibers of the facial nerve (ephaptic transmission) gives rise to the spasm and synkinesis that are typical in patients with HFS. This hypothesis was supported by subsequent electrophysiological studies (e.g., Nielsen, V. K. Pathophysiological aspects of hemifacial spasm. Part I. Evidence of ectopic excitation and ephaptic transmission. Neurology 34: 418–426, 1984) that were interpreted to indicate that peripheral ectopic excitation and ephaptic transmission occurs within the facial nerve fibers of patients with HFS. Ferguson proposed the hypothesis that it is an increased excitability in the facial motonucleus that causes the signs of HFS (Ferguson, J. H. Hemifacial spasm and the facial nucleus. Ann. Neurol. 4: 97–103, 1978). This increased excitability was assumed to be induced by abnormal peripheral nervous activity in the facial nerve. Intraoperative electrophysiological studies in patients undergoing microvascular decompression (MVD) to relieve HFS have supported the latter hypothesis (e.g., Møller, A. R. and Jannetta, P. J. On the origin of synkinesis in hemifacial spasm: Results of intracranial recordings, J. Neurosurg. 61: 569–576, 1984; Møller, A. R. Hemifacial spasm: Ephaptic transmission or hyperexcitability of the facial motor nucleus? Exp. Neurol. 98: 110–119, 1987).

Micro Vascular Decompression (MVD) *of the seventh cranial nerve* at its root exit zone (REZ) from the brainstem has been recognized for the last two decades as being the most effective treatment for HFS. MVD has a high success rate and a low rate of complications when the procedure is performed by experienced surgeons and when the abnormal muscle response and brainstem auditory evoked potentials (BAEP) are being monitored. Although disorders such as trigeminal neuralgia can be controlled, at least for a certain period of time, by medications, especially those of the anti-epileptic type, there is no known medical treatment for HFS.

More recently, the use of *botulinum toxin* in treating HFS was introduced. This treatment has been shown to be helpful in alleviating the spasm in patients with HFS, although its effects are most often transient and there are considerable side-effects, but for some patients, botulinum toxin injections may provide enough relief to avoid surgery, at least temporarily.

The *vascular conflict* that is usually found at the REZ of the facial nerve during operations on patients with HFS has been recognized as being the cause of the disease. The REZ of the seventh cranial nerve is known as a "critical anatomical site," as it corresponds to the junction of oligodendrocyte myelin and Schwann cell myelin.

The probability that vascular compression is directly involved in creating the symptoms and signs of HFS is supported by the observation that vascular decompression of the facial nerve causes the abnormal muscle response to disappear (Møller, A. R. and Jannetta, P. J. Microvascular decompression in hemifacial spasm: Intraoperative electrophysiological observations. Neurosurgery 16: 612–618, 1985) thus indicating that the facial motonucleus is no longer being subjected to abnormal antidromic impulses. With the technology of modern imaging techniques (Magnetic Resonance Imaging, MRI), images are sufficiently refined to demonstrate the neurovascular conflict(s).

June 1996

M. Sindou
Y. Keravel
A. Møller

Acknowledgements

The editors want to especially acknowledge the ANPP Foundation (Paris) and Mrs Hélène OLLAT (M.D.), its scientific director, for their generous support which allowed contributors to meet together in Chinon, France, to prepare this book.

The Editors thank Cleat **Szczepaniak** and Joyce **Beatty** for their superb secretariat assistance. Particular thanks are given to **Cleat Szczepaniak** for her excellent and meticulous copy editing of the entire volume.

Descriptive anatomy of the seventh and eighth nerves

Ph. Mercier[1], **G. Brassier**[2], and **St. Velut**[3]

[1]Laboratoire d'Anatomie, Faculté de Médicine Angers, Service de Neurochirurgie et Universitaire d'Angers, Angers, France
[2]Service de Neurochirurgie, Faculté de Médicine, Université de Rennes, France
[3]Laboratoire d'Anatomie, Faculté de Médicine, Université de Tours, France

Summary

Advances in microsurgery for pathologies of the cerebellopontine angle require excellent knowledge of the anatomy of neural and vascular structures and of neurovascular relationships in this area. This chapter summarizes the authors' personal works as well as those presently found in the literature.

Key words: Microsurgery, anatomy, facial nerve, cochleo-vestibular nerve, arterial vascularization.

Personal anatomical laboratory studies

We studied the cerebellopontine angles (CPA) on both sides in 25 adult cadavers. Following formaldehyde fixation for 48 hours, the specimens were injected by catheterization of the common carotid and vertebral arteries. Red latex was used in 20 of the specimens and chinese ink in the remaining 5 as tracer elements. In some cases, the veins were perfused with a blue-colored latex solution. The calvarium and the cerebrum were removed to expose the tentorium cerebelli. Then the tentorium was sectioned and reflected posteriorly and the cerebellum was retracted to provide a superior view of the CPA. After that, the arachnoidal membrane, the superior petrosal vein, the anterior inferior cerebellar artery (AICA), the seventh (CN VII) and the cochlear vestibular (CN VIII) cranial nerves were examined using 3X to 20X magnification operating microscope (Wild Leitz and Zeiss Opmi). After removing the superior wall of the internal auditory canal with a drill to study the arachnoid of the canal, the cerebellum, with its preserved nerves and arteries, was removed from the skull for examination of the original course and termination of the vessels related to CN VII and CN VIII. The nerves were next freed from their osseous beds by sectioning the cranial nerves flush with the foramina orifice through which they emerged, i.e., in the case of the cochlear vestibulo-facial nerve bundle, at the level of the falciform crest. This made it possible to explore arterial supply to the facial nerve at the level of the brainstem.

I. Neural relationships

CN VII has both a motor and a sensory root, the latter called the nervus intermedius. The two roots appear at the caudal border of the pons, just lateral to the recess between the olive and the inferior cerebellar peduncle, the motor part being the more medial. The vein of the middle cerebellar peduncle often runs between the two roots. The two roots form a 160° angle with their counterpart nerve. The first 2 or 3 millimeters of the motor root, at its origin, seems to adhere to the pons (Fig. 1) and then it crosses the cerebellopontine angle, where its course shifts gradually upward. CN VIII lies immediately to the lateral side of the sensory root. The nervus intermedius usually passes closer to CN VIII than to CN VII as these nerves approach the internal acoustic meatus. The nervous intermedius often consists of several fascicles. In one fifth of cases [14], it is not a separate nerve until it reaches the internal auditory meatus. The intermedius nerve forms a curve around the motor portion of the facial nerve. When it emerges from the pons it is in a lateral-dorsal position but becomes ventral to the facial nerve in the internal acoustic meatus (Fig. 3). The length of CN VII between the pons and the porus is about 12 to 16 mm (mean 13 mm). Salah [15] reported

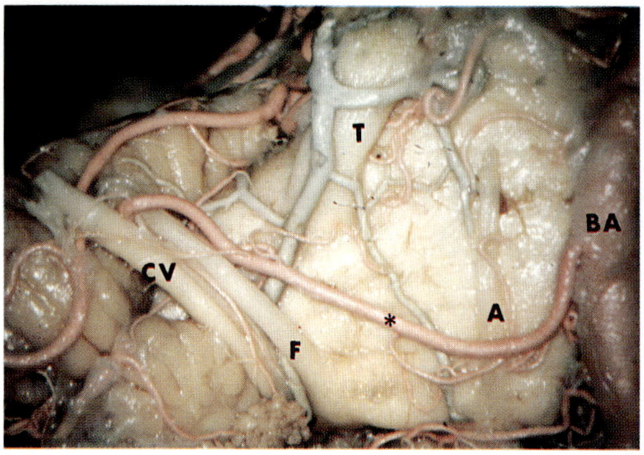

Fig. 1. Right anterior view of the pons. *F* facial nerve; *CV* cochleovestibular nerve; * anterior inferior cerebellar artery; *T* trigeminal nerve; *BA* basilar artery; *A* abducens nerve

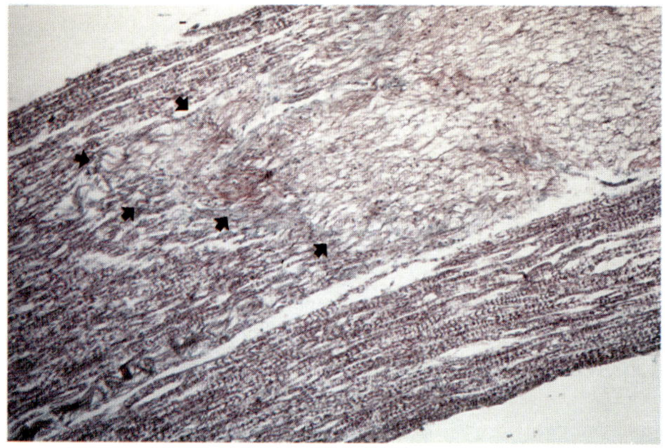

Fig. 2. Photomicrograph of a section of the facial nerve roots (trichrome de Masson). The transition zone, or pial ring, is arch-shaped and characterized by a net diminution of myelin (arrows)

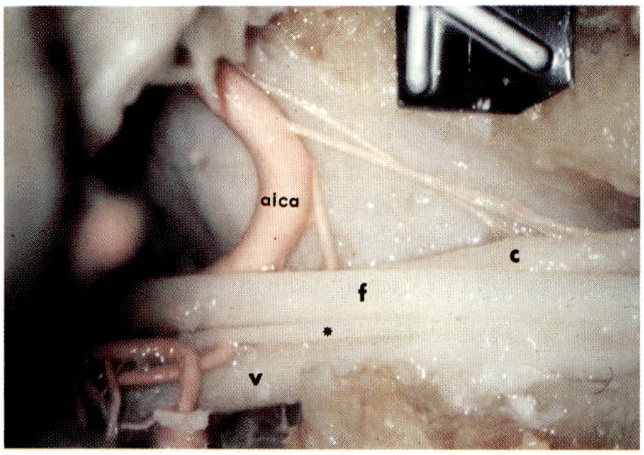

Fig. 3. Right superior view of the internal acoustic meatus. *f* facial nerve; *c* cochlear nerve; *v* vestibular nerve; * intermediate nerve; *aica* anterior inferior cerebellar artery

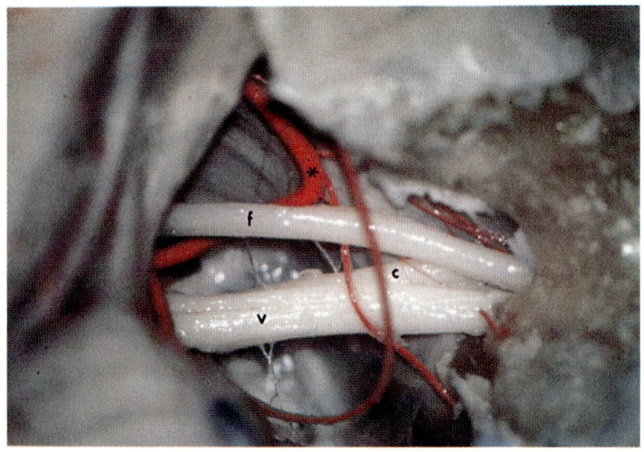

Fig. 4. Right superior view of the internal acoustic meatus. *f* facial nerve; *c* cochlear nerve; *v* vestibular nerve; * anterior inferior cerebellar artery

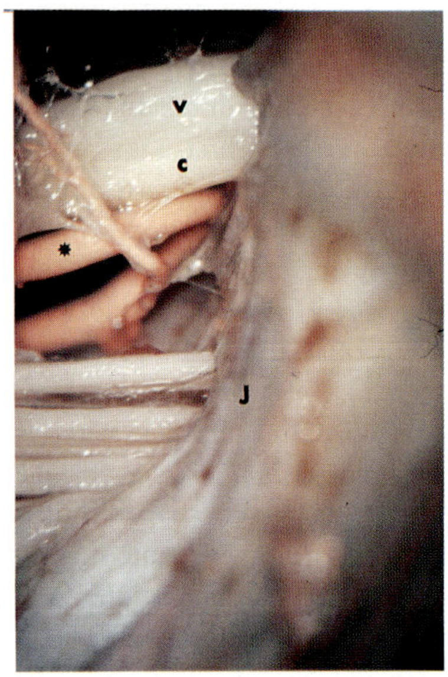

Fig. 5. Right posterior view of the pontocerebellar angle. *c* cochlear nerve; *v* vestibular nerve; * anterior inferior cerebellar artery; *J* jugular foramen with the exit of the glossopharyngeal, the vagus, and the accessory nerves

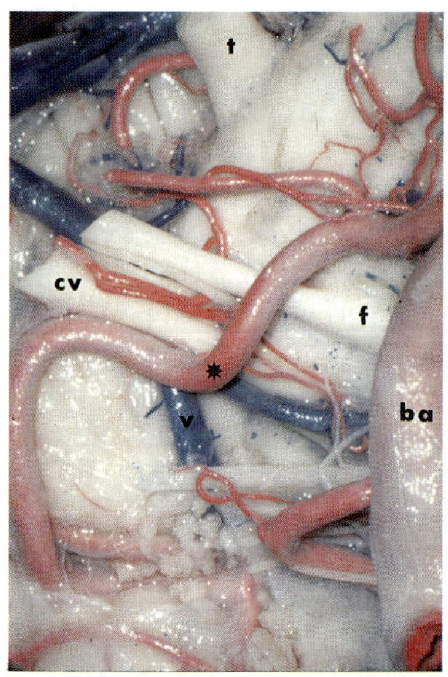

Fig. 6. Right anterior view of the pons. *f* facial nerve; *cv* cochleovestibular nerve; * anterior inferior cerebellar artery; *t* trigeminal nerve; *ba* basilar artery; *v* vein of the middle cerebellar peduncle that courses under the CN VII-VIII nerve complex

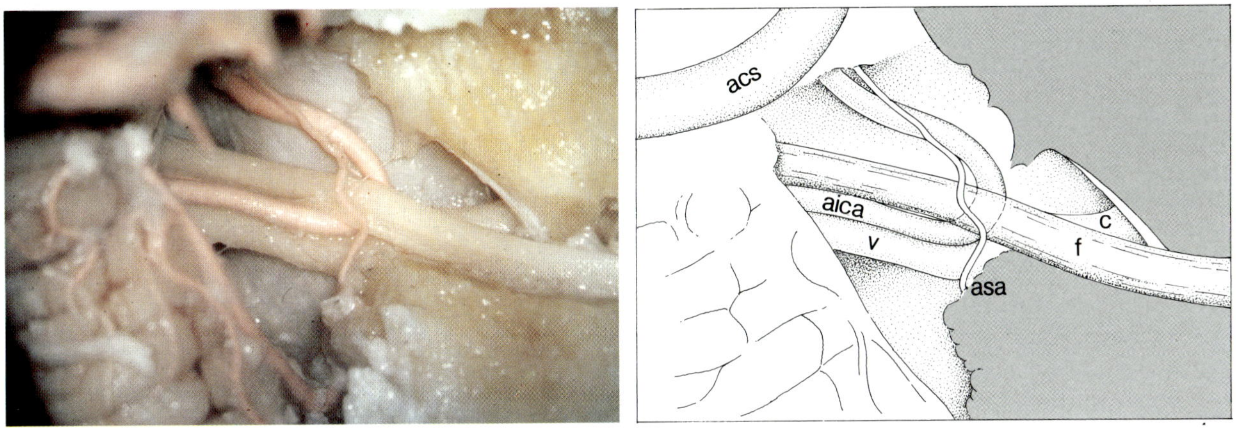

Fig. 7. Right superior view of the acoustico-facial bundle. *f* facial nerve; *C* cochlear nerve; *V* vestibular nerve; *As* subarcuate artery; *aica* anterior inferior cerebellar artery

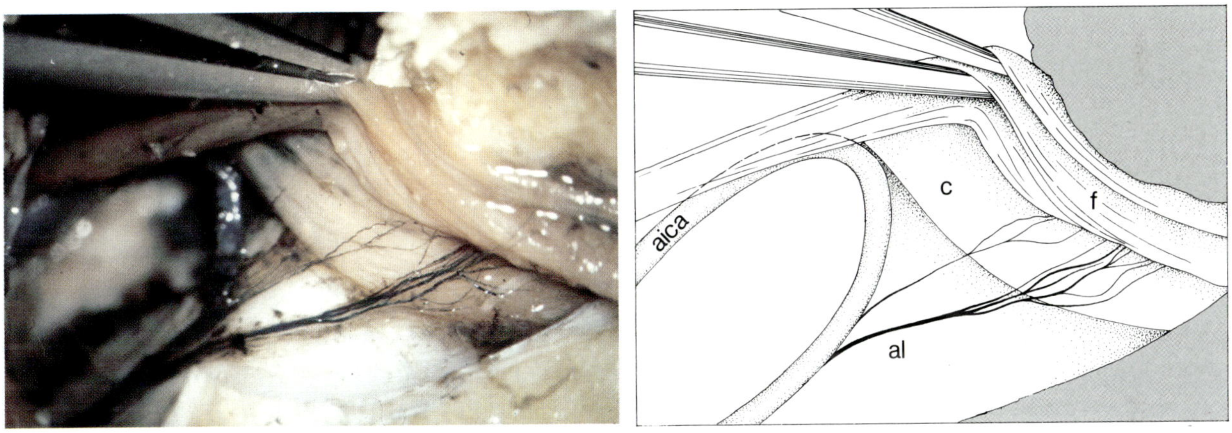

Fig. 8. Right superior view of the internal acoustic meatus. *F* facial nerve; *C* cochlear nerve; *Al* labyrintic artery; *aica* anterior inferior cerebellar artery

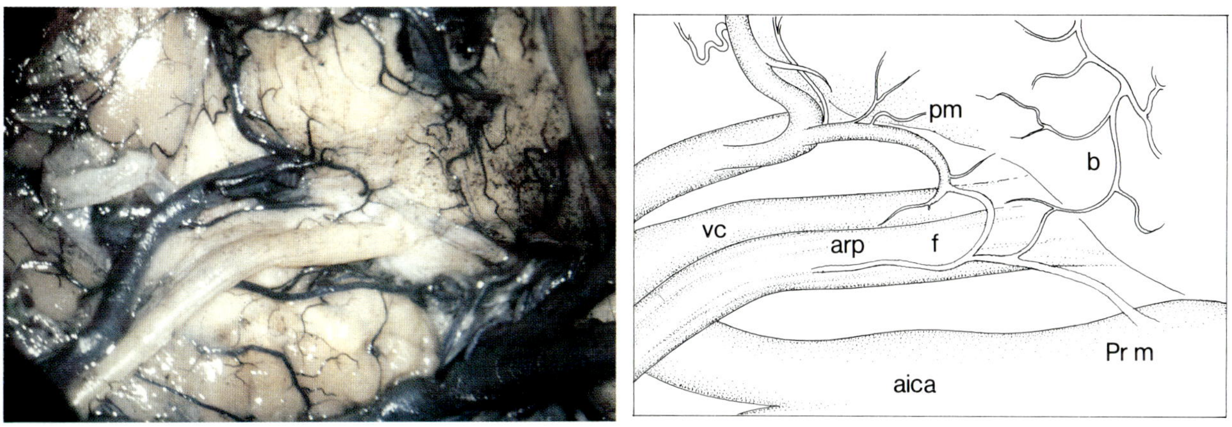

Fig. 9. Anterior view of the facial nerve at the level of the pons. *F* facial nerve; *VC* vestibulocochlear nerve; *arp* proximal radicular artery; *aica* anterior inferior cerebellar artery; *b* basilar branch; *pm* post-meatal AICA branch; *prm* pre-meatal AICA branch

Table 1. Relationship between the loop of the AICA and the VII–VIII in the C.P.A.

	Sunderland 1945	Mazzoni 1970	Salah 1978	Mercier 1980	Ouaknine 1981–82
Loop under the nerves	26%	51%	50,50%	38%	52%
Loop between the nerves	49%	43%	39%	56%	36%
Loop over the nerves	2%	6%	10,50%	2%	9%
No loop	23%			4%	3%

Table 2. Relationship of loops of the AICA with the internal auditory meatus

	Sunderland 1945 242	Mazzoni 1970 100	Boussens 1972 20	Salah 1978 85	Martin 1980 50	Mercier 1980 50	Ouaknine 1981–82 65
Loop outside the meatus	36%	33%	60%	64%	46%	40%	56%
Loop at the orifice	25%	27%	22%	25%	54%	32%	25%
Loop inside the meatus	39%	40%	15%	14%		28%	19%

the length to be between 10 and 13 mm (mean 12 mm) and Lang [4] reported the average length to be between 15 and 50 mm (mean 19.5 mm).

Histological appearance

Tarlov [17, 18] described that a nerve root consists of both a central glial and a peripheral non-glial segment. This transition zone – called "pial ring" – is arch-shaped and is characterized by a plexus of neuroglial fibers and connective tissue and by an important diminution of myelin (Fig. 2). Many of the axons passing through the pial ring may undergo constriction at this level. The pial ring seems to be a variable distance from the brainstem. According to Tarlov, the glial segment of the root of CN VII is between 0.5 and 1.2 mm, and that of both the cochlear and vestibular nerves is even longer (5 to 10 mm).

II. Neurovascular relationships

The anterior inferior cerebellar artery (AICA) arises as a single trunk from the basilar artery (BA) in 78% of cases, as 2 arteries in 18% of cases, and in 4% of cases as 3 arteries within the lowest two-thirds of the BA (medial third 40% and inferior third 60%) [9]. The AICA passes in front (70%), behind (22%), or between (8%) the bundles of CN VI; then the artery runs lateral and slightly downwards (premeatal segment), crosses the cochleovestibular bundle (meatal segment), makes a loop, then gives off numerous collateral branches and turns backwards to reach the cerebellum (postmeatal segment) (Fig. 4). When there are two AICAs or when the AICA is divided into two main branches in the premeatal segment, both of them make a loop at different distances from CN VII and CN VIII. We find loops of the AICA or one of its branches in 96% of our cases. There are three different types of relationships between each loop and the CN VII-CN VIII complex (Table 1): 1) loop under the nerves (38% of our cases) (Figs. 5 and 6); 2) loop between the nerves (56% of our cases); 3) loop over the nerves (2% of our cases); and 4) no loop (4% of our cases). There are three different types of relationships between each loop and the meatus (Table 2): 1) loop outside the meatus (40% of our cases); 2) loop at the porus acusticus (32% of our cases); and 3) loop inside the meatus (28% of our cases). As outlined in these two Tables, our results do not really differ from those of other investigators [2, 5, 8, 12, 13, 15, 16, 17]. In our personal material, in 10 cases a loop of the vertebral artery (4 cases) or of the posterior cerebellar artery (6 cases) was visualized near the origin of the facial nerve. Only Lang [4] noted that the PICA reaches as far as the lower border of CN VII and CN VIII (15 patients, or 50%).

The cerebellar vascular territory of the AICA is very variable and depends on the development of the two other cerebellar branches (the anterior superior artery and the posterior cerebellar artery); in 26% of our cases the AICA was found to be vascularizing only the flocculus, in 36% of our cases the AICA was found to be vascularizing the flocculus and the cerebellar territory close to the horizontal sulcus, and in 38% of our cases the AICA was found to be vascularizing the anterior inferior half of the cerebellum. In the remaining cases, the PICA was found to be vascularizing the flocculus and the cerebellar territory close to the horizontal sulcus and/or the anterior inferior half of the cerebellum. These variabilities in the vascular territory may explain the nonsymptomatic or symptomatic consequences of AICA occlusion [1].

During its course, the AICA gives off numerous branches: the perforating arteries, the subarcuate artery, the auditive artery, and some branches that supply blood to the facial nerve.

The perforating arteries arise from the premeatal or postmeatal segments close to the brainstem and probably supply blood to the nucleus of the facial nerve in the pons.

The subarcuate artery is an important small artery that has been described in detail by Nager [11]. This artery supplies blood to the atrium mastoideum and the ductus semicircularis lateralis. It arises from the premeatal segment (in 58% of our cases), the meatal segment (in 12% of our cases) or the postmeatal segment (in 26% of our cases); in a few cases (4% of our cases), it arises from a labyrinthine artery or a recurrent artery. The subarcuate artery courses laterally and enters the temporal bone in the subarcuate fossa, which is situated 1 or 2 mm above the porus acusticus. As Fisch [3] did, we call any artery going to the bottom of the internal auditory canal a labyrinthine artery. This artery is almost constant and we found it in 96% of our specimens (Fig. 7). Mazzoni [17] found it in 97% of his cases.

In our study we found that all of the auditive (labyrinthine) arteries that arose from the AICA came more frequently from the premeatal segment (42%) or the meatal segment (50%) than from the postmeatal segment (8%). The number of arteries was variable (Table 3). In 62% of our cases, we found that only one of the arteries that arose from the AICA bifurcated into the internal auditory canal. In 36% of our cases, we found two arteries arising from the AICA that bifurcated into the internal auditory canal, and in only 1 case (2%) did we find three arteries that did so (Fig. 8).

Table 3. Number of internal auditory arteries in the internal auditory meatus

	Fisch 1968	Mazzoni 1970	Boussens 1972	Salah 1978	Mercier 1980	Ouaknine 1981
1	45%	51%	30%	86%	62%	29%
2	55%	45%	59%	14%	36%	44%
3		4%	10%		2%	18%
4			10%			9%

III. Vascularization of the facial nerve (according to Mercier [10])

A study of the vascularization of the facial nerve in the cerebellopontine angle and in the internal acoustic meatus showed that there were two sources of blood supply: one at the brainstem and the other at the internal acoustic meatus.

Afferent arterioles at the level of the pons

In a study of 50 cadavers, Mercier et al. [10] found a proximal radicular artery situated on the dorsal surface of the facial nerve where the facial nerve emerges from the brainstem. This artery originated from the confluence of a number of arterioles (arteriolae). One of these arterioles, a collateral branch of the premeatal AICA, arose where the latter left the anterior surface of the pons to course with the facial and vestibulocochlear nerve. This arteriole passed the anterior surface of CN VII and CN VIII as they emerged from the brainstem (Fig. 9). Mercier et al. [10] found this arteriole in 48 of the 50 specimens reported in his study (in 1 case there were two arteries: one of these arteries arose from the caudal portion of the AICA, and the other arose from the rostral portion of the AICA. A second arteriole arose from the third middle portion of the basilar artery and it coursed beneath the AICA onto the anterior surface of the pons, ran behind the abducens nerve, and divided into two smaller arterioles – one traveled to the anterior

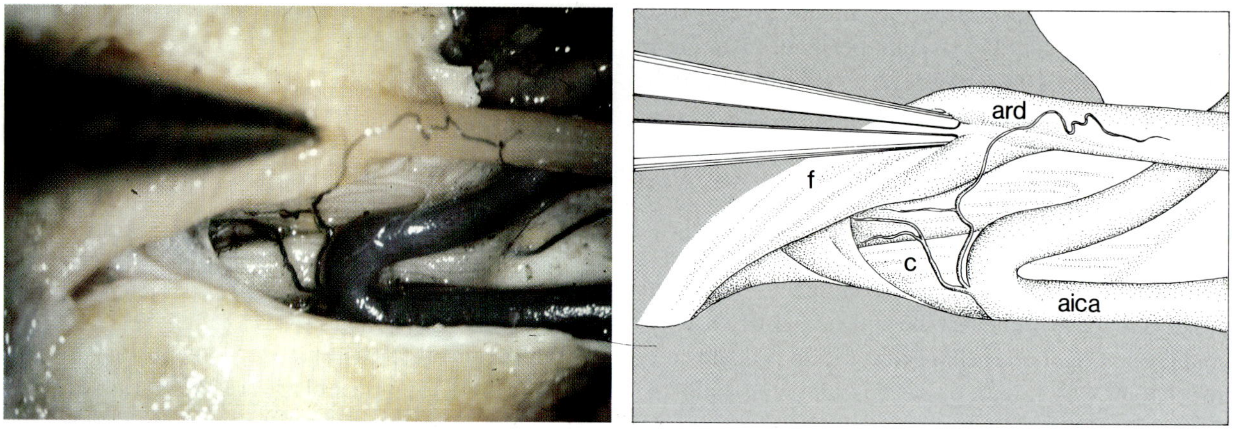

Fig. 10. Left superior view of the internal acoustic meatus. *F* facial nerve; *C* cochlear nerve; *ard* distal radicular artery; *aica* anterior inferior cerebellar artery

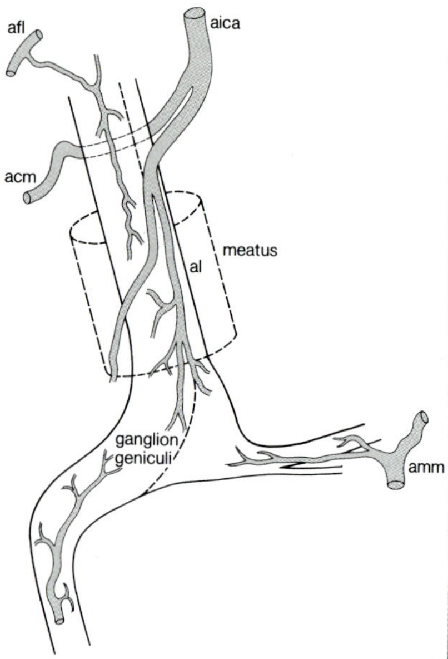

Fig. 11

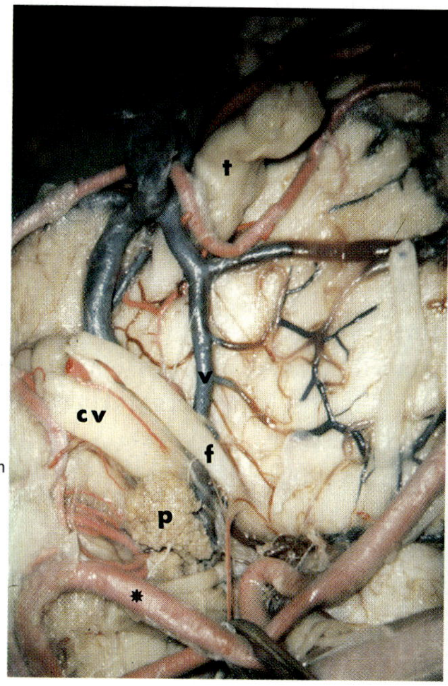

Fig. 12

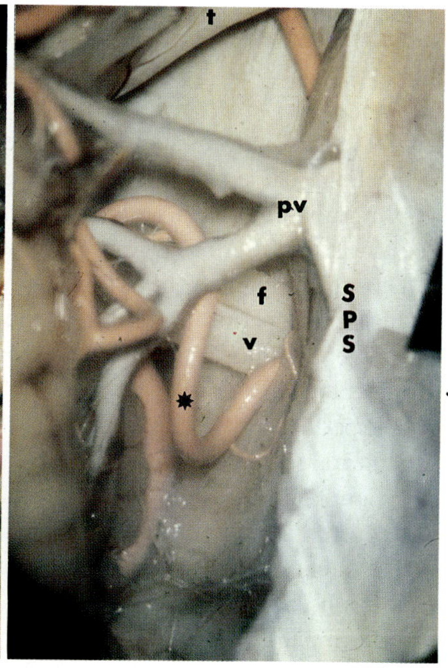

Fig. 13

Fig. 11. Blood supply of the facial nerve. aica anterior inferior cerebellar artery; *acm* middle cerebellar artery; *amm* middle meningeal artery; *al* labyrinthic artery; *afl* artery of the lateral fossa of the bulb

Fig. 12. Right anterior view of the pons. *F* facial nerve; *CV* cochleovestibular nerve; * anterior inferior cerebellar artery; *T* trigeminal nerve; *V* vein of the middle cerebellar peduncle that courses between CN VII and CN VIII; *P* choroid plexus

Fig. 13. Right superior view of the internal acoustic meatus. *F* facial nerve; *V* vestibular nerve; * anterior inferior cerebellar artery; *T* trigeminal nerve; *PV* petrosal vein; *SPS* superior petrosal sinus

surface of the pons and the trigeminal nerve (which it sometimes failed to reach), and the other traveled to the anterior surface of the pons above the bulbar groove and the emerging facial nerve. This second arteriole was present in 43 of 50 cases reported in the Mercier et al. study [10].

A third arteriole, a collateral branch of the post-meatal portion of the AICA, was flush with the pons, where it branched off from the AICA and its perforating branches before reaching the transverse groove of the cerebellum. This arteriole, which was traveling to the facial and the vestibulo-cochlear nerves, divided into 2 or 3 small branches after contact was made with the facial and the vestibulo-cochlear nerves. The arteriole was present in 32 of 50 cases reported in the study by Mercier et al. [10]. A fourth arteriole, a collateral branch of the recurrent artery, originated at the loop of the AICA at the level of the internal acoustic meatus. This arteriole usually traveled along side the vestibulocochlear nerve and then divided when contact was made with the pons. It was present in 19 of the 50 cases reported in the study by Mercier et al. [10]. A fifth arteriole, a branch of the artery to the bulbopontine groove arising from the PICA or from the basilar artery, was present in 16 of the 50 cases reported in the study by Mercier et al. [10]. These five arterioles joined to form the proximal radicular artery. Thus the anastomosis was bi-arterial in 6 cases (12%), tri-arterial in 29 cases (58%), and tetra-arterial in 15 cases (30%) in the 50 cases reported in the study by Mercier et al. [10].

Afferent arterioles at the level of the internal acoustic meatus

Mercier et al. noted that in the 50 cases of their study [10] the afferent arterioles had two different origins:

1. One arteriole arose from either the anterior vestibular artery (arteria vestibularis anterior) or from the artery of the vestibular ganglion (arteria ganglia vestibularis), both of which are branches of the labyrinthine artery. The anterior vestibular artery gave off, at the level of the transverse crest, an arteriole that traveled to the facial nerve and which bifurcated in a "T" configuration, one branch of which anastomosed with the artery of the geniculate ganglion in the facial canal and one (the recurrent branch) which anastomosed with the distal radicular artery. This arteriole was found in 42 cases reported in the study by Mercier et al. [10].
2. A second arteriole originated from either the meatal loop of the AICA or from one of its branches (Fig. 10). Thus this arteriole was a radicular arteriole of the meatus. In 10 cases in Mercier's study [10], the arterioles originated directly from the loop of the AICA; 15 arterioles arose from the labyrinthine artery before the labyrinthine artery divided into its terminal branches. In 3 cases the arterioles arose from the cochlear artery, and in 2 cases the arterioles arose from a meningeal artery.

These branches participated together in the vascularization of the facial nerve (Fig. 11), either by anastomosing with the distal radicular artery coming from the anterior vestibular artery or by dividing into fine capillaries that traveled towards the facial canal (only five of these branches had their origins outside the auditory meatus).

IV. Venous relationship

Numerous veins course over the surface of the brainstem; based on Matsushima's work [16], we think that one of them – the vein of the middle cerebellar peduncle – is particularly close to the CN VII-CN VIII complex; the vein of the middle cerebellar peduncle, which is formed at the inferior margin of the middle cerebellar peduncle by the union of the vein of the cerebellomedullary fissure, the pontomedullary sulcus vein, and the lateral medullary vein, is often seen to ascend between the facial and vestibulocochlear nerves (we have found this to be so in approximately 50% of our cadavers) (Figs. 12 and 13); in the other 50% of our cadavers the vein of the middle cerebellar peduncle is seen to pass laterally between the vestibulocochlear nerve and the flocculus or, more rarely, within the facial nerve. Then, the vein ascends to form one of the medial group of superior petrosal veins.

Conclusion

The present anatomical study shows a loop of the AICA can be found in numerous "normal" cadavers (i.e., those without hemifacial spasm) close to the CN VII-CN VIII complex (see Tables 1 and 2). These loops are located between these nerves and near or inside the meatus, but never at the origin of the facial nerve's dorsal root exit/entry zone. These findings are different from the ones observed in patients with hemifacial spasm, in whom the conflicting loops arising from the AICA and the PICA are located at the very root exit zone of the facial nerve at the pons. When performing a vascular decompression at this level one must be very careful with the perforating arteries that supply the nucleus and the facial nerve at the level of the pons and also with the auditory arteries in order to avoid postoperative facial palsy and hearing loss.

References

1. Atkinson WJ (1949) Anterior inferior cerebellar artery. J Neurol Neurosurg Psychiatry 12: 137–151
2. Boussens J, Caille JM, Piton J, Rozsztes N, Djoumbi E (1970) Contribution à l'étude de l'artère cérébelleuse moyenne et du système artériel du conduit auditif interne. Corrélations anatomo-radiologiques. CR. des séances. 67ème Congrès ORL. Librairie Arnette, Paris, pp 139–142

3 Fish U (1968) L'anatomie chirurgicale du système artériel du conduit auditif interne chez l'homme. Rev Laryngol Rhinol (Bordeaux) 89: 659–671
4. Lang J (1983) Clinical anatomy of the head. Springer, Heidelberg
5. Martin RG, Grant JL, Peace D, Thess C, Rhoton AL Jr (1980) Microsurgical relationships of the anterior inferior cerebellar artery and the facial-vestibulocochlear nerve complex. Neurosurgery 6: 483–507
6. Matsushima T, Rhoton AL Jr, de Oliveira E, Peace D (1983) Microsurgical anatomy of the veins of the posterior fossa. J Neurosurg 59: 63–105
7. Mazzoni A (1969) Internal auditory canal arterial relations at the porus acusticus. Ann Otol 78: 797–814
8. Mazzoni A, Hansen CC (1970) Surgical anatomy of the arteries of the internal auditory canal. Arch Otolaryngol 91: 128–135
9. Mercier Ph (1980) Anatomie Microchirurgicale de l'angle Pontocérébelleux. Thèse, Lyon, p 251
10. Mercier Ph, Cronier P, Mayer B, Pillet J, Fischer G (1982) Microanatomical study of the arterial blood supply of the facial nerve in the ponto-cerebellar angle. Anat Clin 3: 263–270
11. Nager GT (1954) Origins and relations of the internal auditory artery and subarcuate artery. Ann Otol Rhinol Laryngol 91: 51–61
12. Ouaknine GE (1982) Microsurgical anatomy of the arterial loops in the ponto-cerebellar angle and the internal acoustic meatus. In: Samii M, Jannetta PJ (eds) The cranial nerves. Springer, Heidelberg, pp 378–390
13. Ouaknine GE (1982) The arterial loops of the pontocerebellar angle. Adv Oto-Rhino-Laryngol 28: 121–138
14. Rhoton AL Jr (1974) Microsurgery of the internal acoustic meatus. Surg Neurol 2: 311–318
15. Salah S, Bock FW, Perneczky A, Koos WT, Tschabitcher M (1976) Vascular anatomy of the cerebellopontine angle. In: Koos WT, Bock FW, Spetzler RF (eds) Microneurosurgery. Georg Thieme, Stuttgart, pp 69–84
16. Sunderland S (1965) The arterial relations of the internal auditory meatus. Brain 68: 23–27
17. Tarlov IM (1937) Structure of the nerve root. 1. Nature of the junction between the central and peripheral nervous system. Arch Neurol Psychiatry 37: 555–560
18. Tarlov IM (1937) Structure of the nerve root. 2. Differentiation of sensory from motor roots; observations on identification of function in root of mixed cranial nerve. Arch Neurol Psychiatry 37: 1338–1355

Correspondence: Prof. Philippe Mercier, Service de Neurochirurgie, Centre Hospitalier, Universitaire d'Angers, F-49033 Angers Cedex 01, France.

Functional anatomy of the facial nerve

H. Lacombe

Otorhinolaryngology Department, Hopital Delafontaine, Saint-Denis, France

Summary

Embryologic individualization of the facial nerve begins by the fifth week of gestation, but final arrangement occurs by the third month, including communication between the facial nerve and the branches f the trigeminal nerve. In the brainstem the specific nuclei of the facial nerve are located within five columns that correspond to the main functions; however, three quarters of the fibers of the motor component of the facial nerve are of the special visceral efferent type. Fibers' topographical arrangement within the nerve stays controversial in man but seems to follow a partial diffuse type. Acoustico-facial reflex pathways have many clinical implications. Central connections of the facial motonucleus have been mainly demonstrated in animal. Trigeminal communications emphasize the "blink reflex of the orbicularis oculi muscles," which is probably a nociceptive reflex with a complex multisynaptic pathway.

Key words: Facial nerve, embryology, physiology, trigeminal communications.

Introduction

The facial nerve, which is for the most part a motor nerve, includes centrifugal autonomic and centripetal afferent elements, thus providing parasympathetic vegetative and sensory innervation. The present paper does not provide a description of the intratemporal and peripheral portions of the facial nerve. The central portion of the facial nerve, however, will be emphasized in order to present a clearer understanding of its physiological aspects.

Developmental aspects of the seventh cranial nerve

The embryonic development of the facial nerve (CN VII) is associated with the second Hyoid branchial arch.

In the earliest vertebrates the seventh cranial nerve was originally both the motor and sensory nerve of the second gill arch. The evolution towards modern mammals consisted of: 1) the moving of the embryonal homologue into the middle ear, thus making the sensory fibers unimportant and making motor function nearly of primary importance, and 2) the development of individualized true facial muscles, which imply also the evolution of skin [44].

Motor fibers arise mainly from a nuclear group in the special visceral efferent column (SVE) the seventh cranial nerve. The afferent fibers of the seventh cranial nerve develop in much the same way as do the sensory neuroblasts of the eighth nerve within the acoustico-facial primordium, which is composed of a placode, cells of the otocyst, and neural crest elements [21].

The separation between acoustic and facial primordium leading to a distinct facial and cochlear nerve occurs by the fifth week of gestation. Shifting motions of meninges and adjacent structures result in winding and binding curvatures and stretching of the seventh nerve around the abducent nucleus, the otic vesicle, and the inner ear.

The chorda tympani and petrosal nerves are the first branches of the seventh nerve to form. It seems probable that the lingual nerve is first joined by the chorda tympani before its branches reach the zone of the salivary ganglion [16].

In a 12-mm embryo, the geniculate ganglion is well defined and lies rostral to the acoustic ganglion. The nervus intermedius can be recognized in a 14-mm embryo. In a 16-mm embryon, a branch arising from the ventral aspect of the geniculate ganglion joins the undivided glossopharyngeal ganglion, thereby allowing a little latter for communication with the seventh nerve.

In the 8 to 20-mm embryo two main branches (the chorda tympani and the petrosal nerves) are present, with the nerve fibers destined for the zygomatic and temporal regions and for the cervical bundle, all of which lie close to the deep surface of the myoblastic laminae and form the facial muscles.

Distal nerve growth occurs when the embryo is between 20 and 40 mm in size – by the time it grows to 26 mm a thin stapedius branch is developed, as is another tiny branch – the plexus – lateral to the ninth and tenth nerves, thus allowing communication between these two nerves.

In the 60-mm embryo one can see the beginning of a definite arrangement of distal nerve growth by the appearance of an inter-anastomoses of peripheral branches, especially in the infraorbital and perioral regions that communicate freely with branches of the trigeminal nerve. The main facial disposition is definitive by the time the embryo grows to about 80 mm.

There are clinical implications associated with the developments that occur in various developmental fields: for example, the facial canal uncovered by bone, the abnormal course of the seventh cranial nerve, the size of the Fallopian canal [27]. Some congenital pathological findings are interesting from a functional standpoint, for example: 1) the establishment of communication between the trigeminal nerve and the facial nerve that can be seen in a 26-mm embryo; 2) the independent formation of geniculate ganglion and nervus intermedius from motor pathways, which explains the normal tearing and taste that occurs in patients with congenital palsies; and 3) both sixth and seventh nerve palsy seen in patients with Mobius syndrome, although limb abnormalities often associated with this condition cannot be explained by a single unifying theory [4].

Facial nerve nuclei in the brainstem

General disposition among cranial nuclei

In the brainstem, the cranial nerves are distributed in functional areas according to the nature of each nerve fiber. Gaskell in 1886 and 1889 and Herrick in 1913 described 7 columns within the brainstem (Fig. 1) that correspond to a specific category of fibers (the reader is referred to a review of Gaskell and Herrick's work that was done by Nieuwenhuis [32]). The specific nuclei of the facial nerve are located within 5 of these 7 columns. Afferent and efferent areas in the facial nerve are respectively situated in a posterolateral and ventromedial direction.

Three quarters of the fibers of the motor component in the facial nerve are of the special visceral efferent type (SVE) innervating mainly mimic muscles from the second branchial arch. The SVE column contains also the motor nucleus of the fifth nerve and the bulbar ambiguous nucleus of the ninth, tenth, and eleventh cranial nerves.

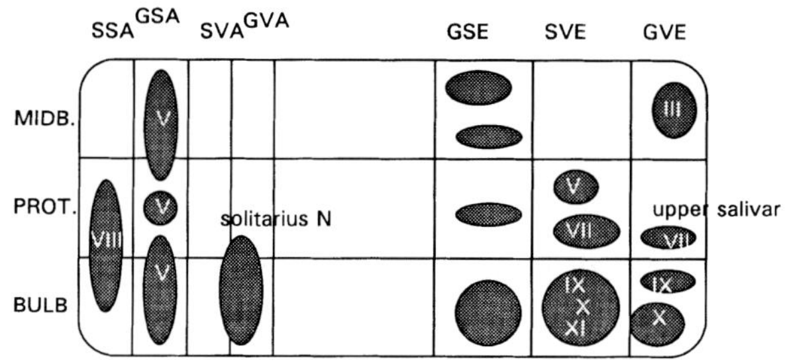

Fig. 1. Functional columns of cranial nerve nuclei in the brainstem

The general visceral efferent (GVE) column contains the facial upper salivary nucleus as well as the Edinger-Westphal (III) nuclei, the inferior salivar (IX) nuclei, and bulbar dorsal (X) nuclei.

The special visceral afferent (SVA) column is mixed with the general visceral afferent (GVA) column in a single bulbar mass called the Solitarius nucleus, which receives gustatory afferent fibers not only from the seventh cranial nerve but also from the ninth and tenth cranial nerves.

The general somatic afferent (GSA) column regroups in the sensory, mesencephalic, superior sensory, and spinal tract of the trigeminal nerve.

Functional arrangement of the seventh nerve nuclei and fibers

The lacrymomuconasal and superior salivar nuclei that produce vegetative fibers are located lateral to the seventh cranial motonucleus within the pontine tegmentum. The intermediate nerve includes sensory fibers that terminate in the solitarius nucleus and other types of fibers that terminate in the superior salivary nucleus. Both types of fibers are intermingled in the cerebellopontine angle (CPA) [36], but separate into two bundles as they enter the brainstem [5].

Facial motor bundle and nucleus

The seventh motor nucleus of the seventh cranial nerve is a column of cholinergic multipolar neurons lying in the ventrolateral portion of the reticular formation of the pons. It is close to the superior olivary

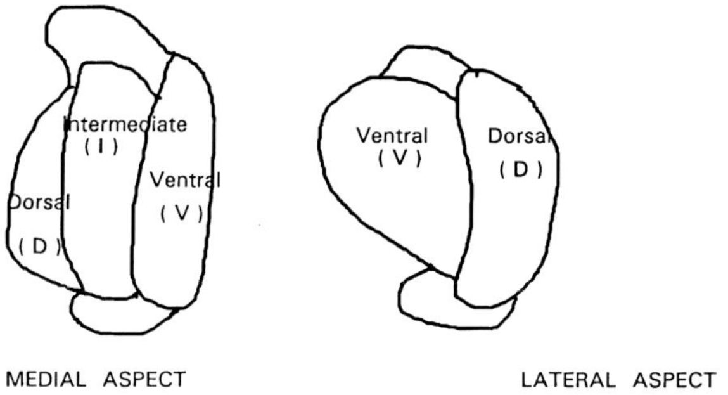

Fig. 2. Illustration of the medial and lateral aspects of the motor nucleus of the facial nerve in man according to Eyries [18]. *D* dorsal; *V* ventral; *I* intermediate. Following this work (serial cuts and Born's anatomical reconstruction techniques), the motor nucleus of the facial nerve was described as roughly triangular in shape. Szentagothai [38] assigned a functional basis to those grouped by stimulation in animal: D = buccinator and buccolabial; V = frontalis and orbicularis; I = auricularis muscles and platysma

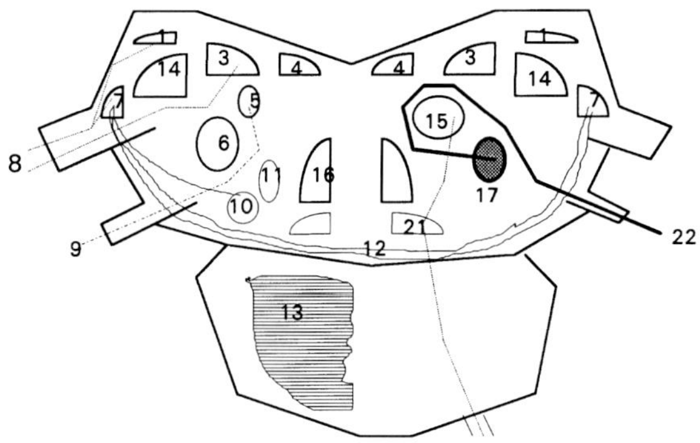

Fig. 3. Horizontal section through cochlear nuclei. **1.** Cochlear dorsal N. **3.** Vestibular N. **4.** Prepositus XII N. **5.** Solitarius N. **6.** V spinal N. **7.** Vental cochlear N. **8.** Vestibulocochlear N. **9.** Intermedius N. **10.** Sup olive N. **11.** Central tegmental B **12.** Trapezoid body **13.** Pontine N. **14.** Inf cereb. ped **15.** VI N. **16.** Med longitude. F **17.** FACIAL NUCLEUS **21.** Medial **22.** FACIAL NERVE

nucleus, and medial to the trigeminal spinal nucleus and the vestibular nucleus. The motor nucleus, which contains about 7000 neurons [42], is divided into three parts (dorsal, ventral, and intermediate) according to a topographical map of various face muscles (Fig. 2) designed by Eyries and Chouard [18]. The exact projection of all face muscles in man is not yet completely known. The upper part of the nucleus that controls the upper face muscles receives fibers from both central hemispheres of the brain.

The exact location of efferent neurons that control the face muscles has been studied by classical neuroanatomical techniques [9]. Radpour and Gacek [35], using horseradish peroxydase (HRP) retrograde labelling techniques in experiments in the cat, proved that the frontalis muscle is the only muscle whose neurons are represented in both the medial and lateral divisions of the motor facial nucleus of the facial nerve, which can explain some failures of reinnervation of this muscle following degenerative nerve pathologies.

Motor fiber pathways

The motor fibers of the facial nerve (Fig. 3) encircle the abducence nucleus, dorsal to the medial longitudinal fasciculus (MLF), project ventrolaterally, and exit the brainstem near the caudal border of the pons in the CPA. The facial nerve contains about 11,600 fibers [25] that course through the temporal bone (intrameatal, tympanic, and mastoid) and exit at the stylomastoid foramen to ramify throughout the parotid gland. Several variations of the course of the facial nerve have been described [13], the main one being a division in the temporal and cervical branches with an intermediate ramus.

The topographical arrangement of fibers in the facial nerve in man is not completely understood as most experimental studies on the facial nerve were done in animals. Classical axonal neuroanatomical degenerative techniques and studies involving retrograde axonal transport with HRP provided the anatomical basis for explaining some clinical observations. In addition, experience acquired as a result of injuries to the facial nerve during middle ear surgery for stapedectomy and from the results of intraoperative stimulation of the seventh cranial nerve during surgery [22] supports the assumption that the facial nerve is organized according to the peripheral distribution of the facial nerve. This assumption is also supported by the positive results of intrafascicular grafting [31] as well as by anatomical [34] and clinical [28] studies. However, studies using the HRP tracer technique in animals [20, 35, 40, 41] indicate that all peripheral branches are distributed throughout the facial nerve at all levels within the seventh cranial nerve in a multifascicular pattern. Moreover, in these studies two groups of sensory fibers were identified: 1) fibers of small diameter (1 to 2 μ) in the intermediate nerve, and 2) myelinated afferent fibers of large diameter that originate in cell bodies in the geniculate ganglion, or afferent fibers from an other source, such as the trigeminal nerve [35].

Finally, considering all the evidence, we may assume that there is a partial diffuse arrangement of fibers in

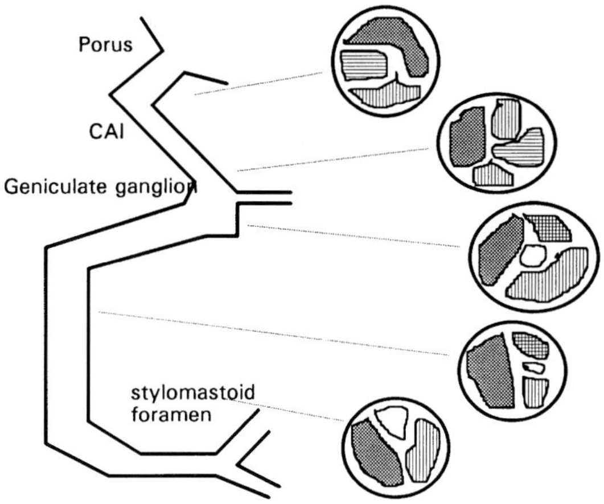

Fig. 4. Intraneural topography

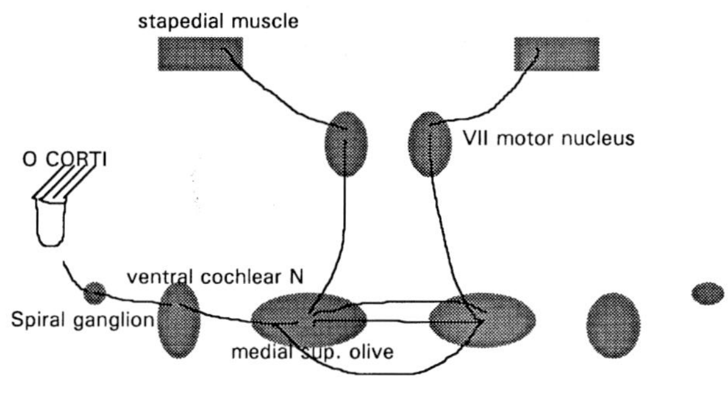

Fig. 5. Stapedial reflex

the facial nerve in man (Fig. 4) that could become more established from the central portion to the distal end of the nerve.

Many clinical implications can be drawn from such observations:

- Seventh nerve lesions in the temporal bone or internal auditory canal result in a global facial weakness rather than a selective one [29].
- A slow-growing compressive lesion such as a vestibular schwanoma rarely results in facial palsy. It has been assumed that the critical number of non-functional facial fibers that can be associated with normal function of the face is 75% [14, 17].
- Following severe facial trauma, random arrangement of fibers within the nerve trunk accounts for the occurrence of misdirected regenerating fibers, thus explaining synkinesis. Mass movements of the face should be correlated to neighboring stimulation of unmyelinated "young" regenerating fibers. However, regenerating axons of immature mammals such as the neonatal rat may be capable of growing back to the appropriate muscle, thus restoring facial motor nucleus somatotopy [41].
- Finally, partial diffuse arrangement of fibers within the nerve trunk explains that primary anastomosis or free grafting on the facial nerve – whatever the process (epineural repair or grafting) – cannot result in an organized reinnervation, regardless of the skill of the surgeon or the chosen biomaterial [12].

Acoustico-facial (stapedius) reflex

Middle ear muscles (stapedius and tensor tympani) are regulators of auditory input to the cochlea. The acoustic stapedius tensor reflex is elicited in man by sound about 85 decibels (dB) above hearing threshold of normal hearing individuals. Tactile or electric stimulations of periauricular areas can also produce a contraction of the stapedial muscle [15]. There is a direct pathway that includes 3–4 neurons (Fig. 5): through primary auditory afferent cells in the ventral cochlea nucleus, with axons in the trapezoid body partially contacting ipsilateral stapedius motoneurons, interneurons of the ipsilateral and contralateral medial superior olive, and stapedius motoneurons [3].

There are indirect pathways that activate the stapedius reflex and that may involve the cells of the red nucleus [3], which are known to respond to sound, and the rubrobulbar tract. The lateral zone of the reticular formation receives fibers from the auditory pathway. Moreover, it should be stressed that parallel to the pathways of the extrapyramidal system the olivocochlear bundle and the stapedius reflex are linked together, since interruption of the former lowers the threshold of the latter [3].

The location of motor neurons in relation to the stapedius muscle has raised a controversy as a result of data obtained from studies that utilized classical retrograde techniques. An HRP study in cat demonstrated their location to be outside the main nucleus of the facial nerve, between the facial and lateral superior olivary nuclei [26].

The acoustico-facial reflex has many clinical applications, mainly because both ipsilateral and contralateral middle ear reflexes are valuable diagnostic and prognostic tools that can be used in patients with conductive hearing loss, retrocochlear disease, and facial palsy [19].

The stapedius reflex is activated by suprathreshold external sounds, which ensures the protection of inner ear sensory receptors by attenuating low-frequency sound pressure. Recently, activation of this reflex has been demonstrated to provide protection against noise-induced hearing loss caused by high-frequency magnetic coil acoustic impulses [8]. The stapedius reflex may play a role in speech processing, since patients with Bell's palsy have impaired speech discrimination [45].

Non-motor fibers

The efferent parasympathetic component of the facial nerve exits the medulla together with the intermediate nerve (Fig. 6). Preganglionic fibers pass from the superior salivary nucleus into the facial nerve and are then distributed: 1) through the greater petrosal nerve to the pterygopalatine ganglion where they synapse (the postganglionic fibers pass to the lacrimal glands), and 2) through the chorda tympani to the lingual nerve, relaying in the submandibular ganglion to the sublingual glands. Chouard [5] found that only the chorda tympani bundle originates in the superior salivary nucleus; whereas the petrosal nerve bundle originates in a lacrymomuconasal nucleus, which is composed of three groups of nerve fibers located in the external part of the radicular fibers.

Central connections are involved in nerve impulses to the salivary nucleus, especially for the secretion of tears, which are not mediated by the pyramidal tract. Fibers from the hypothalamus that are under the influence of higher levels of the brain, such as parts of the cortex, and limbic structures that influence emotions are most likely also involved.

Misrouting of regenerating fibers following severe palsy can explain the crocodile tears syndrome, which manifests as profuse tearing when salivating. This could be explained by parotid secretory fibers sprouting in the lesser petrosal nerve and that enter the empty axon sheaths of secretomotor bundles of the greater petrosal nerve and travel to the sphenopalatine ganglion. The acoustico-facial anastomosis connects the intermediate nerve with vestibular nerve fibers, but these fibers remain in the internal auditory canal, as has been shown using classical neuroanatomical techniques [6]. These fibers may play an important part in the vegetative innervation of the inner ear.

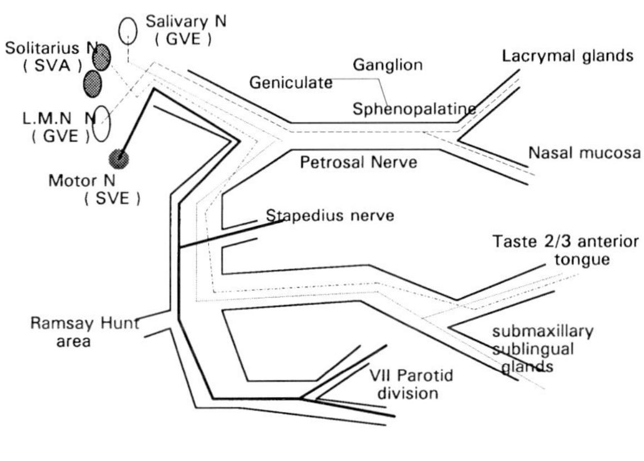

Fig. 6. Systematization of facial nerve components

Special visceral afferent fibers (SVA)

Special visceral afferent fibers, which enable taste from the anterior two-thirds of the tongue, pass through the lingual nerve to the chorda tympani. Their pseudo-unipolar cell bodies lie in the geniculate ganglion where the intermediate nerve enters the geniculate ganglion, and the SVA terminate in the upper part of the nucleus of the tractus solitarius. The latter receives efferent fibers (GVA and SVA) from the ninth and tenth cranial nerves. Only the rostral portion of the tractus solitarius nucleus is afferented by gustative impulses, and is thus named the "gustatile nucleus." This part of the solitarius nucleus is the only portion that sends efferent fibers to the ventro-postero-medial nucleus of the thalamus [2].

General somatic afferent (GSA) fibers

General somatic afferent fibers (GSA) convey sensitivity of the Ramsay-hunt area. They pass to pseudo-unipolar nerve cells in the geniculate ganglion via the auricular branch of ninth cranial nerve. These fibers terminate in the superior sensory (tactile) nerve and spinal tract (pain and thermal sensitivity) of the nucleus of fifth cranial nerve.

Central connections of the facial motonucleus

The motor "face" area

The motor "face" area is situated ventrolaterally in motor cortical regions on the pre- and postcentral fissure, and it receives afferent input from the motor nucleus through the corticobulbar pathway. The projection is bilateral from the lower part of the nucleus, which innervates the muscles of the upper portion of the face (which explains why this portion of the face is spared in patients with central facial palsy). Only some of these corticobulbar fibers directly project on motoneurons, whereas most of them relay in the reticular formation [24]. This occurs especially in the lateral tegmental section of the reticular formation, which is a system of noradrenergic neurons that give propriobulbar projections not only to the nuclei of seventh cranial nerve, but also to those of the fifth, ninth, and twenfth cranial nerves.

Other cortical areas of the face

Besides the motor "face cortical area," many other cortical areas are implicated: 1) premotor and parietal areas; 2) temporal pole of the hemisphere; and 3) the greater part of the temporal cortex, the island, the cingulate area, the hippocampus, and the basolateral part of the amygdala [10]. Extensive studies of the pathways of these other cortical areas have been done in the monkey but they have not been demonstrated in man. Many of these areas project to the hypothalamus and thereby relay expressions of emotions.

Rubrobulbar fibers from upper facial motoneurons

Rubrobulbar fibers from upper facial motoneurons seem to exist in man, but only a few such fibers can be present.

Auditory, secondary, and tertiary fibers involved in the stapedial reflex

Auditory, secondary, or tertiary fibers involved in the stapedial reflex represent other central connections from the facial motonucleus.

Trigeminal communications

The blink reflex

The "blink reflex" of the orbicularis oculi muscles [23] is the main trigemino-facial reflex (Fig. 7). This blink reflex is elicited by electrical stimulation of the supraorbital nerve, which is a branch (V1) of the fifth cranial nerve. Two electrophysiologic components can be observed in the response from the orbicularis oculi muscle. The R_1 component is unilateral and it appears with a latency of about 10 milliseconds. It is an oligosynaptic reflex, whose afferents are sensory fibers of the fifth cranial nerve and efferents are motor fibers

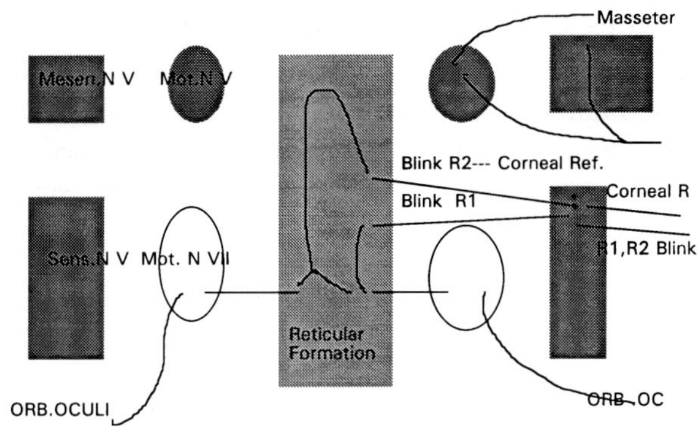

Fig. 7. Organization of the blink reflex

of the seventh cranial nerve. Messina [30] considered this reflex to be a myotatic reflex. The nerve conduction velocity of this reflex indicates that exteroceptive A myelinated fibers of medium size are the fibers that contribute to the efferent pathway of the blink reflex [11, 33].

The R_2 component of the response from the orbicularis oculi muscle occurs with a longer latency and the response is bilateral. It is probably a nociceptive reflex [43] with a complex multisynaptic pathway through afferents that are similar to those of the ascending tracts (the reticulobulbar formation of both motor facial nuclei) of the the R_1 component.

It has been shown that in cases of facial palsy the recovery of the blink reflex precedes that of the stapedial reflex (G. Freyss, unpublished data).

The corneal reflex

The corneal reflex has the same organization as the reflex that provides the R_2 component in the blink reflex response, although afferent fibers for the corneal reflex are most likely myelinated fibers of small size [11].

Superficial communications

The superficial communication that exists between the branches of the fifth and seventh cranial nerves and between the rami of the auriculotemporal nerve and the superior division of the facial nerve are the strongest and most constant of such superficial communication. Many reflex actions of the facial nerve are conveyed through the fifth cranial nerve via such anastomosis. The rami noted above are trigeminal fibers that can be found in branches of the facial nerve, and they may play an important role in mediating facial proprioception and deep sensitivity [1]. This could in some cases explain partial reinnervation and some return of facial function following denervation without grafting [7, 28].

Direct connections from the trigeminal nucleus to the facial nucleus

Direct connections from the trigeminal nucleus to the facial nucleus have yet to be demonstrated on a neuroanatomical level [37] as well as on a neurophysiological level [39].

References

1. Baumel JJ (1974) Trigeminal facial nerve communications: Their function in facial muscle innervation and reinnervation. Arch Otolaryngol 39: 34–44
2. Beckstead RM, Morse JR, Norgren R (1980) The nucleus of the solitary tract in the monkey. Projections to the thalamus and brainstem nuclear. J Comp Neurol 190: 259–282
3. Borg E (1973) On the neuronal organization of the acoustic middle ear reflex. A physiological and anatomical study. Brain Res 49: 101–123
4. Carlson BM (1981) The development of facial muscles and nerves in relation to the mobius syndrome. Otolaryngol Head Neck Surg 89: 903–906
5. Chouard CH (1972) Systeme lacrymo-muco-nasal. In: Chouard CH (ed) Anatomie, pathologie et chirurgie du nerf facial. Masson, Paris, pp 19–21
6. Chouard CH (1975) Acoustico-facial anastomoses in Meniere's disease. Arch Otolaryngol 101: 296–300
7. Conley JJ (1964) Accessory neuromuscular pathways to the face. Trans Am Acad Ophthalmol Otol 68: 1064–1067
8. Counter SA, Borg E (1993) Acoustic middle ear muscle reflex protection against magnetic coil impulse noise. Acta Otolaryngol (Stockh) 113: 483–488
9. Courville J (1966) The nucleus of the facial nerve: The relations between cellular groups and peripheral branches of the nerve. Brain Res 1: 339–354
10. Crosby EC, DeJonge BR (1963) Experimental and clinical studies of the central connections and central relations of the facial nerve. Ann Otol 72: 735–755
11. Cruccu G, Bowsher D (1986) Intracranial stimulation of the trigeminal nerve in man. II. Reflex responses. J Neurol Neurosurg 49: 419–427
12. Crumley R (1980) Spatial anatomy of facial fibers: A preliminary report. Laryngoscope 90: 274–276
13. Davis BA, Anson BJ, Budinger JM (1956) Surgical anatomy of the facial nerve and the parotid gland based upon a study of 350 cervico-facial halves. Surg Gynecol Obstet 102: 385–412
14. De Bischop G, Bence G, Bence Y (1985) Selection of the electrophysiological methods for diagnosis in the facial palsy. In: Portmann M (ed) The facial nerve. Masson, Paris, pp 349–352
15. Djupesland G (1967) Electromyography of the tympanic muscles in man. Int Audiol 4: 34–41
16. Dozin A (1965) Les connexions du ganglion sous-maxillaire chez l'embryon humain. Acta Anat (Basel) 61: 213–258
17. Esslen E (1977) Electromyography and electroneurography. In: Fisch U (ed) Facial nerve surgery. Kugler, Amsterdam, pp 93–100
18. Eyries C, Chouard C (1963) Les origines reelles du nerf facial. Ann Otol Laryngol 80: 775–802
19. Freyss G, Casteran JM (1979) Optimisation de l'utilisation du reflexe stapedien α la distinction des surdites endo et retrocochleaires. Rev Laryngol (Bordeaux) 100: 673–679
20. Gacek R, Radpour S (1982) Fibers orientation of the facial nerve: An experimental study in the cat. Laryngoscope 92: 547–556
21. Gasser RF (1967) The development of the facial nerve in man. Ann Otol Rhinol Laryngol 76: 37–56
22. Kemp LG (1980) Topographical organization of the distal portion of the facial nerve. J Neurosurg 52: 671–673
23. Kimura J (1983) Clinical uses of electrically elicited blink reflex. Adv Neurol 39: 773–786
24. Kuypers HGJM (1958) Cortico bulbar connection to the pons and lower brainstem in man: An anatomical study. Brain 81: 364–388
25. Lang J (1984) Clinical anatomy of the cerebellopontine angle and internal acoustic meatus. In: Pfaltz CR (ed) Adv Oto-Rhino-Laryngol 34: 8–24
26. Lyon MJ (1978) The central location of the motor neurons to the stapedius muscle in the cat. Brain Res 143: 437–444
27. Marquet J (1981) Congenital malformation and middle ear surgery. J Roy Soc Med 74: 27–42
28. Martin H, Helsper JT (1957) Spontaneous return of function following surgical section of the seventh cranial nerve in surgery of parotid tumors. Ann Surg 146: 715–727
29. May M (1973) Anatomy of the facial nerve (spatial orientation of fibers in the temporal bone). Laryngoscope 82: 1311–1329
30. Messina C (1975) On the nature and meaning of the blink reflex early response. Electroenceph Clin Neurophysiol 15: 119–124
31. Millesi H (1977) Technique of free nerve grafting in the face. In: Rubin L (ed) Reanimation of the paralyzed face. CV Mosby Co, St. Louis, pp 124–135
32. Nieuwenhuis R (1974) Topographical analysis of the brainstem: A general introduction. J Comp Neurol 156: 255–276
33. Ongerboer de Visser BW (1983) Anatomical and functional organization of reflexes involving the trigeminal system in man: Jaw reflex, blink reflex, corneal reflex and exteroceptive suppression. Adv Neurol 39: 729–738
34. Podvinec M, Pfaltz CR (1976) Studies on the anatomy of the facial nerve. Acta Otolaryngol (Stockh) 81: 173–177
35. Radpour S, Gacek R (1985) Anatomic organization of the cat facial nerve. Otolaryngol Head Neck Surg 93: 591–596
36. Rhoton AL, Kobayashi S, Hollinshead WH (1968) Nervus intermedius. J Neurosurg 29: 609–618
37. Stewart WA, King RB (1963) Fiber projections from the nucleus caudalis of the spinal trigeminal nucleus. J Comp Neurol 121: 271–286
38. Szenthagothai J (1948) The representation of facial and scalp muscles in the facial nucleus. J Comp Neurol 88: 207–220
39. Tanaka T, Yu H, Kitai ST (1971) Trigeminal and spinal inputs to the facial nucleus. Brain Res 33: 504–508
40. Thomander L, Aldskogius H, Grant G (1982) Motor fibre organization in the intratemporal portion of cat and rat facial nerve studies with the horseradish peroxydase technique. Acta Otolaryngol (Stockh) 93: 397–405
41. Thomander L, Aldskogius H (1985) Facial motor nucleus somatotopy is restored after facial nerve regeneration in neonatal rats. In: Portmann M (ed) Facial nerve. Masson USA, p 210

42. Vanbuskirk C (1945) The seventh nerve complex. J Comp Neurol 81: 303–333
43. Willer JC, Roby A, Boulu P, Boureau F (1982) Comparative effects of electro-acupuncture and transcutaneous nerve stimulation on the human blink reflex. Pain 14: 267–278
44. Wind J (1977) The facial nerve and human evolution. In: Pfaltz CR (ed) Adv Oto-Rhino-Laryngol 22: 215–219
45. Zakrisson J, Borg E, Blom S (1974) The acoustic impedance change as a measure of stapedius muscle activity in man. Acta Otolaryngol (Stockh) 78: 357–364

Correspondence: H. Lacombe, M.D., Otorhinolaryngology Department, Hopital Delafontaine 2, Rue Pierre Delafontaine, F-93205 Saint Denis, France.

Imaging of the normal facial nerve

J. Vignaud[1], **J.-L. Sarrazin**[1], **D. Soulie**[1], **C. Pharaboz**[2], and **Ph. Meriot**[3]

[1]Hopital du Val de Grace, Paris, France
[2]Hopital Begin, Paris, France,
[3]Hopital Morvan, Brest, France

Summary

The imaging of the normal intracisternal and intrapetrosal facial nerve within the internal auditory canal and cerebellopontine angle cistern is described. The facial nerve is best seen using T_2 weighted images obtained in three dimensional Fourier transformation. 0.4-mm thick joint sections in any direction are thus obtained. The facial and cochleovestibular nerves are always seen, and vessels larger than 1-mm thick are analyzed. Their relationship to the facial nerve is seen using two orthogonal projections. Within the facial canal, the facial nerve and the geniculate ganglion normally enhance after gadolinium injection. The facial canal is best seen with high resolution computerized tomography—the entire course of the canal is described as well as the canals of the intrapetrous branch of the facial nerve.

Key words: Facial nerve, facial canal, internal auditory canal, cerebellopontine angle cistern, normal imaging.

Introduction

Knowledge of the normal facial nerve and its neighboring vessels is helpful in understanding the pathological conditions discussed in this report.

I. Facial nerve within the cerebellopontine angle and internal auditory meatus

The facial nerve within the cerebellopontine angle cistern (CPAC) and internal auditory meatus (IAM) is demonstrated by magnetic resonance imaging (MRI).

A precise *delineation requires*:

- *good contrast* between the nerve and the cerebrospinal fluid (CSF): T_2 weighted sequences are mandatory; they image the nerves and vessels in dark grey contrasting with the CSF, which is white. The sequences may be obtained by either spin-echo or gradient-echo techniques [2].
- *high resolution techniques*, by using a matrix 512 × 512 for a field of view of 18 cm. In such a condition, the pixel size is 0.35 mm.
- thin sections: 3 to 0.4 mm, depending on the equipment. If only 3-mm thickness of a section is available, sections must be overlapped in order not to miss a small structure.

The precise study of the relationship between a nerve and its surrounding structures requires sections to be obtained on several planes longitudinally as well as cross-sectionally from the structure to be studied. This is made possible by reformatting images from the data of a series of sections acquired in Two DFT (Two Dimension Fourier Transformation) or from the data of a volume acquired in Three DFT. In such a condition, contiguous sections of 0.4-mm thickness may be obtained in any direction [8, 9].

The vessels are easily demonstrated by the techniques previously described, but MR angiography (MRA) has certain advantages [3]. MRA is performed using gradient-echo T_1 weighted sequences, which image all the vessels in white contrasting with the nerves and brainstem, which are grey, while the CSF is dark grey. Sections are thin (1 mm) and contiguous. However they have rather low resolution due to the size of the matrix (256 × 256) for a field of view 22 × 22 cm wide (pixel size 0.85). On these 'native' sections, on which the angiogram is built, the relationship between the vessels and the nerves is easily studied, but the resolution is too poor to differentiate between the seventh and eighth nerves; and, moreover, for the same reason, reformatted images are fairly unclear. However, new software and techniques are being developed that dramatically improve the quality of MRA images.

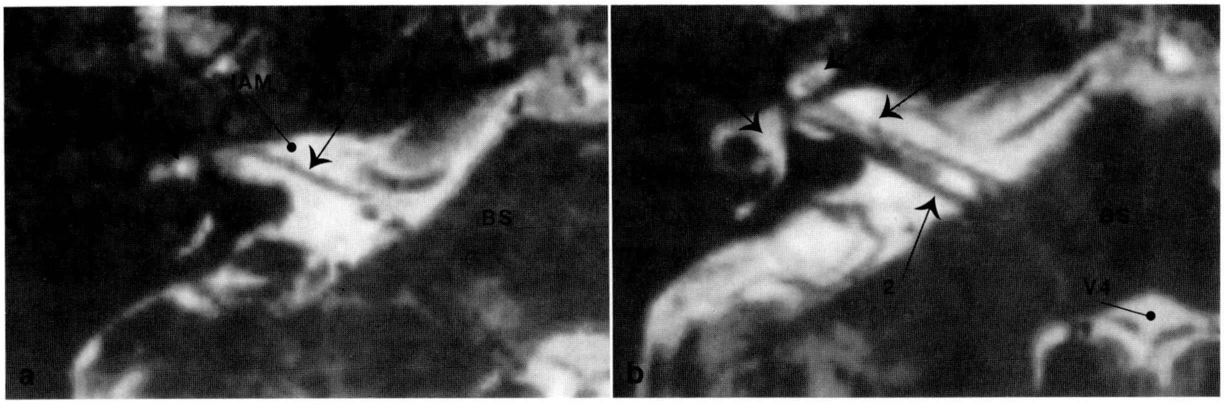

Fig. 1(a-b). Axial 1-mm gradient echo T_2 weighted sequence images through the right cerebellopontine angle (CPA) and inner ear (**a** above the basal turn of the cochlea; **b** level of the basal turn). The facial nerve (*1*) can be followed throughout the CPA and the IAM, above and anterior to the eighth nerve (*2*), with a vascular loop of the AICA (*3*) in the right internal acoustic porus. The cochlea (*4*), the labyrinth (*5*), and the lateral and posterior semicircular canals are also identified thanks to the high signal of the endovestibular fluids. *BS* brain stem; *V4* fourth ventricle; *IAM* internal auditory meatus

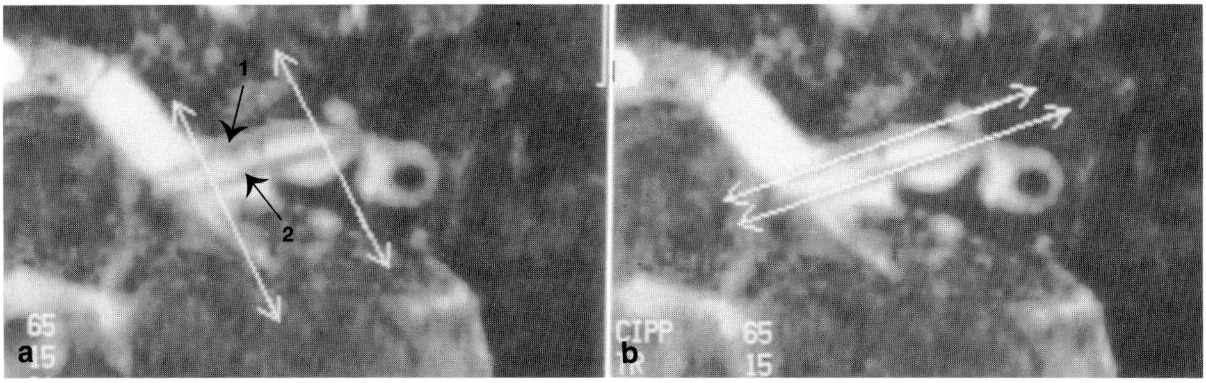

Fig. 2(a-b). Axial 1-mm thin T_2 weighted images focused on the left CPA and inner ear to display two planes of reconstruction chosen by the neuroradiologist. *1* seventh nerve; *2* eighth nerve

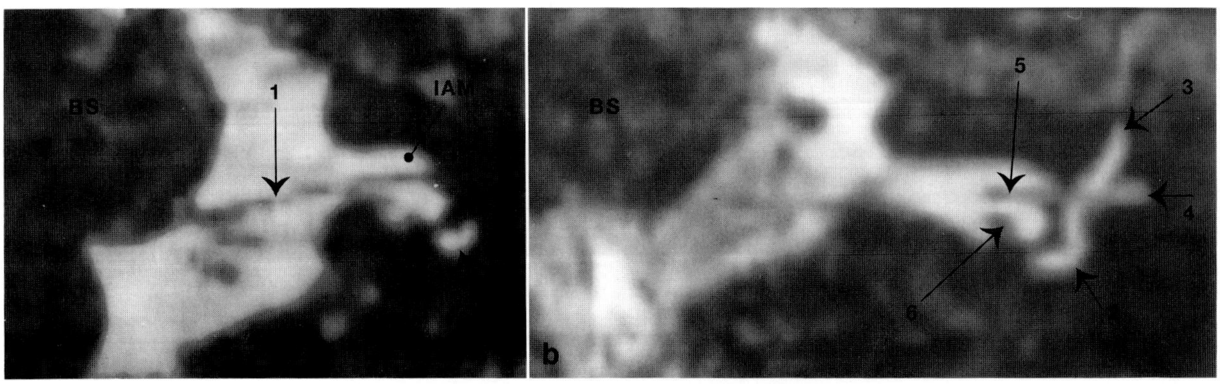

Fig. 3(a-b). Frontal oblique thin T_2 weighted images through a left CPA and inner ear (**a** through the anterior part of the IAM; **b** posterior to **a**. The facial nerve (*1*) is exposed in its entire length in the anterior part of the IAM. Posteriorly the basal turn of the cochlea (*2*), the superior (*3*) and lateral (*4*) semicircular canals are visible. The crista transversalis (*5*) and a part of the eighth nerve (*6*) in the fundus of the IAM can also be recognized. *BS* brainstem; *IAM* internal auditory meatus

a) The facial nerve and its relationship to the cochleo-vestibular nerve

The whole facial nerve can be made visible using MRI as described above [6, 7]. On axial sections, from top to bottom (Fig. 1) one can see it emerging from the inferior lateral aspect of the pons above and anterior to the eighth cranial nerve, running within the cerebellopontine angle cistern (CPAC) along with the eighth nerve and traveling within the internal auditory meatus (IAM) up from the porus to the fundus of the meatus.

From this set of axial sections illustrated in Fig. 1, one can get images of the facial nerve according to various orientations (Fig. 2) and study its entire course as well as its relationship to the eighth nerve. In the CPAC and the IAM the facial nerve runs just above the eighth nerve. At the fundus of the IAM the facial nerve lies above the cochlear nerve. The cresta falciformis separates these two nerves (Fig. 3).

Oblique sagittal sections perpendicular to the meatus show cross-sections of the seventh and eighth nerves. In the CPAC, the seventh nerve runs above and anterior to the eighth cranial nerve. In the IAM a series of sections from aperture to fundus at first shows the facial nerve above the cochleo-vestibular nerve, then above the cochlear nerve, and then lateral to the inferior vestibular nerve (Fig. 4).

b) The facial nerve and its relationship to blood vessels

Using T_2 weighted sequences and high solution MR, all blood vessels thicker than 1 mm in diameter are detectable (Fig. 1b). The anterior and inferior cerebellar artery (AICA) is always visible as are other arteries such as the posterior inferior cerebellar artery (PICA) and the vertebral artery when present in the cistern.

One can assess the presence or absence of blood vessels thicker than 1 mm close to the facial nerve, their course, and their location in the IAM and/or CPAC. Assessment of close contact between vessels and the facial nerve is difficult. To maximize such an assessment, two orthogonal views are required: axial sections and a set of sections perpendicular to the nerve. Axial sections show the relationship between the blood vessel and the lateral aspects of the facial nerve; perpendicular sections show the relationship between the vessel and the superior and inferior aspects of the nerve (Fig. 5). One must be aware of the fact that because the vessels are moving due to arterial pulsations that occur during the acquisition time of the sequence, the resulting image of the vessels is an average of their courses between systole and diastole, and it will thus show blurred contours of the vessels and the visibility of small vessels may be impaired. Cardiac gating should be mandatory to avoid these pitfalls, but this is not yet available for use with the described sequences.

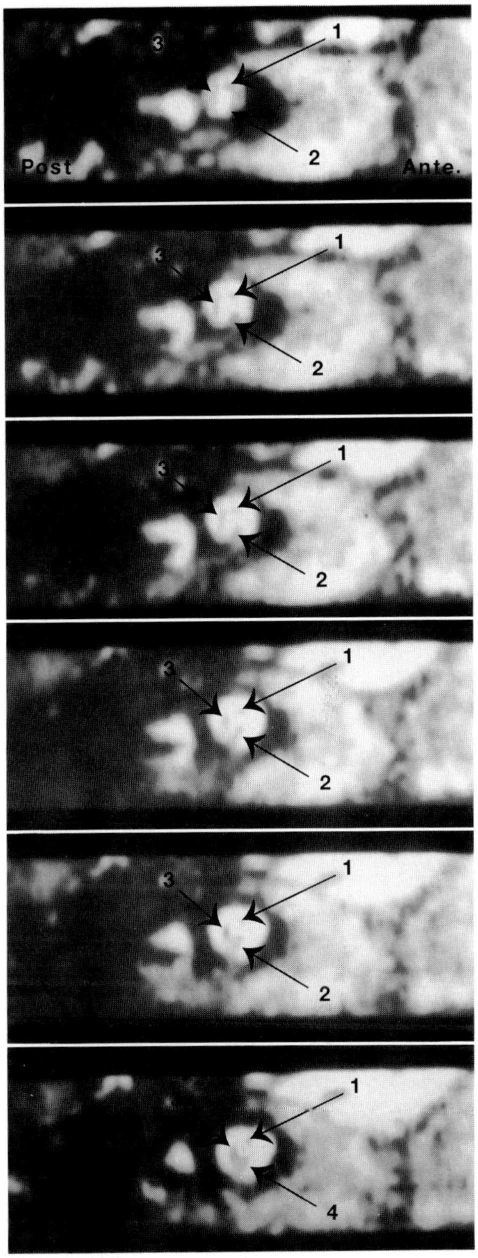

Fig. 4. Sagittal oblique thin T_2 weighted images (reconstruction in a plane perpendicular to the long axis of the IAM from the fundus to the porus). The facial nerve (*1*) is seen above and anterior to the vestibular nerves (*2*) and the cochlear nerve (*3*). Near the porus of the IAM the facial nerve (*1*) lays above the bundle of the cochleovestibular nerve (*4*), which is in a typical crescent shape

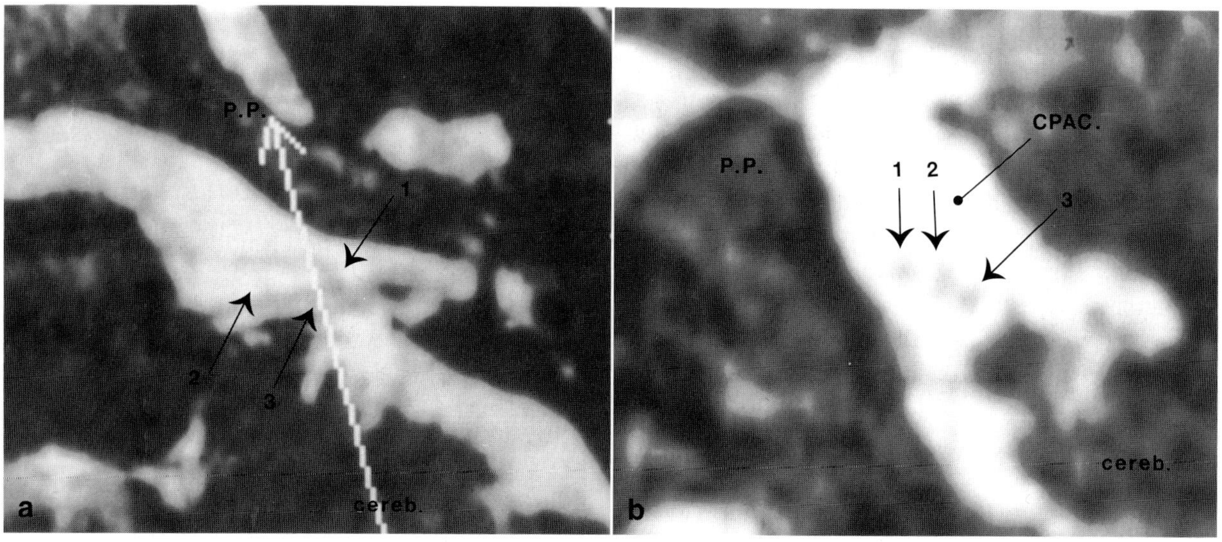

Fig. 5(a-b). Axial thin T_2 weighted images (**a**) and sagittal oblique in a plane perpendicular (⟨ – ⟩) to the axis of IAM and at the level of the porus (**b**). The loop of the AICA (*1*) is well recognized inside the high signal of the cerebrospinal fluid of the CPA (image 5a). The relationship of the loop (*1*) with the facial nerve (*2*) and the eighth nerve (*3*) can be identified on the cross section (image 5b). *PP* petrous pyramid; *cereb* cerebellum; *CPAC* cerebello-pontine angle cistern

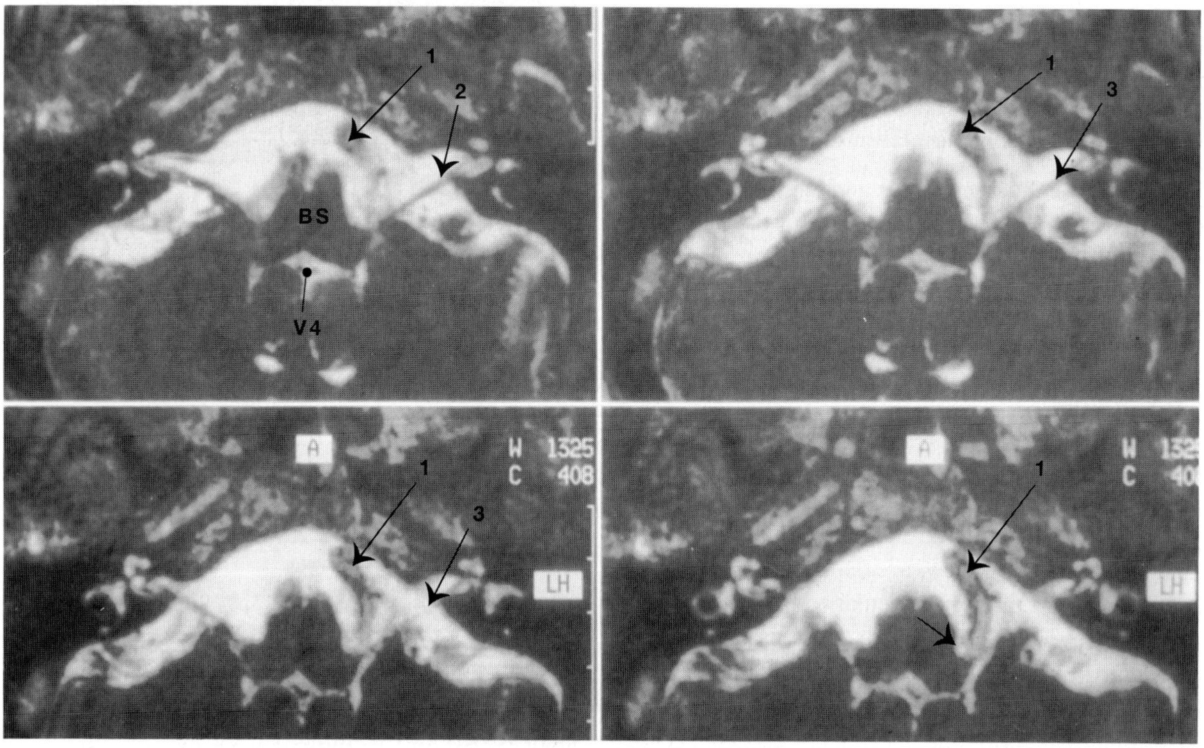

Fig. 6. Set of 4 axial 1-mm thin T_2 weighted images from top to bottom. Left vertebral megadolicho artery (*1*) close to the brainstem (→) and the apparent origin of the seventh (*2*) and the eighth (*3*) nerves. *BS* brainstem; *V4* fourth ventricle

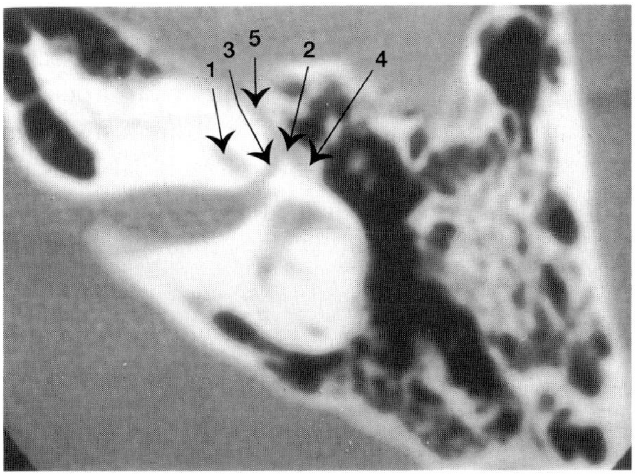

Fig. 7. Axial computer tomography (CT) scan at the level of the superior part of the left cochlea (*1*). The geniculate fossa (*2*) is located in the angle between the canal of the first (*3*) and the second portions (*4*) of the facial nerve. Anteriorly the canal for the superficial petrosal nerves (*5*) can be identified

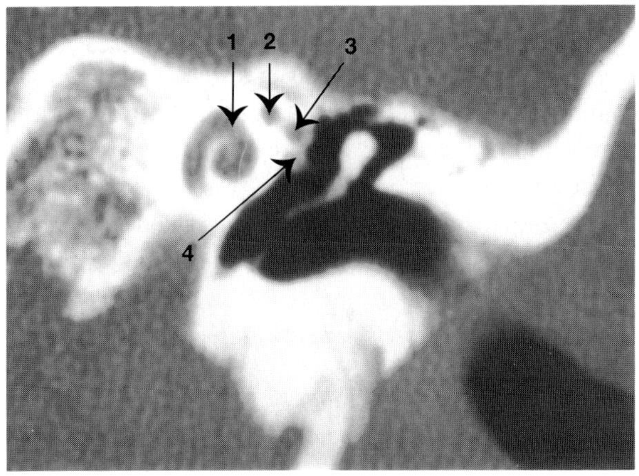

Fig. 8. Frontal CT scan at the anterior part of the left cochlea (*1*). The canals of the first portion (*2*) and the second portion (*3*) of the seventh nerve look like glasses. The round hole of the canal of the tensor tympani (*4*) is located inferiorly

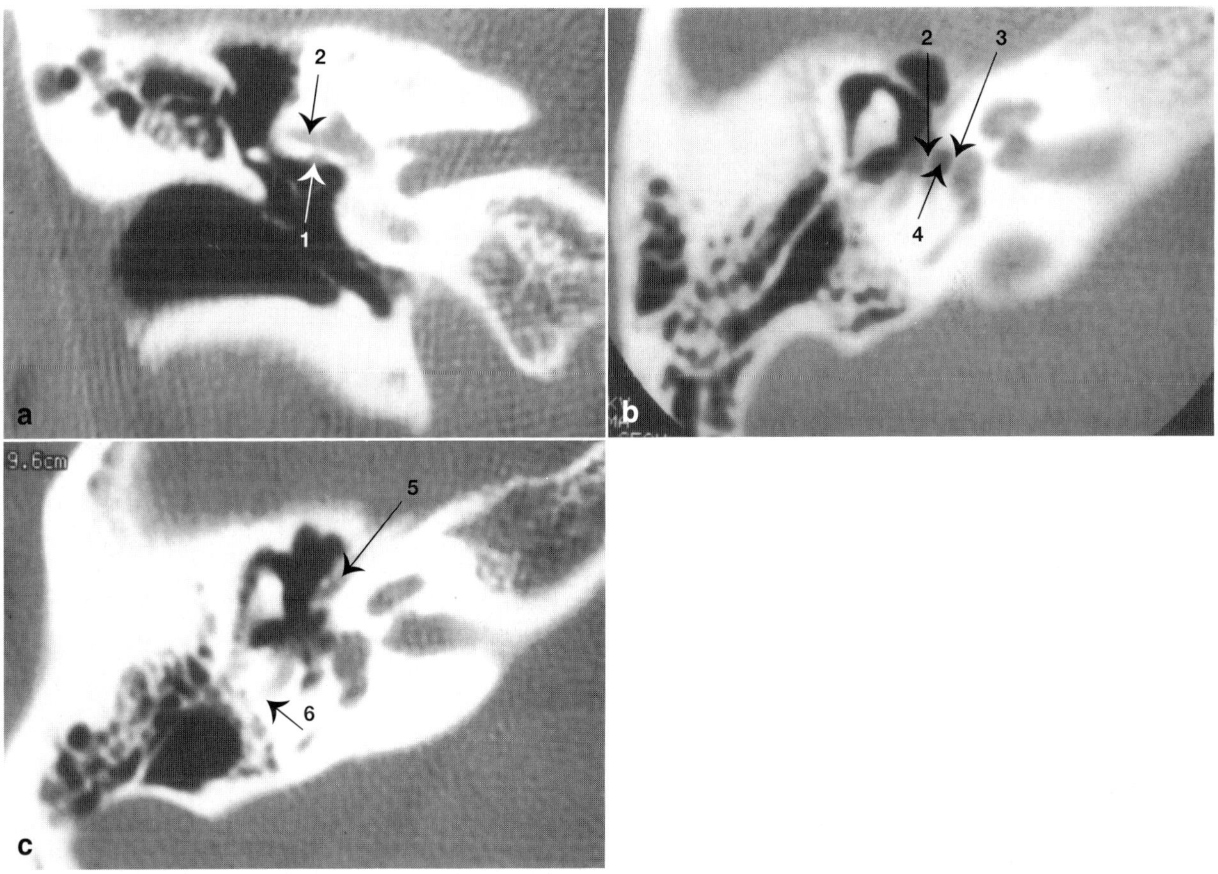

Fig. 9(a-c). CT scans in frontal (**a**) and axial (**b–c**) planes. The canal of the second portion of the facial nerve (*1*) is under the lateral semicircular canal (*2*) and in front of the foot plate of the stapes (*3*); notice the air gap (*4*) between these two structures. Figure 9c is 1 mm below 9b: the canal of the tensor tympani (*5*) must not be misinterpreted as the canal of the second portion of the facial nerve that is above and close to it; the angle between the second and the third portions of the canal of the seventh nerve (*6*) can be seen at the posterior part of the middle ear

Discussion

In our opinion, we can aid a surgeon by precisely mapping nerves and vessels within the cisterns of the cerebellopontine angle and the IAM. We can also assess the presence or absence of vessels with a diameter of more than 1 mm close to the facial nerve, and ascertain their courses and their contacts with the nerve and brainstem; however, we cannot define whether these vessels are responsible or not for a hemifacial spasm, except for dolichomega arteries impinging the brainstem at the origin of the facial nerve (Fig. 6).

II. Facial nerve and facial canal within the petrous pyramid: CT and MRI studies

The facial canal is imaged by *high resolution CT* using a matrix of 512 × 512 for a field of view 9.6 × 9.6 cm wide (pixel size 0.2 mm). The images are displayed using a large window setting (4000 Hounsfield Units). Sections are thin (1 mm) and contiguous. Two orthogonal views are necessary: direct axial sections and either direct coronal sections or reformatted images from the data of the direct axial set of sections.

Results

I. Facial canal

a) The first part of the facial canal

as illustrated in Fig. 7, is seen in axial section above the postero-superior aspect of the cochlea. The geniculate fossa is seen at the tip of an acute angle of the first and second parts of the facial canal. The canal for the superior petrosal nerve extends from the geniculate fossa. In the coronal section illustrated in Fig. 8 the first and second parts of the facial canal are seen as two round openings (mimicking spectacles) that are overlying a third opening—the canal of tensor tympani.

b) The second part of the facial canal

runs under the lateral semi-circular canal and over the oval window. In the coronal sections illustrated in Fig. 9a, it is seen as an opening under the lateral semicircular canal. Its wall is sometimes so thin that it is impossible to assess whether or not there is a physiologic defect. In the axial projection illustrated in Fig. 9b the facial canal is displayed along its long axis, facing the most upper part of the footplate of the stapes, from which it is separated by an air gap. The facial canal must not be mistaken for the canal of tensor tympani, which is seen on the inferior section illustrated in Fig. 9c.

c) The third part of the facial canal

is running downwards within the mastoid. In the coronal sections illustrated in Fig. 10a it is easily identified at the level of the mid-portion of the posterior semi-circular canal. In the axial sections illustrated in Fig. 10b it is seen in cross-section and it is sometimes difficult to identify from the surrounding mastoid cells, especially when they are opaque.

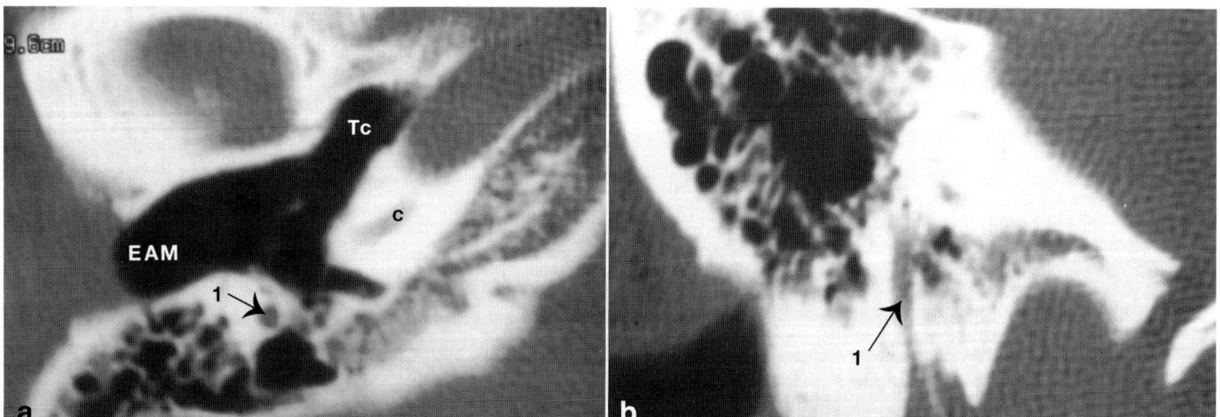

Fig. 10 (a-b). Axial (**a**) and frontal (**b**) CT scans showing the canal of third portion of the facial nerve (*1*) within the mastoid. *EAM* external auditory meatus; *TC* tympanic cavity; *C* cochlea

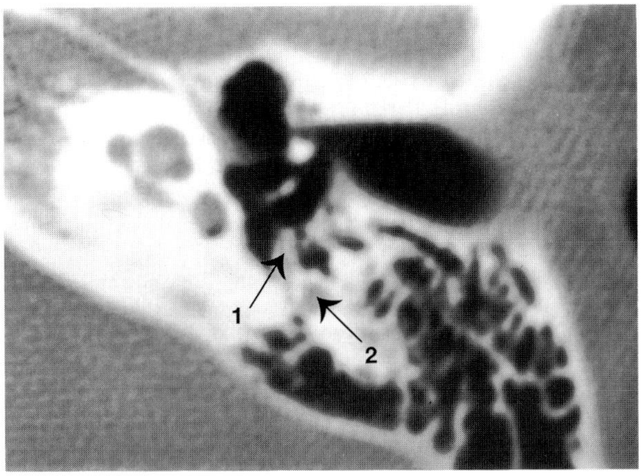

Fig. 11. Axial CT scan of the left ear displaying the canal of the stapes muscle (*1*) inside the canal of third portion of the facial nerve (*2*)

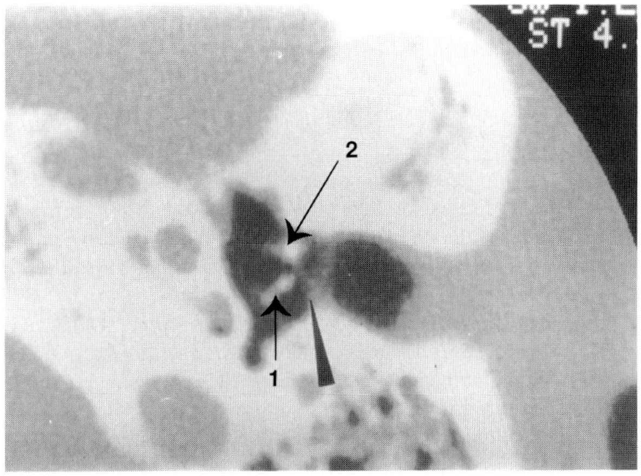

Fig. 12. Axial CT scan. The chorda tympani (⩾) can be visualized going outside the long process of the incus (*1*) and inside the handle of the malleus (*2*)

Anterior to the course of the third part of the facial canal, lies the pyramid of the stapes muscle (Fig. 11). The facial nerve gives to this muscle the stapedial nerve, and lower, the canal of the chorda tympani. On axial sections this canal can be seen as a small opening which, from bottom to top, progressively moves aside the facial canal to enter the tympanic cavity. The chorda tympani itself is seen in the tympanic cavity from posterior to anterior: behind the incus, then between the incus and malleus, and finally anterior to the malleus; in a coronal section it is seen as a small soft tissue dot, and in axial section it is seen as a strip (Fig. 12).

II. Facial nerve

The facial nerve itself within the facial canal is displayed by MRI using T_1 weighted sequences with gadolinium injection [1, 5]. Physiologically, the content of the facial canal, including nerve, geniculate ganglion, and vessels, enhances significantly using this process due to high vascularization within the facial

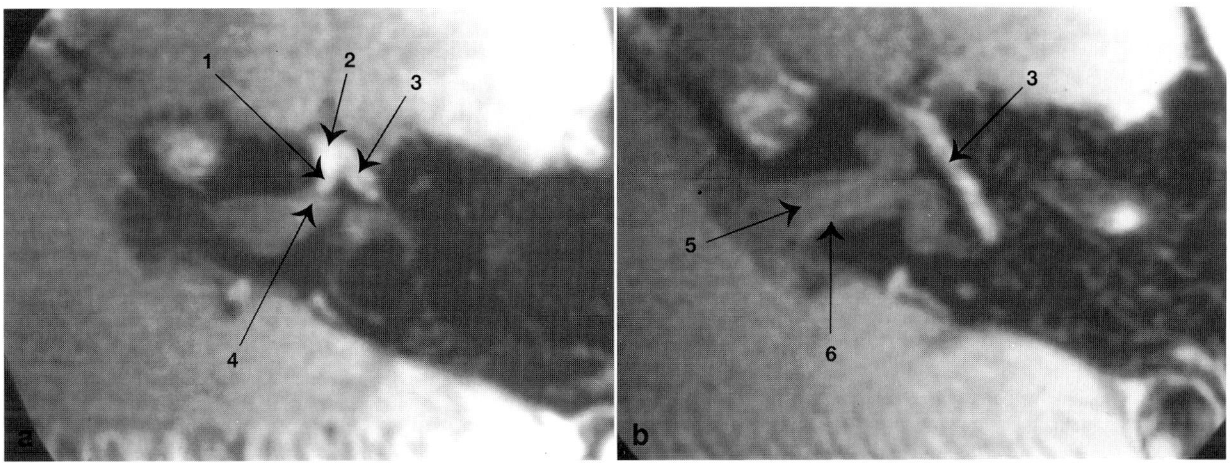

Fig. 13 (a-b). Axial T_1 weighted images of the left ear after injection of gadolinium. The seventh nerve in the first portion (*1*), the geniculate ganglion (*2*) and the second part of the facial nerve (*3*) enhance markedly, unlike the nerves in the IAC (facial (*4*), cochlear (*5*) and inferior vestibular (*6*) nerve), which do not

canal (Fig. 13), whereas the facial nerve never does in normal conditions in the IAM [4].

References

1. Balkany T, Fradis M, Jafek BW, Rucker NC (1991) Intrinsic vasculature of the labyrinthine segment of the facial nerve-implications for site of lesion in Bell's palsy. Otolaryngol Head Neck Surg 104: 20–23
2. Casselman JW, Kuhweide R, Deimling M, Ampe W, Dehaene I, Meeus L (1993) Constructive interference in steady state-3DFT MR imaging of the inner ear and cerebellopontine angle. AJNR Am J Neuroradiol 14: 47–57
3. Felber S, Birbamer G, Aichner F, Poewe W, Kampfl A (1992) Magnetic resonance imaging and angiography in hemifacial spasm. Neuroradiology 34: 413–416
4. Gebarski SS, Telian SA, Niparko JK (1992) Enhancement along the normal facial nerve in the facial canal: MR imaging and anatomic correlation. Radiology 183: 391–394
5. Girard N, Poncet M, Chays A, Florence A, Gignac D, Magnan J, Raybaud C (1993) MRI exploration of the intrapetrous facial nerve. J Neuroradiol 20: 226–238
6. Kim HN, Kim YH, Park IY, Kim GR, Chung IH (1990) Variability of the surgical anatomy of the neurovascular complex of the cerebellopontine angle. Ann Otol Rhinol Laryngol 99: 288–296
7. Martin N, Le Bras F, Krief O, Chedid G, Marsault C, Nahum H (1992) MRI anatomy of the acoustic-facial bundle in vivo. J Neuroradiol 19: 88–97
8. Nagaseki Y, Horikoshi T, Omata T, Ueno T, Uchida M, Nukui H, Tsuji R, Sasaki H (1992) Oblique sagittal magnetic resonance imaging visualizing vascular compression of the trigeminal or facial nerve. J Neurosurg 77: 379–386
9. Nakashima S, Sando I, Takahashi H, Fujita S (1993) Computer-aided 3-D reconstruction and measurement of the facial canal and facial nerve. I. Cross-sectional area and diameter: preliminary report. Laryngoscope 103: 1150–1156

Correspondence: Jacqueline Vignaud, Hopital du Val de Grace, 74 Boulevard de Port-Royal, F-75230 Paris Cedex 05, France.

Neurophysiological study of the facial nerve

G. Freyss and **G. Tailame**

E.N.T. Department, Hôpital Lariboisière, Paris, France

Summary

The facial nerve is often involved in paralysis and spasm, and there are some unique aspects in the evaluation of facial nerve disorders. Electroneurography (ENoG) and computed surface electromyography (EMG) allows an accurate early prediction of the severity of idiopathic facial paralysis, and thus the opportunity to provide an optimal and very successful medical management of its severe forms.

The development of intracranial intraoperative electro- physiological recording and stimulation gave a new dimension to intracranial facial nerve surgery [19]. Such intraoperative monitoring reduced the sequelae of pontocerebellar tumor surgery. Above all, it has contributed to the understanding the mechanisms of the essential hemifacial spasm and for providing optimal surgical treatment of vascular compression of the facial nerve.

Key words: Facial nerve, electromyography, electroneuropathy, blink reflex, magnetic transcranial stimulation, prognosis of facial paralysis.

Introduction

Techniques of electrophysiological explorations have been undergoing steady improvement, and the results of such developments have been reported at various symposia that have focused on the facial nerve [6, 15, 23, 27]. The facial nerve has some unique characteristics:

- with regard to its electrophysiology, the proximal segment of the nerve is not feasible.
- and with regard to therapeutics, the efficiency of medical treatments of both paralysis and hemifacial spasm has been controversial for a long time.

It is important to take practical precautions to preserve the function of the facial nerve when operating on adjoining lesions that affect the facial nerve intracranially (tumors of the cerebellopontine angle or vascular compression, as well as lesions of the facial nerve itself). For this purpose the use of intraoperative neurophysiologic monitoring is important, but most classical electrophysiological techniques offer only inadequate results.

The development of special methods for intracranial intraoperative monitoring of the facial nerve has improved the preservation of facial function in operations in which the facial nerve is involved.

The integration of electrophysiological monitoring into different operations has had several beneficial implications:

1) intraoperative monitoring of the facial nerve has helped to protect the facial nerve throughout the course of operations to remove tumors of the cerebellopontine angle.
2) the results of investigations that were done using intraoperative recordings from the facial nerve and facial muscles during operations to relieve hemifacial spasm have advanced our understanding of the pathophysiology of hemifacial spasm and the mechanism of synkinesis, have supported evidence of vascular compression being the cause of pathology, and have elucidated the role of abnormalities in the facial motonucleus.

In idiopathic facial paralysis, medical treatment with corticosteroids, when prescribed ultraprecociously at high dosages, offers noteworthy efficacy. Such treatment is exclusively intended for severe cases of Charles Bell's paralysis, implying unacceptable sequellae. Corticosteroids can be modulated according to individual prognoses by means of electroneurography examination, which allows the early follow-up of patients. However, for patients with facial paralysis following intracranial surgery (acoustic neuroma removal), which is probably due to nerve ischemia, there is no agreement on an effective medical treatment.

Electromyography

Electromyography (EMG) is the recording of electrical activity from muscles, e.g. motor unit potentials from voluntary and involuntary muscle contractions and spontaneous activity of the muscle fibers. There is a distinct difference between the electrical activity recorded from normal muscles, from denervated muscles, and from diseased muscles (myopathy). There are two ways to record muscle activity, namely via needle electrodes or via surface electrodes.

1) EMG Recordings using needle electrodes

Technique

For diagnostic purposes, bipolar needles are used. For studies of face muscles, such electrodes should be inserted in the orbicularis oris muscles and not in the mentalis muscle (which has bilateral innervation). For intraoperative recording of facial EMG, two monopolar needles are inserted in the orbicularis oris and orbicularis oculi muscles 1-cm apart. When the needles are inserted in these muscles, specific reactions can be evaluated: normal muscles at rest are electrically silent; during voluntary muscle contraction motor unit discharge frequency increases with increasing strength of the contraction (interference pattern: amplitude 50–1500 μV) (Fig. 1); if the face (or a portion of it) is paralyzed, as long as a few action motor units can be recorded, even when there are no visible contractions of the facial muscles at all, it may be assumed that the lesion has not yet reached the point that would result in severe degeneration of the facial nerve. If a few action motor units can be recorded after the seventh day from the onset of the paralysis, severe degeneration of the facial nerve will not occur [5].

The main drawback of recording EMG in this way for evaluating facial nerve function is that isolated motor units can give a positive response. Thus a few intact fibers that may give a response would lead the clinician to assume that the prognosis for recovery is good, whereas in reality most of the nerve trunk may be severed. We have found that recording from surface-integrated EMG is a better choice, because such recordings represent the activity of the entire facial nerve.

Fibrillation Potentials: Denervated muscles produce spontaneous electrical potentials that are of low amplitude (10–200 μV). These potentials do not appear until 10–20 days after onset of the paralysis. In idiopathic facial palsy, prognosis cannot sufficiently be substantiated by needle electrode EMG recordings before the end of the third week, which is much too late to be practically useful. This is why we have not used needle EMG in cases of idiopathic facial paralysis for more than 15 years.

Electromyographic findings are pathognomonic for essential hemifacial spasm [4]. Typically, EMG recordings show synchronized activity of the motor units of all facial muscles involved and high-frequency firing of motor units of up to 350/sec. This is in contrast to the maximum firing level of 50 to 70/sec in normal musculature (Fig. 2).

Symptomatic hemifacial spasm (that is not essential hemifacial spasm) may be due to the presence of tumors involving the facial nerve (acoustic neuroma, cholesteatoma, and chemodectoma of the temporal bone). Symptomatic hemifacial spasm lacks the high-frequency repetitive character and the regularity of essential hemifacial spasm. In blepharospasm the EMG discharge pattern is quite different, as the firing of the involved motor units is asynchronous and the discharge rate is within normal limits.

In post-paralytic synkinesis, EMG reveals a perfect synchrony of the discharging motor units in the in-

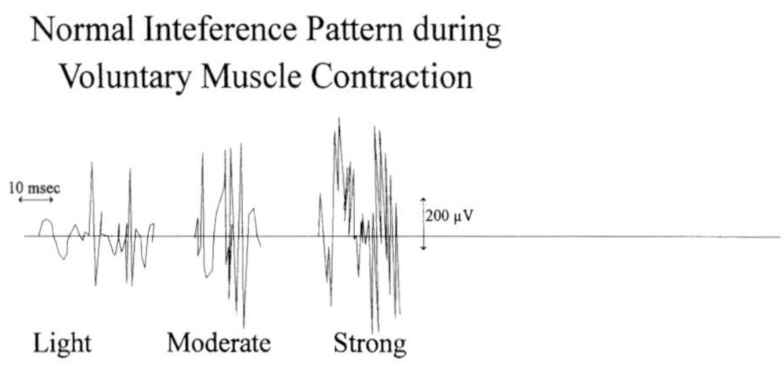

Fig. 1. Needle EMG in the orbicularis oculi muscle

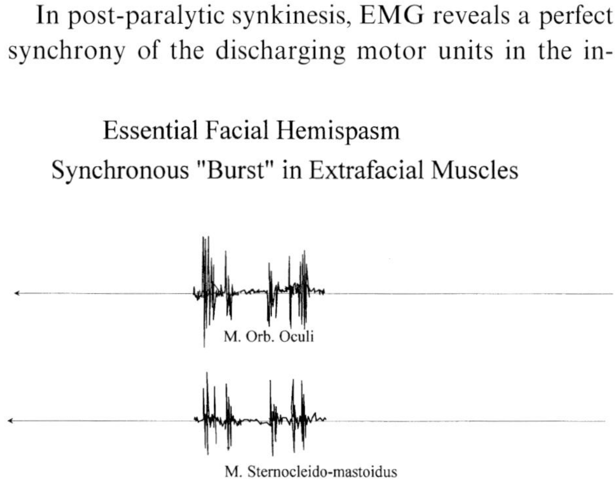

Fig. 2. Needle EMG recording (according to Laskawi [15], modified, semi-schematic)

volved muscle and provides electrophysiological proof that the sprouts of a single regenerating axon can innervate different groups of facial muscles.

2) EMG Using surface electrodes

During maximum voluntary contraction of face muscles, all elementary motor units are active and the EMG recordings represent activity that is generated in all muscles situated in, under, or near the recording electrode [16]. This allows a much more quantitative signal processing.

Technique

Following skin preparation, the EMG recording surface electrodes are applied to the skin overlying the muscle(s) from which the recordings are to be done, and the electrode is connected to the amplifier. In our institution we use the sensory kit of Medelec, firmly held on the zygomatic muscle by the patient. The recorded EMG activity is then rectified and integrated. Raw data and integrated data are always displayed simultaneously. Amplifier settings are: amplitude amplifications, 50 mV/division; bandpass filtering, 16 to 800 Hz, 12 dB/octave; observation window, 10 sec, 1 sec/division. Maximum contraction should last at least 2 sec. Results are expressed as the maximum of integrated amplitude, and measurements are done at rest and during maximum zygomatic contraction, thus avoiding recording simultaneous masseter muscle contractions. Results are expressed in absolute amplitude (in mV), and not as the percentage of the EMG potentials that are recorded from the normal side. This is because integrated EMG recorded from the normal side is not always normal in the first days after onset of the paralysis. Using an absolute measure enhances the reproductibility of the measurements. At rest, noise should be less than 10 μV [22], normal maximum amplitude is >450 μV, 250 μV corresponds to a mild paralysis, 60 μV is associated with a clinically complete paralysis, and if the response is under 35 μV, an early deterioration of the ENoG is indicated, and that is associated with a poor prognosis for recovery and severe paralysis is likely to result. An early improvement in the EMG recording announces a good recovery.

Electroneurography (ENoG)

ENoG plays an important role in the early diagnosis of the severity and prognosis of Bell's palsy. Described by Esslen [4,5] and popularized by U. Fisch [6], ENoG is a particular form of evoked electromyography.

Technique

In our institution, we use a Medelec MS 6 electromyograph. The facial nerve is electrically stimulated, using a bipolar ball electrode, placed over the nerve trunk under the lobus auricularis, with the cathode located distally. The stimuli are square waves of 0.1-ms duration (longer durations are painful). A minimum number of stimulations are used, beginning at 4 mA (constant current) on the normal side, repeated if necessary at a low frequency (0.5 Hz) at 10 mA intensity and, if there is no response, the gain of the recording amplifier is increased. We use a recording window of 30 ms (3 ms/division) for oscilloscopic observation as well as for oscillographic recording. Before the application of the stimulus and placement of the recording electrodes, the skin is cleaned and abrased with skin preparation paste. The ground electrode for the recording is placed on the forearm. For recording compound muscle action potentials we use surface electrodes (we use a Medelec $AgCl_2$ metallic sensory recording kit) placed on the zygomatic muscle on the nasomalar sulcus. The electrodes have a low impedance. The two recording electrodes should be placed at the same distance from the stimulating cathode. Such placement (a line through the electrodes should be perpendicular to a line through the bipolar stimulating probe) is critical for obtaining a maximum response wave. If necessary, the bipolar stimulation probe or the sensory recording electrodes should be slowly rotated.

The amplifier gain should be set to 1000 μV/division. This gain must be increased up to 200 μV/division if no response is noted at 10-mA stimulus intensity. The recorded responses are band-filtered 16–3200 Hz (12 dB/octave slope).

The peak-to-peak amplitude of the biphasic response is measured, and results of the ENoG is expressed as a percentage of the response from the normal side. This very important test is not easy to perform. It is best done using a tandem approach with the patient placed next to a clinician in the same room. Patients with thick subcutaneous fat or with enlarged parotids are difficult to test, and in children we are obliged to use the Hilger's test.

The great advantage of using ENoG is that it provides quantitative results. The fiber-optic cathode oscilloscope screen of the Medelec equipment directly provides a paper recording of the potentials. The output of the Medelec unit can also be connected to an analog-to-digital converter in a microcomputer so that the signal can be digitally processed.

The drawback of using ENoG is that the stimulation point is distal rather than proximal to the lesion. This means that only after the axoplasmatic flow is blocked does the response to the stimulation decrease (thus with a lag of approximately 72 hours). This is why we use surface electromyography (EMG) in addition to ENoG for precise clinical testing.

Clinical significance (Figs. 3 and 4)

Precise prognosis must include the consideration of the fact that ENoG expresses a very dynamic time-dependent process with a time lag (Figs. 3 and 4), i.e., the prognosis is dependent on the absolute value of ENoG as related to the time delay between the onset of facial paralysis and the evaluation for possible treatment. "The earlier during the first 14 days the response of the ENoG potential drops to 10% or less of normal, the worse the prognosis" [5]. In 1975, Pialoux et al. [22] created a template that graphically expressed the prognosis of treatment of facial nerve disorders with accuracy, taking into account ENoG values and time delays between the onset of facial paralysis and the evaluation for possible treatment (Fig. 5). Extensive use of this template confirmed the high efficiency of ENoG in predicting graphically the prognosis of a patient if this test was used between the third and seventh days after onset of facial paralysis. The prognosis is confirmed by a second recording done 5–7 days later that gives the velocity of the decrease in the ENoG amplitude (slope): this slope is very steep for severe forms of facial paralysis and is associated with poor

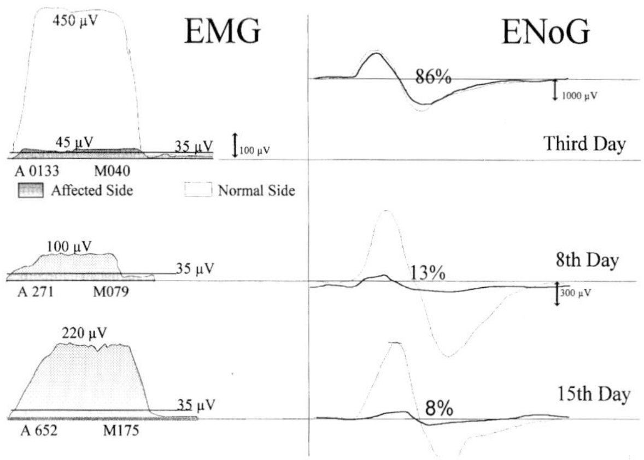

Fig. 3. Serious facial paralysis recorded in the early 1970's. The final result was acceptable – complete motor recovery, but with associated synkinesis. Notice that the early EMG was $>35\,\mu V$ (total clinical facial paralysis) and then the early increase of EMG amplitude is associated with the return of clinical function; this is in contrast with a continuous decrease in the amplitude of ENoG values in the ENoG recording. This patient had only infiltrations

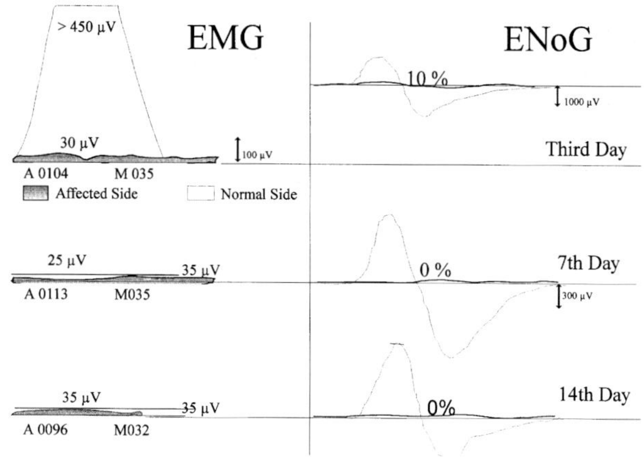

Fig. 4. Recording of a very severe facial paralysis in the early 1970's, before the use of high doses of cortisone as treatment. Notice the total absence of any EMG response that occurred very early in the recording, which was associated with an early rapid decrease in ENoG values. The patient had decompressive surgery on the fifteenth day following onset of facial paralysis and finally had an incomplete recovery and significant synkinesis. In 1994 these sequellae would be considered unacceptable

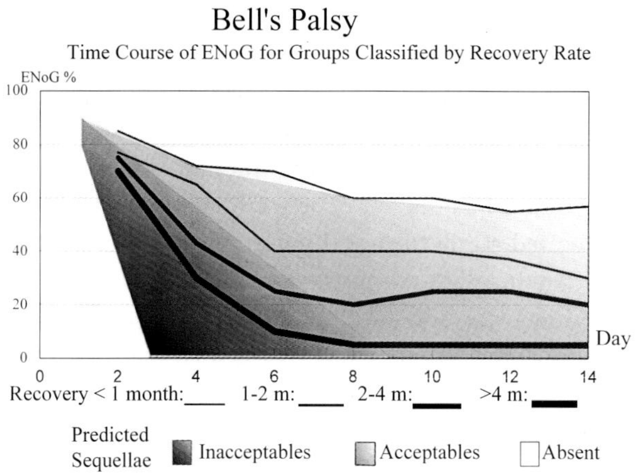

Fig. 5. Updated template: Projection of Tojima's results [29] on our original template [22]. Notice that the fast drop in ENoG values apparently stopped on the eighth day following onset of facial paralysis, which was due to efficient medical management. (This is in contrast with our previous recordings done in 1975 [22], cf Figs. 4 and 5)

recovery (incomplete recovery of facial movement and, particularly, severe synkinesis); when the ENoG amplitude goes down slowly it is associated with good recovery of facial paralysis. In these cases a paradoxal decrease in the ENoG amplitude could often be seen to contrast with an increase in EMG amplitude and clinical test scores tests, which showed a reappearance of voluntary movements. An important factor is that the first exam should be done early, and if the patient is only seen for the first time 15–20 days after the onset of facial paralysis, the efficiency of the template is low. Such patients have been seen too late to benefit from medical management. This well-established situation should clearly be improved.

The high efficiency of early treatment with high doses of cortisone is well expressed in the inflexion of the prognostic curve and by the early return of facial function (this treatment is associated with complete recovery within 1–2 months). An important goal in the treatment of facial paralysis is that the ENoG curve should not go under 40%, as this is the limit associated with total recovery and absence of synkinesis [17, 29]. Improvements in both the ability to make early prognoses and in the efficiency of medical management have led us to the following strategy: The use of corticosteroids has totally renewed the treatment of idiopathic facial paralysis (isolated paralysis of sudden onset, without audio-vestibular modifications). The effectiveness of corticosteroids is dose-dependent: in severe forms of idiopathic facial paralysis, very high doses, such as those recommended by Stennert [27], give better results than does, for instance, Synacthen[R]. Treatment with Synacthen,[R] however, is effective only within the first ten days following onset of facial paralysis.

Most of our patients with a clinical total facial paralysis were seen between the third and seventh day following onset of the facial paralysis. If there is a change in the ENoG recording or if the EMG response is $< 35\,\mu V$ (which in most cases is followed by a fast decrease in ENoG values), the treatment would be that proposed by Stennert [27]. If EMG is $> 35\,\mu V$ and the ENoG recording is normal, we use Synacthen[R] 1 mg/day up to the twelfth day.

Patients seen in the first hours frequently have an incomplete paralysis (which could lead to a misleading prognosis): they receive 1 mg/day of Synacthen[R] and have control of their facial muscles within three days. If the paralysis remains partial (palsy), we stop the treatment. If the paralysis worsens and is associated with a normal ENoG recording, we continue the treatment up to the twelfth day. If an early ENoG recording shows an abnormality, we opt for a Stennert's maximum treatment [27].

In patients seen at a later stage, i.e., after the fifteenth day, we could not prove the effectiveness of the corticosteroid treatment.

Herpes zoster-oticus has a more severe prognosis. In young patients without contraindications, we use Stennert's treatment associated with antiviral drugs. In elderly patients, we use standard Synacthen[R] treatment, which suppresses zosterian pain and favors vestibular rehabilitation (a vestibular destruction is associated in half of these cases). In other contraindication cases (very old patients and pregnant women), we only do facial nerve vascular pedicle infiltrations using Xylocaine.[R]

Children

In most children (with the exception of those with herpes zoster-oticus), facial paralysis is associated with a good prognosis. Most of the time such children don't need aggressive treatment. Surface EMG and a low-intensity Hilger's test can be done in most children.

Traumatic facial paralysis

Neurosurgical patients are easily tested using Hilger's device at bedside. An early or a very fast decrease in the responses indicates the necessity of subsequent facial nerve surgery.

Appearance of a facial paralysis after middle ear surgery

A very early prognosis can be made as soon as the patient is totally awake. A total absence of a voluntary response in the integrated EMG recording ($< 35\,\mu V$) is a good indication of an anatomical lesion of the facial nerve.

Hilger's test

Hilger's facial neurostimulator is a very portable and easy-to-use device. With this neurostimulator the facial nerve trunk or its branches are stimulated, and the threshold of the current intensity that produces the visible (clinically) twitching of the corresponding muscle is measured. This test is easily used in children and at bedside in comatose patients. Following simple skin preparation, a ground electrode is applied on the back of the neck and a monopolar handheld probe is placed on the branches of the facial nerve. The temporal branch is stimulated at mid-distance between the side-whiskers and eyebrow, and the mandibular branch is stimulated at the mandibular notch where the mandibular branch of the facial nerve crosses the lower rim of the mandible at the interior rim of the masseter. Very short stimulations are applied, beginning at 3 mA (to the superior facial branch) and at 5 mA (to the inferior branch). We usually do not test the facial trunk in children (too painful). Only the gross threshold must be determined. Serial tests before the twentieth day are necessary.

An early disappearance of any response before the seventh-to-tenth day can usually be associated with a severe prognosis. The accuracy of this test has, however, been questioned [1]. Blumenthal and May [1] described the use of the amount of muscle twitch in response to supramaximal stimulation using the same device. We, the authors, have no personal experience with this technique.

Magnetic stimulation of facial nerve

Magnetic stimulation enables a painless exam of the facial nerve by stimulating the proximal nerve ending across the lesion. This allows comparison of the response to proximal stimulation with that obtained distally from the site of the lesion. Such a comparison is essential for the determination of the ratio of blocked/degenerated fibers. A strong impulse of magnetic field is generated by electric current that flows through a coil, and this magnetic field can induce electrical neural tissue, such as a peripheral nerve, depending on the position of the coil. Potosching and Stennert [24] showed new ways to assess facial nerve dysfunction using such magnetic stimulation. Recently, Glocker et al. [9] gave an exhaustive view of the time-course and relevance of electrophysiological parameters in 97 patients with Bell's palsy.

Technique

Glocker et al. [9] positioned a coil occipitally, with the lowest point of the coil over the mastoid, which allowed supramaximal transcranial stimulation of the facial nerve.

Schmid et al. [25] demonstrated that the stimulation site was within the proximal segment of the facial nerve canal.

The compound action potentials [9] produced by this stimulation were compared with the results of ENoG in the same patient.

Results

In healthy subjects, Magstim evokes responses with a shape and amplitude similar to those recorded by ENoG and an increased latency of 0.8 ms [9].

The typical finding with Magstim in patients with Bell's palsy is the early absence or marked amplitude reduction in the evoked muscle response, as compared to that obtained by ENoG. Moreover, with the stimulus intensity of Magstim just sufficient to evoke a supramaximal response on the unaffected side, a muscle response on the affected side is not obtained. This situation persists during the first few months after the onset of the paralysis [9].

These authors concluded that the finding that Magstim does not yield a prognostic clue in Bell's palsy is very important to the clinician, and they believe that an accurate prognosis can be provided with the use of ENoG recordings.

It is of interest to note that the site of maximum lesion observed with Magstim (proximal segment of the facial nerve canal) is the same as that described surgically by Fisch [6] (maximum swelling) and, more recently, through MRI imagery by Kohsyu et al. [13] (gadolinium enhancement of the facial nerve) in patients with Bell's palsy.

In patients suffering from tumors in the cerebellopontine angle, Wolf et al. [32] found Magstim of the facial nerve to be valid in preoperative examinations (2/3 of Wolf's patients had elongated latencies) and in psychological preparation of the patient in predicting the outcome of facial function after surgery.

The blink reflex

The blink reflex is a trigemino-facial reflex used to measure the length of time it takes for an electrical stimulus applied to the supraorbital nerve at the forehead to result in a blink of the eyes. The afferent limb of this reflex arc is the trigeminal nerve that conducts nerve impulses to the trigeminal nucleus in the brainstem that connects to the facial motonucleus. The efferent limb is the facial nerve [28, 30].

Standard technique

A stimulating electrode is placed on the forehead at the supraorbital nerve. The stimulus is a square wave of 100–200 μs duration with an intensity varying from 1 to 14 mA (constant current), delivered at a low pseudorandom rate. The reflex response is EMG activity recorded simultaneously and bilaterally from the orbicularis oculi muscles by using concentric needle electrodes. In pathological cases, recordings are also made from other facial muscles (the mentalis and the orbicularis oris). In normal relaxed people, the reflex response is recorded only from the orbicularis oculi muscle and it consists of (Fig. 6):

- an early component, R_1, which is highly reproducible, with a biphasic or triphasic shape and that could follow a frequency stimulation increase up to 2 Hz. This component has a latency of 10.4 ms (SD = 0.4) [17]. This component can only be recorded on the stimulated side.
- a late component, R_2, which is prolonged, multiphasic, and highly variable in shape, amplitude, and delay. This component's latency is 25–30 ms [18] and corresponds to the blinking movement, and it occurs both ipsilaterally and contralaterally.

The R_1 component is generated through the reflex arc in the ipsilateral portion of the brainstem and it has a direct connection between the trigeminal pathway and the facial motor nucleus. The R_2 component is presumed to be mediated through polysynaptic interneurones in the lateral reticular formation of the brainstem. This late response adapts rapidly to repeated stimulations if they are regular.

In normal individuals, during stable sustained contractions of the facial muscles, both an R_1, R_2 response could be recorded from other facial muscles when these were voluntarily contracted muscles, with these two components having the same duration, latency, and shape as when recorded from the orbicularis oculi muscle [23].

The normal blink reflex is abolished during anaesthesia in man [19, 20, 21], but not in animals [7].

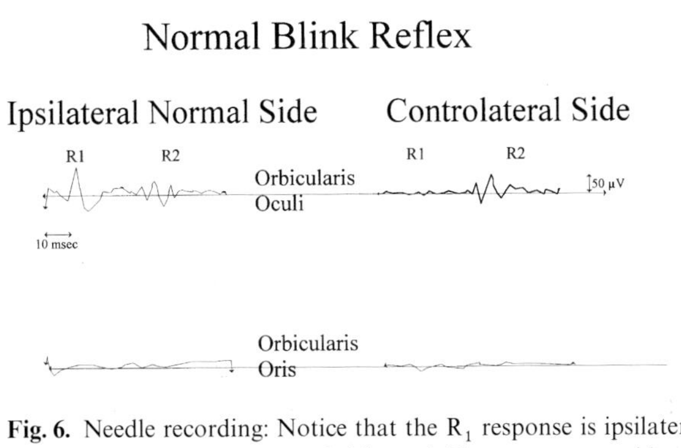

Fig. 6. Needle recording: Notice that the R_1 response is ipsilateral only, and that the R_2 response is bilateral. The responses could only be recorded in auricular oculi muscles and not in other facial muscles

Animal model

The blink reflex has been studied in several animal species such as the monkey [31], the cat and the rat [7].

Pathology

The clinical interest in the blink reflex in aiding the diagnosis of various lesions of the trigeminal nerve, pons, and medulla [8, 10, 18] has been considerably reduced due to the development of magnetic resonance imagery (MRI), and the use of the blink reflex as a prognostic tool in facial paralysis [11, 18] is overshadowed by the efficiency and the simplicity of electroneurography (ENoG).

Because the blink reflex involves the entire length of the facial nerve (including the facial motonucleus), it offers a way to explore pathologies that involve the intracranial portion of the facial nerve and the facial motonucleus, such as that related to essential hemifacial spasm or synkinesis. We will focus on the modification of the R_1 component, because this component is a very stable, reproducible, and is the result of an oligosynaptic reflex wave whose synapse is in the facial motor nucleus.

Synkinesis (Fig. 7) of facial muscles often manifests after severe peripheral nerve paralysis following a delay of 3 to 4 months, and then it is often the most apparent sequelae of this severe facial paralysis. Synkinesis is more apparent in the areas of the orbicularis oculi and oris muscles. These associated movements are very fast when they are induced by a voluntary or spontaneous blink. The synkinesis could easily be recorded by inducing a blink reflex response by directing an air puff at the eye. In such cases, ipsilateral stimulation (blink) induces a reflex response with both components (R_1 and R_2) appearing not only in the orbicularis oculi muscle but also in many other facial muscles of the spastic hemiface [17]. The importance of this spread of activity that represents synkinesis is that it is related to the degree of degeneration of the facial nerve. When degeneration is studied in the acute stage, on the

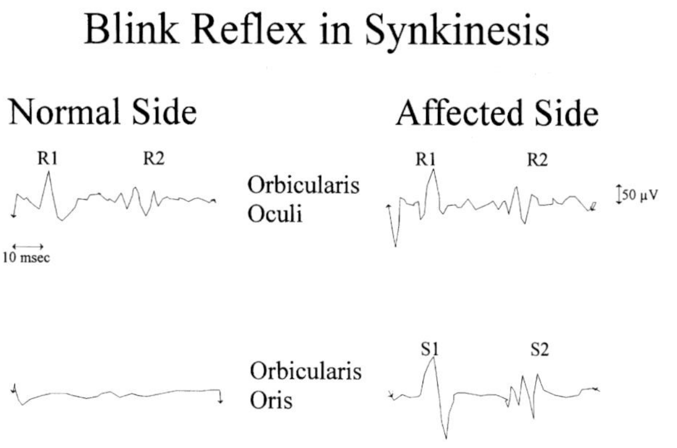

Fig. 7. An abnormal blink reflex recorded in a patient with post-paralytic synkinesis (according to Maeyama [17]). Notice that R_1 response is recorded on both sides (crossing) and that the responses could be recorded in many muscles on the affected side (lateral spread)

fifteenth day, by the modifications of the ENoG recordings [17], 100 percent of patients with totally abolished ENoG recordings (=0) had synkinesis. There was no synkinesis if the amplitude of the ENoG response remained higher than 40 percent. The latency of the R_1 component was slightly increased in such patients, with mean values of 12 ms (SD 1.4) in the orbicularis oculi muscle, 13.6 ms (SD 2.0) in the orbicularis oris muscle [17], and 14.4 ms (SD 0.4) in the mentalis muscle [23]. The R_1 components could be recorded bilaterally after stimulation of the normal side (thus an abnormal R_1 response).

In patients with essential hemifacial spasm twitching occurs irregularly and is not accompanied by voluntary and reflex movements of the face. If a spasm could not be visually seen on the patient's face, the investigators could often record the spasm by asking the patient to make an extended, maximum contraction of his or her entire face (which is frequently followed by spontaneous hemifacial spasm). In essential hemifacial spasm, Møller and Jannetta [20] noted that the blink reflex could be elicited intraoperatively on the affected side, despite the use of inhalation anesthetics, that the amplitude increased (facilitation) after a brief stimulation at a high rate, and that the response spread to the mentalis muscles (synkinesis) (lateral spread of the blink reflex). Finally, a particularly important finding was that vascular decompression suppresses this abnormal blink response and that the response elicited by electrically stimulating one branch of the facial nerve while recorded from muscles that are innervated by another branch (the lateral spread) disappears instantaneously during the operation when the offending vessel is moved off the nerve and it reappears if the blood vessel is allowed to fall back on the nerve [20, 21]. (See this book, Chapter by Møller "Pathophysiology of Hemifacial Spasm").

An extensive study of the facilitation of the R_1 component of the blink reflex on repetitive stimulation was done in normal individuals and in patients with synkinesis and essential hemifacial spasm [23]. In a study by Laskawi et al. [15] an abnormal blink reflex response was documented in 40 percent of the patients [15] with signs of synkinesis (a pathological spread of the blink reflex response), and a bilateral early component (R_1) after stimulation of the affected side. This abnormal bilateral R_1 response was not always present when elicited from the pathological side.

Especially interesting is the fact that such an abnormal blink reflex has been observed after anastomosis of the cranial nerves VII–XII [23], and it has been compared with abnormalities (involuntary discharges in innervation areas of other motor cerebral nerves, the spinal accessory nerve (CN XI), and the trigeminal and hypoglossal nerves (CN XII) observed in patients with essential hemifacial spasm [15]. This finding could hardly be explained by an isolated peripheral facial nerve lesion and it indicates a more centrally-located mechanism.

More recently, Darrouzet et al. [3] discussed the importance of the blink reflex in predicting facial function risk.

Intraoperative facial monitoring

The likelihood of successful preservation of facial function following removal of an acoustic neuroma has been improved by the development of intraoperative monitoring techniques.

Techniques

There are a number of techniques presently being used for intraoperative monitoring [12]. At our institution, we use an NIM 2^{R*} (intraoperative monitoring system) with monopolar stimulation. Recording needle electrodes are placed in the orbicularis oris and orbicularis oculi muscles (2 needles placed 1 cm apart) with the ground electrode placed on the forehead. We find it best to use a monopolar cathode stimulator to map the vicinity of the facial nerve with regard to tumor mass. However, when trying to separate the facial nerve from adjacent neural structures, a bipolar insulated stimulator is more selective [2].

Results

EMG recordings indicate two major factors: At rest, pseudorandom muscle activity measures 30–50 μV, and mechanical irritation of the nerve during surgery causes an increase in EMG activity (burst) that lasts for a few ms. This brief episode of activity, which is associated with specific surgical maneuvers, aids the surgeon to avoid causing damage to the nerve. Prolonged tonic EMG activity, which can be heard as a "staccato" sound, may reflect significant neural injury due to excessive traction, irrigation, etc. [14].

Electrical stimulation with a handheld probe elicits an electromyographic (EMG) response. The threshold for eliciting an evoked EMG response provides an indication of the functional status of the nerve. At the beginning of the operation, a 0.05 mA stimulation could provide a response that has an amplitude as high as 1000 μV. At the end of the operation, after the tumor has been removed, the ability to elicit an EMG response from low-amplitude stimulation of the facial nerve near the brainstem is a reasonable predictor of postoperative intact facial function [14, 26]. If a stimulation of 0.3 mA induces a response that is more than 800 μV, a good prognosis can be expected. The final shape of the facial nerve after tumor removal is also important [14].

For further information on intraoperative facial monitoring during hemifacial spasm surgery see Møller [21] and his Chapter in this book, "Pathophysiology of Hemifacial Spasm."

Progress

In addition to the methods described above, new electrophysiological techniques are still being developed. Such new techniques promise to provide computerized digital analysis in either the temporal or the spectral domain. The techniques being developed also utilize modelling techniques [16]. However, their application to intraoperative monitoring of the facial nerve has yet to be validated.

Acknowledgement

*Xoned Company, Jackson, Florida.

References

1. Blumenthal F, May M (1986) Electrodiagnosis. In: May M (ed) The facial nerve. Thieme, New York, pp 241–262
2. Dankle JA, Wiegand DA (1994) Investigation of a coaxial bipolar nerve stimulator for intraoperative motor nerve monitoring. Laryngoscope 104: 619–622
3. Darrauzet S, Wang T, Eshapasse T, Guerin J, Duroux S, Bebear JP (1994) Valeur pronostique du réflexe de clignement dans la chirurgie du neurinome de l'acoustique. Communication aux Journées multirégionales d'otolaryngologie, Lyon, vril. J Franc Otolaryngol 43: 251–253
4. Esslen E (1957) Der Spasmus facialis, eine Parabiose Erscheinung. Dtsch Z Nervenh 176: 149–172
5. Esslen E (1977) Electromyography and electroneurography. In: Fisch U (ed) Facial nerve surgery. Proceedings of the Third International Symposium on Facial Nerve Surgery. Kugler, Amsterdam, pp 93–100
6. Fisch U (1977) Managment of Bell's palsy. In: Fisch U (ed) Facial nerve surgery. Kugler, Amsterdam, pp 393–394
7. Fligny I, Lamas G, Poignonec S, Couturier J, Soudant J, Willer JC (1993) Mise en évidence et analyse électrophysiologique du réflexe de clignement chez le rat. Intérêt de ce modèle expérimental. Ann Oto-Laryngol (Paris) 110: 470–473
8. Furata S, Hirota J, Obata E, Ohyama M (1990) Influence of brain tumors on the blink reflex. In: Castro D (ed) The facial nerve. Proceedings of the Sixth International Symposium on the Facial Nerve (held in Rio de Janeiro, Brazil, 1988). Kugler and Ghedini, Amsterdam, pp 143–145
9. Glocker FX, Magistris NR, Rössler KM, Hess CV (1994) Magnetic transcranial and electrical stylo-mastoidal stimulation of the facial motor pathway in Bell's palsy: Time-course and relevance of electrophysiological parameters. Electroenceph Clin Neurophysiol 93: 113–120
10. Hanner P, Badr G, Rosenhall U, Edström S (1986) Trigeminal dysfunction in patients with Bell's palsy. Acta Oto-Laryngol (Stockh) 101: 224–230
11. Henrion P (1988) Etude pronostique de la paralysie faciale périphérique et de ses séquelles par le réflexe trigémino-facial et facio-facial et par la neurographie. A propos de 461 paralysies. Thèse, Paris (Dir. Molina-Negro). Fac Méd Paris-Lariboisière
12. Kartush J, Bouchard K (1992) Intraoperative facial nerve monitoring: Otology, neurotology and skull base surgery. In: Kartush J (ed) Neuromonitoring in otology and head and neck surgery. Raven Press, New York, pp 99–120
13. Kohsyu H, Aoyagi M, Tojima H, Tada Y, Inamura H, Ikarashi T, Koike Y (1994) Facial nerve enhancement in Gd-MRI in patients with Bell's palsy. Acta Oto-Laryngol (Stockh) [Suppl] 511: 165–169
14. Lacombe H, Keravel Y, Peynegre R, Esharagha A (1993) Intérêt du monitoring du facial sur la fonction faciale dans la chirurgie translabyrinthique des neurinomes de l'acoustique. Ann Oto-Laryngol (Paris) 111: 89–94
15. Laskawi R, Stennert E, Limberg C (1990) Electrophysiological investigations in patients with hemifacial spasm. In: Castro D (ed) The facial nerve. Proceedings of the Sixth International Symposium on the Facial Nerve (held in Rio de Janeiro, Brazil, 1988). Kugler and Ghedini, Amsterdam, pp 465–467
16. Lucas MF (1986) Contribution à l'étude du signal d'EMG de surface. Modélisation, identification, classification. Thèse de Dr Ingénieur, Nantes, Fac. des Sciences
17. Maeyama H, Aoyagi M, Tojima H, Inamura H, Kohsyu H, Koike Y (1994) Electrophysiological study of the pathology of synkinesis after facial nerve paralysis. Acta Otolaryngol (Stockh) [Suppl] 511: 161–164

18. Molina P, Bertrand RA, Hardy J (1977) The trigemino-facial reflexes. In: Fisch U (ed) Proceedings of the Third International Symposium on Facial Nerve Surgery. Kugler, Amsterdam, pp 107–128
19. Møller AR, Jannetta PJ (1985) Microvascular decompression in the hemifacial spasm: Intraoperative electrophysiological observations. Neurosurgery 16: 612–618
20. Møller AR, Jannetta PJ (1986) Blink reflex in patients with hemifacial spasm. Observations during microvascular decompression operations. J Neurosurg 72: 171–182
21. Møller AR (1990) Pathophysiology of hemifacial spasm. In: Castro D (ed) The Facial Nerve. Proceedings of the Sixth International Symposium on the Facial Nerve (held in Rio de Janeiro, Brazil, 1988). Kugler and Ghedini, Amsterdam, pp 469–471
22. Pialoux P, Freyss G, Beauvillain de Montreuil C (1975) Quelques développements récents des examens électriques appliqués à l'étude des paralysies faciales. Ann Oto-Laryngol (Paris) 92: 205–212
23. Poignonec S, Lamas G, Aidan D, Willer JC, Soudant J (1993) Exploration électrophysiologique de l'hémispasme facial. Ann Oto-Laryngol (Paris) 110: 385–391
24. Potosching C, Stennert E (1990) Magnetic stimulation: A new possibility in the assessment of facial nerve dysfunction. In: Castro D (ed) The facial nerve. Proceedings of the Sixth International Symposium on the Facial Nerve (held in Rio de Janeiro, Brazil, 1988). Kugler and Ghedini, Amsterdam, pp 183–189
25. Schmid UD, Møller AR, Schmid J (1992) Transcranial magnetic stimulation of the facial nerve: Intraoperative study of the effect of stimulus parameters on the excitator site in man. Muscle and Nerve 15: 829–836
26. Silverstein H, Willcox TO Jr, Rosenberg SI, Seidman MD (1994) Prediction of facial nerve function following acoustic neuroma resection using intraoperative facial nerve stimulation. Laryngoscope 104: 539–544
27. Stennert E (1982) New concepts in the treatment of Bell's palsy. In: Graham N, Gramm MD, House W (eds) Disorders of the facial nerve. Raven Press, New York, pp 313–317
28. Tamai Y, Ywamoto YM, Tsujimoto T (1986) Pathways of the blink reflex in the brain of the cat. Interneurons between the trigeminal nuclei and the facial nucleus. Brain Res 199: 19–25
29. Tojima H, Aoyagi M, Inamura H, Koike Y (1994) Clinical advantages of electroneurography in patients with Bell's palsy, within two weeks after onset. Acta Otolaryngol (Stockh), [Suppl] 511: 147–149
30. Willer JC, Lamour Y (1975) Etude électrophysiologique du réflexe de clignement chez le macaque. CR Acad Sc (Paris) 281 (série D): 563–566
31. Willer JC, Lamas G, Poignonec S, Fligny I, Soudant J (1992) Redirection of the hypoglossal nerve to facial muscles alters central connectivity in human brainstem. Brain Res 594: 301–306
32. Wolf SR, Schneider W, Berg M, Haid CT, Wigand ME (1994) Facial nerve involvement in acoustic neuromas : examination with transcranial magnetic single- and bistimulation. In: Proceedings of the Eighteenth Barany Society Meeting (held in Uppsala, Sweden, June 6–8, 1994). Acta Oto-Laryngol (Stockh) (In press)

Correspondence: Georges Freyss, M.D., Professor of Oto-laryngology (Paris), E.N.T. Department, Hôpital Lariboisière, 3, rue Ambroise, F-75010 Paris, France.

(Primary) hemifacial spasm: epidemiological data

A. Vighetto and **C. Vial**

Botulinum Toxin Outpatient Clinic, Hopital Neurologique Pierre Wertheimer, Lyon, France

Summary

Epidemiological and clinical analyses of hemifacial spasm (HFS) are presented and pertinent literature is reviewed. A group of 61 patients with HFS treated with botulinum toxin (BT) was studied, and a structured questionnaire took into account: age at onset (range: 18–77, mean: 51.1 years) and age at time of initiation of treatment (range: 22–82, mean: 58.1 years), sex distribution (showing a female predominance: 70%), side distribution (showing a predominant involvement of the left side of the face: 67%), initiation and evolution of HFS, personal and family history, symptoms associated with HFS, and response to treatment given before BT. Data on age, sex, and side distributions on these 61 patients were compared to those obtained in a group of 50 patients with HFS who underwent operation to perform vascular decompression. All of the parameters that were analyzed in patients with HFS were compared to those obtained in patients with blepharospasm (BSP). Thus, 57 patients with BSP treated with BT were age-matched with a similar number of the patients with HFS (belonging to the group of 61 patients).

Key words: Hemifacial spasm, botulinum toxin, treatment, epidemiology.

Introduction

Hemifacial spasm (HFS) is a benign chronic involuntary movement of one side of the face, characterized by twitching, tonic spasm, and synkinesis of the muscles innervated by the facial nerve. The term "hemifacial spasm" will be used in this chapter to describe patients with primary hemifacial spasm, i.e. that which fulfills the three following criteria: a) that it is not a sequela to ipsilateral facial palsy, b) that its evolution is chronic and that the disease is self-limiting, and c) that investigations are normal, except for the presence of a vascular compression of the seventh nerve at its root exit zone (REZ) in the posterior fossa, as evidenced by computer topography (CT-scan) or magnetic resonance imagery (MRI).

Clinical work that was pioneered and described by Gowers [22], Brissaud [8], and Babinski [4] has led to the recognition that HFS differs from other facial movement disorders. As early as 1875, Schultze [39] described a pathological case of HFS that involved a compression of the facial nerve by a vertebral artery aneurysm, but this anatomical explanation had remained ignored for years. HFS had been dismissed for a long period of time, up to the seminal paper by Ehni and Woltman [13] and the book written on the topic by Wartenberg [45]. The reasons were probably related to the benign nature of HFS, its limited functional consequences in comparison with other facial movement disorders, its unsettled pathogenesis, and the lack of an effective treatment, all of which caused the medical community at that time to avoid involvement and thus discouraged patients to seek medical care for such a condition.

Now, more clinical and demographical information is available. Major therapeutic advances have been described for large series of patients afflicted with this condition, such as Jannetta's influential papers describing vascular cross-compression [26, 27] as well as studies by Huang et al. [23], Iwakuma et al. [24], and Sindou et al. [41]. More recently, medical treatment of HFS using botulinum toxin has been described [1, 7, 11, 12, 14, 16, 18, 21, 25, 28, 31, 32, 36–38, 42–44, 46], prompting a wealth of demographical information.

HFS is a rare condition. The only epidemiological information can be found in a survey done in Rochester and Olmstead County, Minnesota, between 1960 and 1984 that was reported in the Mayo Clinic Register [3]. In this report the mean annual incidence rate of HFS is estimated to have been $0.74/10^5$ for males and $0.84/10^5$ for females, whereas the mean annual prevalence rate ranged between $7.4/10^5$ for males and $14.5/10^5$ for females, with the highest rates in individuals over age 40. Extrapolation of these prevalence figures to the French population yields an approximate number: 5000 HFS patients in France. A comparison from the same source of data would indicate that the incidence of HFS could be estimated to be about 6 times lower than the incidence of trigeminal neuralgia [29] and 30 times lower than the incidence of Bell's palsy [30].

The following discussion will be based upon information gathered from a series of 61 consecutive patients treated at the Botulinum Toxin Outpatient Clinic of the Pierre Wertheimer Hopital Neurologique, and from a survey of the literature.

Materials and methods

Two groups of patients with HFS seen at our institution were selected for analysis as was a control group of patients with blepharospasm.

The *first group* (group HFS I) of 61 patients was selected between August 1990 and April 1994 at the Botulinum Toxin Outpatient Clinic. This cohort represented all of the patients we had examined and treated in our clinic within that time range who had a diagnosis of HFS, as defined by the above outlined criteria. All of these patients had had an extensive work-up, including CT-scan and MRI, prior to being referred to us. Between November 1993 and April 1994, all these 61 patients were documented prospectively using a structured questionnaire specifically designed for the study and completed by the two authors. The acquired information came from questions asked of the patients, patients' records sent by their general practitioners or the consulting neurologists, the results of neurological examinations, and the inspection of radiological charts. Besides a demographic information section, the questionnaire included: a) detailed time information, regarding age at onset of HFS, age when starting botulinum toxin treatment, and age at the latest visit; b) clinical information, including side of HFS, and type and location of initial symptoms; c) course of illness information, comprising pattern of evolution over time, specific determination of initial event that triggered the HFS, and worsening or alleviating factors of the spasms; d) personal and family history of dystonia and other movement disorders and/or of somatic and psychiatric diseases; e) recording of associated signs and symptoms; and f) description and results of previously administered treatments. From this group all patients but 2 were subjected to at least one treatment with botulinum toxin.

A *second group* (group HFS II) comprised 50 patients with HFS operated on to perform vascular decompression at the Pierre Wertheimer Hopital Neurologique in Lyon, France, by the same neurosurgeon (M. Sindou). These same 50 patients are the subjects of a report in another chapter in this book (Sindou et al.). They are analyzed here only for demographic data and to allow a comparison between a "medical" cohort (group HFS I) and a "surgical" cohort (group HFS II) of patients treated in the same institution.

A *third group* (group BSP) comprised 57 patients with blepharospasm (BSP). Blepharospasm is characterized by bilateral involuntary contractions of the orbicularis oculi muscles that result in a functional impairment that can be quite distressing to the patient. This disease is considered to be a focal dystonia and therefore represents a quite different pathophysiological condition than does HFS. This group was designed to provide a case-control study of HFS and blepharospasm in order to better analyze features of and risk factors for HFS.

The 57 patients (in group BSP) were selected from patients with blepharospasm who were treated at our institution with botulinum toxin in order to be matched for sex and current age (to within five years) with a similar number of patients from group HFS I (this study-group of patients with HFS I was called group HFS Ia). There were actually 4 patients (the youngest ones) from group HFS I that were not considered for this comparison between the two conditions, because we were not able to find in our files age-matched patients with blepharospasm. Patients from group BSP were subjected to the same structured questionnaire as were patients in group HFS I.

Results

Age of patients

In group HFS I the *age at onset* ranged from 18 to 77 years, with a mean value of 51.1 years (Table 1), and no difference was noted between males and females. The majority of the patients (50 percent of females and 66 percent of males) experienced the onset of HFS in their fifth and sixth decades (Fig. 1). In only 4 patients did the spasms begin before age 30. *Patient age at time of initiation of treatment with botulinum toxin* ranged from 22 to 82 years, with a mean value of 58.1 years (Fig. 2). In 62 percent of the patients, the *time from disease onset to treatment with botulinum toxin* was less than 5 years, but extremes in the whole population were ranging between 6 months and 20 years (Fig. 3).

Table 1. Descriptive data of hemifacial spasm as derived from the literature (only series having more than 20 patients and which provided enough descriptive data are included here). Some of the statistics presented have been recalculated from the original data given by the authors. NA = not available

Authors	Number	Sex: F/M	F/M ratio	Age at onset	Age at visit/treatment (years)	Time from onset (years)	Type of study	Side: Lt/Rt ratio
Ehni and Woltman 1945	106	64/42	1,5	mean = 45 (SD = 12) range = 17–70	NA	NA	clinical study	equivalent ?
Auger 1979	23	12/11	1,1	NA	mean = 57	range = 1–25 mean = 5,6	neurophysiology	11/12
Jannetta 1981	229	150/79	2	NA	median decade = 50–60	mean = 5	surgery	137/91 and 1 bilat
Iwakuma et al. 1982	110	77/33	2,3	range = 11–69	range = 18–75	range = 3 months–20 yrs	surgery	53/57
Nielsen 1984	62	41/21	1,9	NA	mean = 54 range = 31–77	range = 2–16	neurophysiology	32/30
Esteban and Molina-Negro 1986	53	39/14	2,8	NA	mean = 52,7 range = 24–81	range = 3,5–50 (mean = 5,7)	neurophysiology	NA
Dutton and Buckley 1988	60	40/20	2,0	NA	Female mean = 63,8 range = 38–88 Male mean = 58 range = 30–79	NA	Bot. Toxin	NA
Biglan et al. 1988	24	NA	NA	NA	mean = 64 range = 23–85	NA	Bot. Toxin	NA
Auger and Whisnant 1980	20	12/8	1,5	range = 30–72	NA	NA	epidemiology	7/13
Taylor et al. 1991	130	78/52	1,5	NA	mean = 60,4 range = 20–86	mean = 6,9	Bot. toxin	NA
Elston 1992	73	42/31	1,3	NA	NA	NA	Bot. Toxin	44/29
Huang et al. 1992	310	143/167	0,9	NA	mean = 53,4 range = 25–76	mean = 4,9 range = 1–30	surgery	168/142
Flanders et al. 1993	65	40/25	1,6	NA	mean = 54,3 range = 25–76	range = 1–30 (mean = 6,4)	Bot. Toxin	39/26
Jedynak et al. 1993	54	34/20	1,7	mean = 51	mean = 59 range = 26–83	NA	Bot. Toxin	28/26
Soulayrol et al. 1993	43	NA	NA	NA	mean = 63	NA	Bot. Toxin	NA
Bénillouche 1993	75	46/29	2	NA	mean = 64, 1 (SD = 11,5) range = 28–91	range = 2mo–31 (mean = 6,2)	Bot. Toxin Bot. Toxin	39/36 39/36
Present series 1994	61	43/18	2,4	mean = 51,1 (SD = 13,2) range = 18–77	mean = 58,1 (SD = 13,4) range = 22–82	range = 6mo–30 (mean = 6,9)	Bot. Toxin	41/20

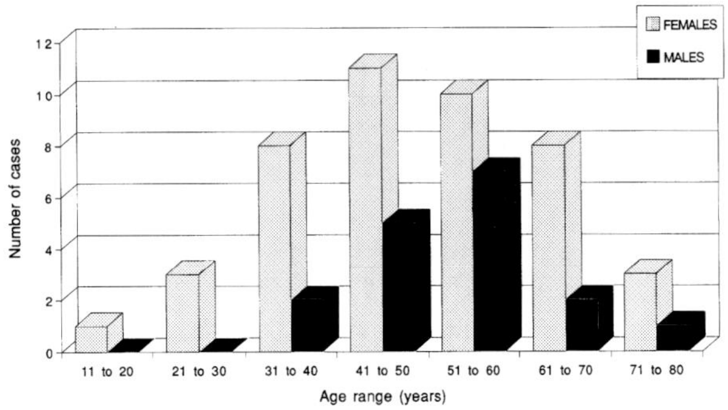

Fig. 1. Age distribution (years) of female and male patients at onset of HFS (group HFS I)

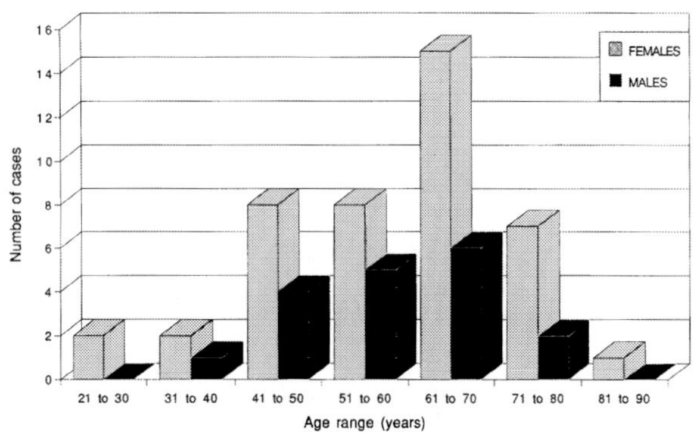

Fig. 2. Age distribution (years) of female and male patients when first treated with botulinum toxin (group HFS I)

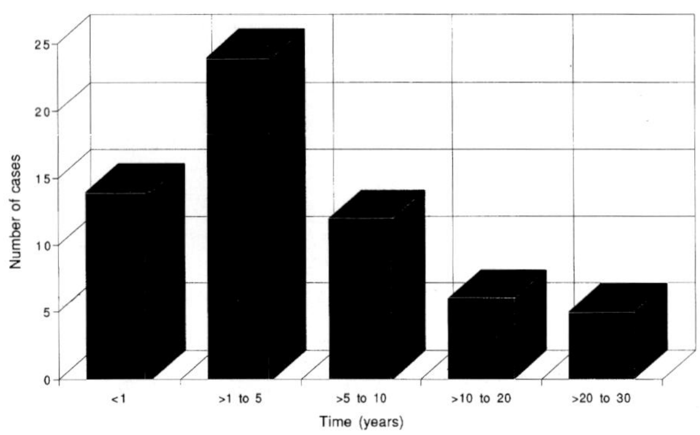

Fig. 3. Time range (years) from onset of hemifacial spasm to initial treatment with botulinum toxin (group HFS I)

In group HFS II, the *age at time of surgery* ranged from 23 to 78 years, with a mean value of 50 years.

Sex of patients

Group HFS I comprised 43 females and 18 males (Table 1). Female predominance, expressed in terms of F/M ratio in Table 1, was 2.4. Similarly, group HFS II comprised 31 females and 19 males, yielding a F/M ratio equal to 1.6.

Side of hemifacial spasm

In group HFS I, the left side of the face was affected in 41 patients (67 percent) and the right side was affected in 20 patients (33 percent). This left-sided predominance was more pronounced among males (14 of 18 patients, corresponding to 78 percent) than among females (27 of 43 patients, corresponding to 63 percent). None of the patients in our series had a bilateral hemifacial spasm. In group HFS II, the left side of the face was affected in 31 patients (62 percent) and the right side was affected in 19 patients (38 percent).

Initiation of hemifacial spasm

Localization of abnormal movements at onset could be determined in 50 patients in group HFS I. Most patients (35/50, that is 70 percent) reported that initial twitches occurred in the periocular region. Some patients could even localize more precisely the first symptoms to the inferior part of the orbicularis oculi muscle. However, some patients reported that the spasm began in the perioral region (7/50, that is 14 percent), and some others reported that the spasm began on the entire one side of the face (8/50, that is 16 percent).

A *triggering initial event* was reported in 14 patients (23 percent) in group HFS I, which usually was an emotional event: acute stress in 7 patients, the death of a spouse in 5 patients, and onset of a severe depression in 1 patient. In 1 patient, HFS had manifested during pregnancy.

Evolution of hemifacial spasm

The evolution pattern in most patients was chronic and progressive. The facial spasms were initially intermittent, barely visible, and localized to a few muscular fibers. Over time, the spasms tended to become more permanent, more intense, and more diffuse. However, in some patients, worsening of the spasms was transient, in close relation with emotional stress and fatigue. Worsening in some patients was also subjective, resulting from psychological intolerance to the disease. In other instances, the spasms remained stable over the years. The intensity of the spasms was affected by external or internal factors in almost all patients in group HFS I. Factors that consistently triggered spasms were reported in 24 of 61 patients (39%), some of whom reported more than one. These factors were (in a decreasing order of frequency): normal life events that cause emotional frustrations (13 patients), efforts involving visual fixation, such as reading (6 patients), changing body position, such as lying down in bed or turning to a particular side (6 patients), social interactions (5 patients), touching the affected side of the face (2 patients), and driving, hearing noise, and drinking alcohol (4 patients). A few patients (6/61, that is 10%) indicated idiosyncratic "tricks" that could temporarily alleviate the spasms: resting in a quiet room (4 patients), putting mild pressure on the affected side of the face (2 patients), or simply using mental effort (1 patient).

Personal and family history

Two patients in group HFS I reported a concomitant history of focal dystonia, represented by laryngeal dystonia and writer's cramp. The most common chronic somatic condition in the patients in group HFS I was high blood pressure. Considering only those patients in group HFS I who had had previously documented hypertension and who had received treatment for hypertension, this condition was present in 15 of these patients (25 percent). Less frequently, we found vascular diseases (e.g., stroke, angina pectoris) (6 patients), migraine (6 patients), cancer (5 patients), thyroid dysfunction (2 patients), diabetes mellitus (2 patients), eye diseases (1 patient), and other miscellaneous conditions (9 patients).

In group HFS I, there was a relatively high incidence of psychiatric illness. Thus, taking into account only psychiatric conditions antedating the onset of HFS with subsequent chronic treatment, we had 13 patients with depression, 8 patients with anxiety, and 1 patient with chronic psychosis. Thus in our population of group HFS I there was a prevalence rate of 36 percent with psychiatric problems.

In 4 patients in group HFS I the family history indicated neurological disorders, which included Bell's palsy (1 patient), Parkinson's disease (1 patient), and hemifacial spasm (2 patients). In the latter cases of familial HFS, each of the 2 patients had one relative (a maternal aunt and a daughter) who had also been afflicted with the disorder.

Symptoms associated with HFS

In the majority of patients in group HFS I, HFS was the only symptom, even in those whose HFS took a long time to evolve. Neuro-otological signs and symptoms were found in only 13 patients (21 percent), as indicated on non-clinical evaluation. These signs and symptoms were mostly vertigo, dizziness, tinnitus, or hearing loss (one or several of these symptoms were present in 6 patients). A vascular-like facial pain, resembling cluster headache, on the same side as HFS was reported by 5 patients. One patient had an ipsilateral deficit of the fifth and eighth nerves, corresponding to surgical sequelae from a previous vascular decompression done in another institution. Only 1 patient gave a description of a clicking noise in the ear, a symptom related to spasmodic contraction of the tensor tympani muscle.

Therapeutic trials before botulinum toxin

In patients in group HFS I, several unsuccessful medical treatments had been tried prior to botulinum toxin injections in our institution. These treatments included the administration of carbamazepine (23 patients), benzodiazepines (10 patients), antidepressant agents (8 patients), neuroleptic (4 patients) and anticholinergic drugs (3 patients), and baclofen (2 patients). Surgical procedures were performed in 3 patients, including 2 who underwent microvascular decompression.

Comparison between data obtained in patients with HFS (group HFS Ia) and patients with blepharospasm (group BSP)

Mean age was not different between the 2 groups (group HFS Ia: 61.4 years; group BSP: 61.0 years) at the time of this study, but the *time from disease onset to treatment with botulinum toxin* was shorter in group BSP: mean delay was 7.3 years (SD = 7.5) in group HFS Ia and 3.4 years (SD = 4.2) in group BSP, the difference being significant at $p < 0{,}001$ (Fig. 4). Six patients in group HFS Ia had a remission but none did in group BSP. A *triggering initial event* was indicated more frequently in group BSP (25 patients) than in group HFS Ia (13 patients). In the former group, triggering events were principally the introduction of a neuroleptic treatment (9 patients) and an emotional stress or depression (8 patients), but other factors were

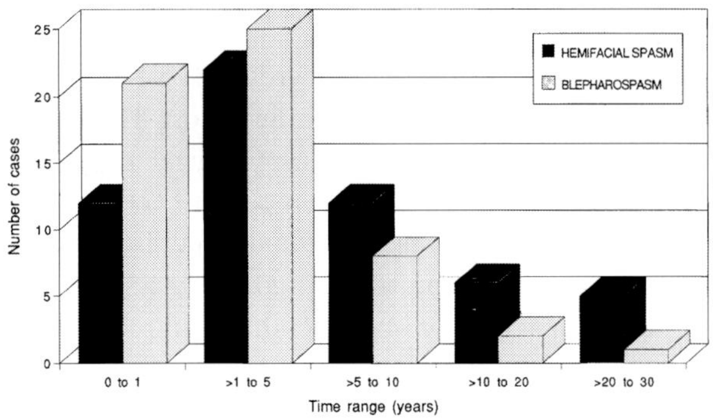

Fig. 4. Time range (years) from onset of disease to treatment with botulinum toxin in both hemifacial spasm (group HFS Ia) and blepharospasm (group BSP)

occasionally found, such as a general surgery procedure (3 patients) and ocular disease (2 patients). *Worsening factors* were described more frequently by patients with blepharospasm (50/57) than by patients with HFS (23/57). The factors most often noted by the patients were fatigue, stress, light exposure, reading, or driving. Similarly, *alleviating factors* were much more common in patients with blepharospasm (20/57) than in patients with HFS (5/57). In the former group, such alleviating factors consisted mainly of physical or psychological rest.

There was evidence of a much higher rate of *personal history* for dystonia in group BSP (25/57) than in group HFS Ia (2/57). In group BSP, the dystonia was mostly manifested in Meige's syndrome (18 patients), and less frequently in laryngeal dystonia (4 patients), parkinsonism (4 patients), or writer's cramp (3 patients). Similarly, a family history of movement disorders was more often noted in group BSP (7 patients) than in group HFS Ia (3 patients). A personal history of somatic non-neurological diseases was nearly equal in terms of hypertension for these two groups (BSP: 14 patients; HFS Ia: 15 patients), as it was for vascular problems (BSP: 5 patients; HFS Ia: 6 patients) and for migraine (BSP: 6 patients; HFS Ia: 5 patients). However, eye diseases were more frequent in group BSP (9 patients) than in group HFS Ia (1 patient). Psychiatric illness was significantly more prevalent in group BSP (36 of the total 57 patients in this group had such illnesses: 25 patients had depression; 7 patients had anxiety; 4 patients had psychosis) than in group HFS Ia (21 of the total 57 patients in this group had such illnesses: 12 patients had depression; 8 patients had anxiety; 1 patient had psychosis). With regard to *medical treatments before botulinum toxin* therapy, in group BSP there was a higher incidence of treatment with antidepressants (20 versus 8 patients) and neuroleptic drugs (16 versus 3 patients), and a lower incidence of treatment with carbamazepine (3 versus 21 patients).

Thirteen patients in group HFS Ia experienced other neurologic symptoms, but none in group BSP had neurologic symptoms other than movement disorders.

Discussion

Age, sex, and side

Our experience is that primary HFS is a disease whose onset begins mostly between the ages of 41 and 60 years, with a mean *age at onset* of 51 years. However, in the present study there was a considerable variation in the age at onset that ranged from 18 to 77 years. Comparative data are surprisingly scarce, and we found only 2 studies [13, 28] that provide information on age at onset of large cohorts of patients with HFS. These studies reported mean values of age at onset of 45 and 51 years, respectively. However, there are occasional reports of HFS starting before 30 years of age [13, 40]. Our series comprised 4 young patients with HFS, the youngest being 18 years old at onset of HFS. Ehni and Woltman's study [13] of 106 patients with HFS included 3 young patients whose HFS began before 30 years of age. It has been reported that HFS can occur in infancy [40], but none of our patients had had an onset of symptoms in infancy. As shown in Table 1, more information is available concerning *age when patients are enrolled for treatment*. In most of the series covered in Table 1, as in our present study, the mean age at initiation of treatment with botulinum toxin ranged between 52 and 64 years [6, 7, 12, 18, 28, 42, 43], although there were still considerable individual variations that ranged between 18 and 91 years. In some studies listed in Table 1 [23, 27] the HFS patients selected for surgery were younger than those selected for medical treatment, thus possibly reflecting a selection bias in these cohorts. This selection bias has also been evidenced in our experience at our Institution, as the mean age of the patients in group HFS II (surgical group) is 8 years younger than the mean age of the patients in group HFS I (medical group). The finding that the delay from onset of HFS to medical or surgical treatment of these patients was significantly longer than it was for patients with blepharospasm is interesting, and the difference may be related to the fact that the functional impairment that results from blepharospasm is more severe than that which results from HFS.

Most investigators of HFS have found a female predominance for the condition (the ratio between female and male is 1.1/2.8; see Table 1) [2, 3, 6, 12, 13, 16–18, 24, 27, 28, 34, 43]. The only known exception in the literature comes from Huang's report [23] that is based on a surgical recruitment of 310 patients and shows a 54 percent male predominance for the condition. This finding may have a racial basis because Huang et al.'s 1992 report [23] differs from other publications in that the series population comprises only Chinese patients; however, a more likely explanation is offered by the authors themselves: a selection bias due to recruitment that predominantly comprised hospitalized veterans of war. In our series, we found a rather high ratio of 2.4 of female over male. This female predominance in HFS cannot be explained by age-biased selection, since we found that the higher female predominance in HFS is homogeneous throughout all ages.

The question as to whether one particular *side of the face* is preferentially involved in HFS has been debated. Indeed, a number of published reports (see Table 1) [2, 6, 24, 28, 34], following the very first one [13] on the subject, indicate no significant difference between right and left-sided hemifacial spasm. However, some publications, each involving a large series of more than 65 patients, show a significant preference towards involvement of the left side of the face ranging between 54 and 72 percent of the patients [16, 18, 23, 26, 27]. This is in agreement with our findings of a left-sided predominance in HFS (67 percent of patients in our present study). It seems that this left-sided predominance in HFS may be more marked in males than in females. In a study based on 75 patients with HFS, belonging to a total group of 173 patients who had HFS or blepharospasm [6], there is only a slight left-sided predominance (52 percent) when the sub-group of 75 patients is considered, but when only male patients were considered, the left-sided predominance was 72 percent. We also found in our series of patients that left-sided predominance was more marked in males (78 percent) than in females (63 percent). The reasons for such an asymmetrical involvement and a putative sexual influence are unclear. It has been suggested that the left-sided predominance in HFS could reflect an embryological predisposition in the relative position of the facial nerve and blood vessels in the root exit zone on the left side [15]. Newton and Mani [33] suggested that the variability in the size of the vertebral arteries, with the one on the left side often being larger than the one on the right side, might be the cause of this left-sided predominance in HFS. However, these anatomical factors do not explain the male predominance. In addition, this postulation does not exclude a more "central" explanation in terms of a putative predominance of the right hemisphere on emotional control and facial expression.

Bilateral hemifacial spasm is very rare [35]. Ehni and Woltman [13] described 6 patients out of a series of 106 with supposedly primary hemifacial spasm, in whom a unilateral facial spasm became bilateral after a delay that ranged from 1 to 15 years. Jannetta reported 1 such patient in a series of 229 with HFS [27]. Our series did not include any patients with bilateral HFS.

It is interesting to compare the results on HFS patients for age, sex, and side distribution with results from studies on *trigeminal neuralgia*, which is another condition related to vascular cross-compression. Sindou et al. [41] described a surgical series studied in our institution that comprised 120 patients with trigeminal neuralgia who were operated on after unsuccessful medical treatment. Sixty percent of these patients underwent operation in their sixth or seventh decade. Only a slight female predominance (52%) was found, and of those, 60 percent had preferential involvement of the right side. Thus, the epidemiological data on trigeminal neuralgia seem to differ from those involving HFS regarding all of the parameters that were discussed above.

Initial symptoms

It is well recognized that in patients with HFS, the spasms usually begin as slight intermittent unilateral twitching of the orbicularis oculi muscle and the localization of the first symptom corresponds to the inferior orbicularis oculi muscle [11, 27]. Progressively over months or even years, these abnormal movements become more severe and more persistent, and spread down over all the muscles of facial expression, with the possible exception of the frontalis muscle. These data are in accordance with relatively rare studies that have focused on the location of initial symptoms. Ehni and Woltman [13] found that in 90 of 99 patients, in whom information on location of initial symptoms was available, the eyelid muscles were primarily affected. Similarly, Auger and Whisnant [3] noted that twitching in the orbicularis oculi muscles was the first sign of HFS in 19 of their series of 20 patients. Esteban and Molina-Negro [17] estimated that in 46 of their 53 patients abnormal contractions began in the lower eyelids. In our series, such information was available for 50 patients: in 35 patients (70 percent) the orbicularis oculi muscle was primarily affected, as evidenced by twitching of the eyelids or tonic spasm. However, some patients (7 or 14 percent in our series) indicated an initial involvement of the lower face. According to Jannetta [27], the HFS of these "atypical patients," whose contractions progress upward and frequently involve the frontalis muscles, may have a different pathophysiologic basis. Finally, 8 of our patients (16 percent) in the present study indicated that the initiation of their HFS occurred simultaneously in the lower and upper regions of the face.

Initial event

As mentioned earlier, the onset of HFS may sometimes be triggered by a physical or emotional event. Although these precipitating factors have not been systematically investigated in previous works, in our experience it seems that nearly 25 percent of patients with HFS link the initial onset of their HFS to an emotional event or to pregnancy. Similarly, Ehni and Woltman [13] noted that in 5 of their series of 106 patients there was a relationship between the onset of HFS and a psychological factor. These clinical facts are important in pathophysiologic terms, as they seem to indicate that abnormal activity in the facial nucleus, whatever its cause, can be modulated by psychological factors.

Factors influencing spasms

Ehni and Woltman [13] systematically investigated factors modulating the intensity of spasms. Spasms can increase due to a number of factors, which differ among patients but which are dominated by mental events. Such factors are mainly anxiety, fatigue, facial voluntary movements, excessive use of eyes, and/or being under observation. In the present study, we corroborated these findings by showing that 39 percent of patients experience a worsening factor at some time during the course of their HFS. On the other hand, in about 20 percent of patients relaxation may transiently have a favorable influence on their spasms [13]. Some patients may learn trick maneuvers, such as putting mild pressure on their facial musculature [44] to alleviate the symptoms, but the effectiveness in controlling the spasms is low and in the present series the proportion of patients who were able to control their spasms in this way did not exceed 10 percent. In only 6 patients in our study did we find that the spasms were influenced by changes in posture, but Jannetta [27] estimated that 50 percent of HFS patients may be able to worsen or ease their spasms by changing the head and body position.

Time course

The evolution of HFS is usually described as being chronic and progressive since the onset of the spasms. Over a period of time, the spasms extend and increase in intensity, resulting in a feeling of aggravation. HFS usually persists during sleep [13, 28]. Several publications indicate the possibility of remission [2, 3, 13, 19, 20, 28]. Although some patients may experience a total remission that lasts for weeks or even years, often giving the impression of a cure, remissions from HFS are always temporary, at least for patients who come for medical care. Sometimes these remissions are anecdotally reported: Gardner and Sava [19] noted 1 patient, as did Geller et al. [20]; Auger [2] noted 3 of 23 patients; Auger and Whisnant [3] noted 3 of 20 patients; Jedynak et al. [28] noted 2 of 54 patients; and Ehni and Woltman [13] noted as many as 9 of 106 patients. Some of these remissions were attributed to emotional or physical events, particularly undergoing general anesthesia. In our present series, we found 8 of 61 patients who had a remission for more than 6 months. At least one factor associated with remission was present in 4 of these 8 patients: 2 patients underwent a surgical procedure to treat their hemifacial spasm, one of which was a microvascular decompression procedure; 1 patient was pregnant; and 1 patient had an improvement in his severe depression.

Associated symptoms

In most patients, facial spasm is the only symptom of HFS. The symptom most often associated with HFS in the literature is moderate ipsilateral facial weakness. Ehni and Woltman [13] reported that 16 of 106 patients in their study had moderate ipsilateral facial weakness, Auger [2] noted 7 of 23 patients, Jedynak et al. [28] noted 24 of 54 patients, Auger and Whisnant [3] noted 4 of 20 patients, and Huang et al. [23] noted 32 of 310. The highest statistic in this regard was reported by Iwakuma et al. [24] who noted 51 of 110 patients, but half of these 110 patients had a facial nerve block previous to their clinical evaluation. None of the patients in our present series was considered to have facial weakness. This discrepancy may be more presumable than real and could be related to definition criteria. Actually, some of our patients had facial asymmetries, occurring either spontaneously or during strong eye-blinking, but we considered these asymmetries as being secondary to spasm and synkinesis, and not related to a genuine facial deficit. Vertigo or ipsilateral impairment of hearing are relatively frequently noted symptoms of HFS: Ehni and Woltman [13] noted 16 of 106 patients with one of these symptoms, Huang et al. [23] noted 15 of 320 patients, Jedynak et al. [28] noted 3 of 54 patients, and in our present series we noted 6 of 61 patients. Associating HFS to ipsilateral trigeminal neuralgia has more direct pathophysiologic significance. This association, which was coined 'tic convulsif' by Cushing [10], is rare. Ehni and Woltman [13] reported this syndrome in only 3 of 106 patients, Huang et al. [23] noted 2 of 320 patients, and Auger [2] noted 1 of 23 patients, but in this latter case trigeminal neuralgia was on the side contralateral to the side with HFS. No case of tic convulsif was found in our cohort, but this may also reflect a population bias due to a medical recruitment. There are a few reports of tic convulsif associated with hypertension that demonstrate that vascular compression of the tenth nerve can cause hypertension (e.g., Ballantyne et al. [5]). Some patients report a clicking noise in the ear [2], as did 1 patient in our present series. To our knowledge, the incidence of headache and facial pain has not been evaluated. Five patients in our present series noted that they had facial pain on the same side as the HFS, and 6 patients complained of migraine headaches, giving an 18 percent prevalence of headache and facial pain in our series. Ehni and Woltman [13] reported that 30 of 106 patients had headaches of various types, including 16 with migraine.

Personal and family history

The influence that personal and family history has on various conditions affecting patients with HFS has not been addressed to any great extent in the literature. A study designed to investigate the relationship of hypertension to vascular disease would be valuable because of its possible origin in vascular conflict. Hypertension is often found in patients with HFS. However, hypertension does not seem to have a stronger incidence in patients with HFS than it does in the rest of the population. In our present series we found hypertension in 25 percent of our patients and vascular diseases in 10 percent, and we noted nearly the same incidence in age-matched patients with blepharospasm. Ehni and Woltman [13] indicated that in their study 41 of 106 patients had evidence of atherosclerosis, and they noted only a very slight increase in the incidence of hypertension in their patients with HFS compared to normals (and only in those who were younger than 50 years of age). Similarly, Jedynak [28] reported a 22 percent incidence of hypertension and vascular diseases. Interestingly, the prevalence of hypertension we found in our patients with HFS was comparable to the 22.5 percent noted by Sindou et al. [41] in their series of patients with trigeminal neuralgia.

Psychiatric problems antedating the onset of HFS are frequently noted and unexplained. We were impressed with the high prevalence of psychiatric problems in our series (36 percent), although the figure is higher for patients with blepharospasm. Other studies have yielded lower percentages, but to our knowledge no systematic evaluation of psychiatric pathology has been done. Jedynak [28] reported a psychological impact of HFS in 44 percent of the HFS patients in his study, but Ehni and Woltman [13] indicated a "psychoneurotic" state in only 6 of 106 patients in their study.

We have been unable to find any studies in the literature on personal and family history of dystonia or other movement disorders. Surprisingly, in our present series we found 2 patients that had dystonia in addition to HFS as well as 4 patients who had a positive family history of dystonia. Of the latter, 2 patients also had a family history of HFS. In cases of familial HFS, evidence has been presented that the origin of such HFS can be found in both an autosomal transmission and a vascular conflict [9].

References

1. Adenis JP, Smolik I, Maes S (1990) Traitement des spasmes faciaux par la toxine botulinique A. J Fr Ophtalmol 13: 259–264
2. Auger RG (1979) Hemifacial spasm: Clinical and electrophysiologic observations. Neurology 29: 1261–1272
3. Auger RG, Whisnant JP (1990) Hemifacial spasm in Rochester and Olmsted County, Minnesota, 1960 to 1984. Arch Neurol 47: 1233–1234
4. Babinski J (1905) Hémispasme facial périphérique. Rev Neurol (Paris) 13: 151–158

5. Ballantyne ES, Page RD, Meaney JFM, Nixon TE, Miles JB (1994) Coexistent trigeminal neuralgia, hemifacial spasm, and hypertension: Preoperative imaging of neurovascular compression. J Neurosurg 80: 559–563
6. Benillouche P (1993) Traitement du blépharospasme et de l'hémispasme facial par la toxine botulique A. Etude rétrospective de 173 patients. Thèse de Doctorat en Médecine, Université Claude Bernard Lyon I
7. Biglan AW, May M, Bowers RA (1988) Management of facial spasm with Clostridium botulinum toxin, type A (Oculinum). Arch Otolaryngol Head Neck Surg 114: 1407–1412
8. Brissaud E (1895) Tics et spasmes cloniques de la face: Vingt-quatrième leçon. In: Meige H (ed) Leçons sur les maladies nerveuses, Paris, Salpétrière 1893–1894. Masson, Paris, pp 502–520
9. Coad JE, Wirtschafter JD, Haines SJ, Heros RC, Perrone T (1991) Familial hemifacial spasm associated with arterial compression of the facial nerve. J Neurosurg 74: 290–296
10. Cushing H (1920) The major trigeminal neuralgias and their surgical treatment based on experience with 332 gasserian operations. Am J Med Sci 160: 157–184
11. Digre K, Corbett JJ (1988) Hemifacial spasm: Differential diagnosis, mechanism, and treatment. In: Jankovic J, Tolosa E (eds) Advances in neurology, vol. 49: Facial dyskinesias. Raven Press, New York, pp 151–176
12. Dutton JJ, Buckley EG (1988) Long-term results and complications of Botulinum A toxin in the treatment of blepharospasm. Ophthalmology 95: 1529–1534
13. Ehni G, Woltman HW (1945) Hemifacial spasm. Review of one hundred and six cases. Arch Neurol Psychiatry 53: 205–211
14. Elston JS (1986) Botulinum toxin treatment of hemifacial spasm. J Neurol Neurosurg Psychiatry 49: 827–829
15. Elston JS (1988) Botulinum toxin therapy for involuntary facial movement. Eyes 2: 12–15
16. Elston JS (1992) The management of blepharospasm and hemifacial spasm. J Neurol 239: 5–8
17. Esteban A, Molina-Negro P (1986) Primary hemifacial spasm: A neurophysiological study. J Neurol Neurosurg Psychiatry 49: 58–63
18. Flanders M, Chin D, Boghen D (1993) Botulinum toxin: Preferred treatment for hemifacial spasm. Eur Neurol 33: 316–319
19. Gardner WJ, Sava GA (1962) Hemifacial spasm—a reversible pathophysiologic state. J Neurosurg 19: 240–247
20. Geller BD, Hallett M, Ravits J (1989) Botulinum toxin therapy in hemifacial spasm: Clinical and electrophysiologic studies. Muscle and Nerve 12: 716–722
21. Gonnering RS (1986) Treatment of hemifacial spasm with botulinum A toxin. Results and rationale. Ophthal Plast Reconstr Surg 2: 143–146
22. Gowers WR (1888) A manual of diseases of the nervous system. P. Blakiston, Philadelphia
23. Huang CI, Chen IH, Lee LS (1992) Microvascular decompression for hemifacial spasm: Analyses of operative findings and results in 310 patients. Neurosurgery 30: 53–57
24. Iwakuma T, Matsumoto A, Nakamura N (1982) Comparison of three different operative procedures in 110 patients. J Neurosurg 57: 753–756
25. Jankovic J, Schwartz K, Donovan DT (1990) Botulinum toxin treatment of cranial-cervical dystonia, spasmodic dysphonia, other focal dystonias and hemifacial spasm. J Neurol Neurosurg Psychiatry 53: 633–639
26. Jannetta PJ, Abbasy M, Maroon JC, Ramos FM, Albin MS (1977) Etiology and definitive microsurgical treatment of hemifacial spasm. J Neurosurg 47: 321–328
27. Jannetta PJ (1981) Hemifacial spasm. In: Samii M, Jannetta PJ (eds) The cranial nerves. Springer, Heidelberg, pp 484–493
28. Jedynak CP, Palfi S, Vidailhet M, Kullmann B (1993) Traitement du spasme hémifacial par la toxine botulique. Rev Neurol (Paris) 149: 202–206
29. Katusic SK, Beard CM, Bergstralh EJ, Kurland LT (1990) Incidence and clinical features of trigeminal neuralgia, Rochester, Minnesota, 1945–1984. Ann Neurol 27: 89–95
30. Katusic SK, Beard CM, Wiederholt WC, Bergstralh EJ, Kurland LT (1986) Incidence, clinical features and prognosis in Bell's palsy, Rochester, Minnesota, 1968–1982. Ann Neurol 20: 622–627
31. Kraft SP, Lang AE (1988) Cranial dystonia, blepharospasm and hemifacial spasm: Clinical features and treatment, including the use of botulinum toxin. Can Med Assoc J 139: 837–844
32. Mauriello JA, Aljian J (1991) Natural history of treatment of facial dyskinesias with botulinum toxin: A study of 50 consecutive patients over seven years. Br J Ophthalmol 75: 737–739
33. Newton TH, Mani RL (1974) The vertebral artery. In: Newton TH, Potts DG (eds) Radiology of the skull and brain. Angiography. CV Mosby, St Louis, pp 1659–1709
34. Nielsen VK (1984) Pathophysiology of hemifacial spasm: I. Ephaptic transmission and ectopic excitation. Neurology 34: 418–426
35. Rosso ALZ, Mattos JP, Fogel LM, Novis SAP (1994) Bilateral hemifacial spasm. Mov Disord 9: 236
36. Ruban JM, Pellissier de Feligonde O, Benillouche P (1993) Analyse de l'efficacité de la toxine botulique A dans le traitement du blépharospasme et de l'hémispasme facial. A propos de 160 cas. Ophtalmologie 7: 481–482
37. Saraux H (1988) Traitement des blépharospasmes et des hémispasmes faciaux par injection de toxine botulique. J Fr Ophtalmol 11: 237–240
38. Savino PJ, Sergott RC, Bosley TM, Schatz N (1985) Hemifacial spasm treated with botulinum A toxin injection. Arch Ophthalmol 103: 1305–1306
39. Schultze F (1875) Linksseitiger Facialiskrampf in folge eines Aneurysma der Arteria vertebralis sinistra. Arch Pathol Anat 65: 385–391
40. Shaywitz BA (1974) Hemifacial spasm in childhood treated with carbamazepine. Arch Neurol 31: 63
41. Sindou M, Amrani F, Mertens P (1990) Décompression vasculaire microchirurgicale pour névralgie du trijumeau. Neurochirurgie 36: 16–26
42. Soulayrol S, Caperan A, Penot-Ragon C, Beaulieu JP, Gastaut JL (1993) Traitements par injections locales de toxine botulique en neurologie. Presse Méd 22: 957–963
43. Taylor JDN, Kraft SP, Kazdan MS, Flanders M, Cadera W, Orton RB (1991) Treatment of blepharospasm and hemifacial spasm with botulinum A toxin: A Canadian multicentre study. Can J Ophthalmol 26: 133–138
44. Tolosa E, Marti MJ, Kulisevsky J (1988) Botulinum toxin injection therapy for hemifacial spasm. In: Jankovic J, Tolosa E (eds) Advances in neurology, vol. 49: Facial dyskinesias. Raven Press, New York, pp 479–491
45. Wartenberg R (1952) Hemifacial spasm, a clinical and pathophysiological study. Oxford University Press, New York
46. Yu YL, Fong KY, Chang CM (1992) Treatment of idiopathic hemifacial spasm with botulinum toxin. Acta Neurol Scand 85: 55–57

Correspondence: A. Vighetto, M.D., Botulinum Toxin Outpatient Clinic, Hopital Neurologique, 59 Boulevard Pinel, F-69003 Lyon Cedex, France.

Hemifacial spasm and other hemifacial abnormal movements: Clinical aspects

S. Palfi[1] and **C. P. Jedynak**[2]

[1]Service de Neurochirurgie Hopital H. Mondor, Créteil, France
[2]Service de Neurochirurgie Centre médico-chirurgical FOCH, Suresnes, France

Summary

This chapter describes clinical aspects of Hemifacial spasm (HFS), based on a review of 72 patients with HFS included in a study of subcutaneous botulinum toxin treatment. The semeiology of these patients with HFS appeared to be stereotypical and consisted of a mixture of uncontrollable twitching and/or sustained contractions limited to the facial territory. Of the 72 patients (age range: 26–83 years), 64% were female. HFS occurred predominantly on the left side (52% against 45% on the right side and 3% on the both sides of the face) without provocative circumstances in most of the cases. Three groups have been characterized according to the extent and the intensity of spasm: mild (8%), moderate (80%) and severe (12%). The 'severe' group appeared to be accompanied by a long evolution of HFS, slight facial weakness and conjunctival irritation. Alternative bilateral spasm, "tic convulsif", familial forms and secondary spasms are described in the second part of this manuscript and presented as particular aspects of HFS. Finally, and in order to better understand clinical aspects of HFS, other hemifacial abnormal movement disorders are also reported and discussed as differential diagnoses of HFS.

Key words: Hemifacial spasm, hemifacial abnormal movement.

Introduction

Hemifacial spasm (HFS) is a disorder characterized by involuntary, episodic twitches of muscles innervated by the facial nerve [4, 5].

This chapter reviews on the first part, the clinical manifestation of HFS illustrated by a study of 72 patients. The second part concerns other facial movement disorders and discusses how to distinguish them from HFS.

Part one

Clinical aspects of hemifacial spasm

Seventy-two patients with primary HFS were referred to the authors for treatment with botulinum toxin, following previous examination in other institutions. Criterion for inclusion in this study was that the patient have a clinical hemifacial spasm, as verified from our examination. Patients with spasms secondary to a facial palsy were excluded. The first patient of this study was examined in September 1986 and the last patient examined in March 1991.

Method of study

A questionnaire, designed and based on the given data and on our observations of the first five patients we examined, was systematically filled out for every patient seen thereafter. Three groups of patients were defined according to the extent and the intensity of the spasm : Group 1, which included cases of HFS that almost exclusively involved the orbicularis oculi; Group 2, which included cases of the most common form of HFS, i.e., between mild and severe; and Group 3, which included cases of very severe forms of HFS that produced complete eye closure, a maximal deviation of the mouth, a prominent nasolabial groove, and a strong contracture of the platysma.

Five patients were studied using electromyography (EMG) recordings from surface electrodes placed symmetrically on the orbicularis oculi muscles to record these muscles spontaneous activity, as well as the synkinesis.

Clinical manifestations

Of the 72 patients we examined, 64% were female. The mean age of these patients at initial presentation was 53 years range 26 to 83 years. The disease was predominant in patients between the ages of 40 and 70 years, occurring most frequently in the oldest. The first manifestation of HFS occurred at least seven years before our initial examination.

HFS occurred in 52% of the cases on the left side, in 45% of the cases on the right side, and only 2 patients demonstrated a spasm on both sides of the face. None of the patients in this study presented with "tic convulsif" (see Part two).

The semeiology of these patients' HFS appeared to be simple and stereotypical. The patients'spasm consisted of a various mixture of twitching and sustained contractions. Minor spasm are, for the most part, simple twitching, whereas severe spasm are more sustained. Some patients described an irregular and rapid series of muscle twitches, often followed by a sustained contraction lasting a few seconds. The spasm exclusively involved the territory of the facial nerve and it nearly always began with twitches in the region of the lower eye lid becoming more intense and progressively spreading to the inferior facial territory, including the platysma, within a few years. The frontalis muscle was often spared from involvement. However, we often observed what Babinski [1] described as a "synergie paradoxale" the spasmodic closure of the eye accompanied not by a low position of the eyebrow, but rather paradoxically by its raising (co-contraction of the orbicularis oculi and the frontalis muscles). When the spasm grew more intense, it caused a complete closure of the eye, a strong pulling of the corner of the mouth, and a contraction of the platysma. In 6 patients, a auditory sensation (a popping, motor boat-type noise) occurred synchronously with the spasm. Eight percent of the patients in our study were designated Group 1 (mild HFS), 80% were designated Group 2 (moderate HFS), and 12% were designated Group 3 (severe HFS).

The evolution of the disorder was slow, progressive, and debilitating. Only 2 patients experienced a remission, 1 patient for 2 months and other for 1 year. There appeared to be a correlation between the duration of the evolution of the HFS and its intensity. However, this could not be statistically verified. The HFS of all of our patients in Group 3 (severe HFS) had evolved over more than five years. Among the 70, no patient in our study experienced a single day without spasms. However, some patients noted lulls in spasmodic activity, lasting from a few minutes to an hour or more. These lulls were prolonged for the patients who had mild HFS, and were short and rare for the patients who had severe HFS.

Provocative circumstances

Some of our patients noted that occasionally speech, chewing, or grimacing triggered the spasm, which was prolonged and repeated after such facial movements, but generally the spasms occurred spontaneously without cause. Some of patients were in the habit of wearing dark sunglasses, complaining that bright light triggered their spasm; However, we found from experimentation that a bright artificial light did not provoke a spasm in any of our patients. A few patients in our study claimed that pressure exerced on an area directly below the earlobe on the affected side of the face inhibited the spasm. Some patients noted that plenty of sleep and relaxation had a beneficial effect, whereas others complained of increased spasm following extended periods of sleep.

Associated symptoms

A very mild facial weakness was observed in 30 of the 72 patients (41%) in this study. This facial weakness was manifested by an incomplete closure of the eye on the spasm side upon the execution of the order to close both eyes tightly. Slight facial weakness was observed in patients with severe forms of HFS. This slight facial weakness was clearly noticed before treatment with botulinum toxin (see Jedynak et al. [12]). Hearing was impaired on the spasm side in 15 patients (21%). Three patients (4%) had total deafness on the affected side. Conjunctival irritation was observed in 17 patients (23,5%) , especially in those who had the severe forms of HFS.

Effect of the will

In all patients in our study, the spasm was absolutely uncontrollable. When asked by the examiner to purposefully inhibit closure of the eye, the patient was unable to do so. The patient was also unable to provoke the spasm voluntarily nor was he or she able to mimic a spasm. Fatigue and emotion were prevalent factors in the majority of the patients in our study, although some of these patients claimed that their fatigue and emotional status were not related to their spasm.

Effect of the sleep

Some patients reported that at night, before drifting off to sleep, the spasm was disturbing. Some other patients reported being awakened from sleep. Of the 14 patients in our study who were observed during sleep, the persistence of spasm was observed in 10 of them.

Functional aspects

Functional problems were manifested in some of the patients when, for example, reading (43%) and driving (50% of those in our study who were drivers). Among the 23 patients who worked, 17 experienced emotional difficulties, especially those who dealt with the public: 1 travelling salesperson and 2 sales assistants lost their jobs due to such difficulties.

Psychological implications

The psychological consequences of having HFS were estimated by the individual patients: 55% reported no psychological consequences, and 45% reported being psychologically affected by the image they presented or thought they presented to others. Three of the 72 patients suffered from depression, which necessitated specific treatment and was directly attributed to the spasm and its social and professional consequences.

EMG Results

EMG recordings in individual patients showed that the continuous contraction of the unilateral orbicularis oculi muscle could not be perceived by the patient. The spasmodic contraction of this muscle was larger and, although brief, much longer than a natural blink. The spasm was seen to occur spontaneously and sometimes we observed synkinetic contractions of the eye during mouth movement. In other cases, the spasm continued beyond the deliberate movement of the inferior part of the face.

Treatment before botulinum toxin

Previous to this study, nine (13%) of our patients had been treated with carbamazepine, with the results being either weak or ineffective in 34%; twenty one (30%) of our patients had been treated by clonazepan [10], with the results being either weak or ineffective in 80%; eight (11%) of our patients had been received tricyclic antidepressants, which provided more positive results than that obtained for the patients noted above who were treated with various medications.

Part two

In addition of the 72 patients described in this previous study, we found particular aspects of HFS and hemifacial abnormal movement disorders that can be taken for essential HFS. We describe first unusual aspects of HFS and other abnormal movement disorders based on literature data.

Particular aspects of HFS

Alternative bilateral spasm

In 1992, a case of alternate bilateral spasm was reported in the literature [21]. This patient, whose spasms were related to a mid brain lesion due to multiple sclerosis, could partially controlled his spasms by will.

"Tic convulsif"

Cushing [3] used the term "tic convulsif" to describe the simultaneous manifestation of HFS and trigeminal neuralgia on the same side of the face, although the onset of each disorder begins at different times. Treatment with diphenylhydantoin and carbamazepine produces a prompt relief of the pain of patients with "tic convulsif", but does not have noticeable effect on the HFS. Trigeminal pain and facial spasm are generally symptomatic and have the same causes: e.g., multiple sclerosis, tumour of the posterior fossa, or vascular malformation [8, 17, 18, 20].

Familial forms of hemifacial spasm

Familial forms of HFS have been reported in the literature [2, 7]. Within the same family, HFS affects the same side of the face and the mode of transmission is autosomally dominant.

Secondary spasms

The clinical aspect of the type of hemifacial spasms that follow a peripheral facial palsy is quite similar to that of a primary spasm: both are in the same location, both have the same sustained contractions, and both have the same bursts of completely involuntary activity. However, the synkinesis that accompanies secondary spasms is different from that which accompanies primary spasm [14]: the synkinesis in the secondary spasms is constant and occurs with every facial movement. Secondary spasms have more contractures and fewer twitches and they are often associated with a unilateral eye watering when salivating.

Hemifacial abnormal movement disorders

Focal seizures [19]

We had the opportunity to observe a case of focal status epilepticus that involved only a few muscles the elevator angulioris and the nasalis muscles of one side of the face (thus, simulating a hemifacial spasm). A venous infusion of diphenylhydantoin caused the continuous motor activity to stop.

Facial tics

Facial tics, which are characteristically sudden and brief, are frequently seen in children [11]. Although tics can often be observed simply by looking at the face, they do not have the same intensity as HFS. Their locations vary, and they are often repetitious in a particular way in the same region of the face. The principal characteristic of facial tics is that patient is able to prevent it for at least one minute. Then, the effort to control the tics fails and they return with greater intensity.

Masticatory spasms

Masticatory spasms occur in the masseter muscle, which is innervated by the trigeminal nerve, and they are accompanied by hemifacial atrophy [13]. This atrophy involves a progressive loss of fat and subcutaneous tissue on one side of the face. Masticatory spasms are nearly always continuous. Each spasm lasts less than one second, are exacerbated by chewing, and, as in HFS, persist during sleep.

Blepharospasm and oro-mandibular dystonia (Meige's Syndrome)

Blepharospasm and oro-mandibular dystonia (Meige's Syndrome) usually involve the face bilaterally. Both are forms of focal dystonia and, as in HFS, are usually seen in the elderly. Blepharospasm is seldom asymmetric but it is easily distinguished from facial spasm by its particular characteristics: it always involves the opposite side of the face a little; it is partially controllable at will; no synkinesis is present.

Parkinson disease

In Parkinson's disease, the drug levodopa may induce abnormal facial movements when maximum dosage is administered. These facial movements may be unilateral or prevalent on one side.

Pathological facial myokymia

Pathological facial myokymia is easily distinguished from fasciculations, which are brief, irregular twitches in different parts of facial muscles; myokymia is a slower contraction that involves small bands of muscles and occurs more continuously while transmitting a ripple to the overlying skin. The causes of myokimia are primarily multiple sclerosis, and, more rarely, gliomas, astrocytomas of the pons, or pontine metastasis. Lesion are localized just above the facial nuclei on the corticobulbar fibers, which are homolateral and uncrossed. However, near the level of the seventh motor nuclei, a group of fibers breaks away and decussates to terminate in the contralateral facial nuclei, particularly in the section of the nucleus that innervates the lower facial muscles. Facial myokimia may result in increased excitability of the facial motor neurons by a release of higher control [6, 9, 16].

Hemifacial paroxystic contractures

The same etiologies are the basis for attacks of hemifacial paroxystic contractures. We had the opportunity to observe such a case regarding a 3 year old girl whose unsuccessful treatments for focal seizures began at the age of 3 months of age. A previous case report by Langston and Tharp [15] provided the diagnosis of a ganglioneuroma of the brainstem before operation. Surgery was performed and the facial contractures disappeared.

Acknowledgement

The authors wish to thank Steven Gendell and Christopher Rains for collaboration.

References

1. Babinski J (1905) Hemispasme facial periphérique. Nouv Iconogr Salpetriore 18: 419–424
2. Carter J, Patrinely J, Jankovic J, McCrary J, Boniuk M (1910) Familial hemifacial spasm. Arch Ophthalmol 108: 249–250
3. Cushing (1920) The major trigeminal neuralgias and their surgical treatment. Am J Med Scien 160: 157–184

4. Digre K, Corbett JJ (1988) Hemifacial spasm: Differential diagnosis mechanism and treatment. In: Jankovic J, Tolosa E (eds) Facial dyskinesias. Raven Press, New York. Adv Neurol 49: 151–176
5. Ehni G, Woltman HW (1945) Hemifacial spasm. Arch Neurol Psychiatry 53: 205–211
6. Espinosa R, Lambert E, Klass D (1967) Facial myokymia affecting the electroencephalogram. Proc Mayo Clin 42: 258–270
7. Friedman A, Jamrozik Z, Bojakowski J (1989) Familial hemifacial spasm. Mov Disord 4/3: 213–218
8. Gardner WJ (1962) Concerning the mechanism of trigeminal neuralgia and hemifacial spasm. J Neurosurg 19: 947–957
9. Gutmann L, Thompson H, Martin J (1969) Transcient facial myokymia. J Am Med Assoc 209: 389–391
10. Herzberg L (1985) Management of hemifacial spasm with clonazepan. Neurology 35: 1676–1677
11. Jankovic J, Fahn S (1986) The phenomenology of tics. Mov Disord 1/1: 17–26
12. Jedynak CP, Palfi S, Vidailhet M, Kullmann B (1993) Traitement du spasme hemifacial par la toxine botulique. Revue Neurolog 149/3: 202–206
13. Kaufman MD (1980) Masticatory spasm in facial hemiatrophy. Ann Neurol 7/6: 585–587
14. Kim P, Fukushima T (1984) Observations on synkinesis in patients with hemifacial spasm. J Neurosurg 60: 821–827
15. Langston JW, Tharp BR (1976) Infantile hemifacial spasm. Arch Neurol 3: 302–303
16. Matthews WB (1966) Facial myokymia. J Neurol Neurosurg Psychiatry 29: 35–36
17. Maurice-William RS (1973) Tic convulsif: The association of trigeminal neuralgia and hemifacial spasm. Postgrad Med J 49: 742–745
18. Pulsinelli WA, Rottenberg DA (1977) Painful tic convulsif. J Neurol Neurosurg Psychiatry 40: 192–195
19. Sicard M, Bollak S (1912) L'hemispasme facial d'origine corticale cérébrale Revue Neurologique 24: 742–743
20. Thiebaut F, Isch-Teussard C, Ebtinger-Jouffroy J (1960) Hemispasme facial dans la sclerose en plaques: Etude clinique et Electromyographique. Revue Oto-Neuro-Ophtalmologioque 32: 162–166
21. Van de Biezenbos J, Horstink M, Van de Vlasakker C, Van Engelen O, Van Eikema Holmes O, Barklof F (1992) A case of bilateral alternating hemifacial spasms. Mov Disord 7/1: 68–70

Correspondence: Dr. Stéphane Palfi, CMC FOCH, 40 rue de Worth, F-92150, Suresnes, France.

Pathophysiology of hemifacial spasm

A. R. Møller

Department of Neurological Surgery, University of Pittsburgh School of Medicine, Pittsburgh, Pennsylvania, U.S.A.

Summary

The results of studies in patients undergoing microvascular decompression to relieve hemifacial spasm have provided considerable evidence that the symptoms and signs (spasm and synkinesis) of this disorder are results of changes in the function of the facial motonucleus. Results of animal experiments show that similar signs may develop after chronic electrical stimulation of the facial nerve or after the facial nerve has been injured slightly (by placing a chromic suture around it) and a blood vessel brought into close contact with the nerve. Injury alone or a close contact with a blood vessel alone does not cause the development of such signs.

There is considerable evidence that vascular compression of cranial nerves (V, VII, VIII, IX, and X) occurs frequently without causing any noticeable symptoms or signs of hemifacial spasm. This support the hypothesis that vascular compression alone does not cause any noticeable symptoms but that another factor is also necessary. It is not known what that other factor may be. It could be a slight injury of the respective nerve or a predisposition in the respective nucleus or both. Since vascular compression seems to be necessary (although not sufficient) to cause symptoms, microvascular decompression is an effective treatment, since the other factor(s) do not seem to cause any noticeable symptoms or signs.

Key words: Animal models, microvascular decompression, facial nucleus, hyperactivity.

Introduction

The pathophysiology of hemifacial spasm (HFS) is not completely understood, despite the fact that extensive experience over the past 20–30 years has shown that HFS can be cured permanently by microvascular decompression (MVD) of the facial nerve where it exits the brainstem [1–8] (and for a recent review see Møller [9]). Reports from several institutions where MVD to relieve HFS is routinely performed show similar results, namely a success rate for cure of HFS between 85 and 95% [9]. In these cases there is no reported evidence of a natural recurrence of HFS, as there is for other disorders that are caused by vascular compression of a cranial nerve root, such as trigeminal neuralgia [10, 11].

Two hypotheses have been proposed to explain the characteristic signs – spasm and synkinesis – of hemifacial spasm [12]. One hypothesis postulates that the symptoms and signs of HFS can be explained by the development of a crosstalk between individual nerve fibers of the facial nerve at the location of the vascular compression [13]. This hypothesis postulates that such ephaptic transmission between denuded motor axons causes the synkinesis as well as the spasm [14, 15]. It is assumed that aberrant neural activity is generated at the location of the cross-compression, which is believed to generate the spasm in patients with HFS.

The other hypothesis, usually associated with work by Ferguson [16], claims that the signs and symptoms of HFS are a result of hyperactivity of the facial motonucleus. It is assumed that this hyperactivity causes both the spasm and the synkinesis, and that it develops as a result of the vascular compression (or irritation) of the root of the facial nerve.

Throughout the past decade considerable research efforts have been devoted to unraveling the pathophysiology of HFS. Studies have been performed in awake patients with HFS [15, 17–21] as well as in patients undergoing MVD operations to relieve HFS [22–30]. More recently, experiments in animals have shown that it is possible to create signs similar to those in patients with HFS by causing an artificial irritation of the facial nerve [31–35]. Thus the abnormal muscle response, synkinesis, and involuntary contractions of facial muscles that are the signs of HFS may develop in animals as a result of a combination of vascular irritation and slight injury to the facial nerve [34, 35] or by chronic electrical stimulation of the facial nerve [31–33].

The results of studies in awake human and in patients who were undergoing MVD operations to relieve HFS as well as the results of experiments in animals have indicated that the pathophysiology of HFS is more complex than was assumed by the original hypotheses. On the basis of such studies, the development of HFS, which usually occurs rather slowly, is assumed by some investigators [22, 28, 36, 37] to depend on neural plasticity, and it has been suggested that a mechanism similar to the kindling phenomenon [38, 39] is involved in the development of HFS [22]. It has also been suggested that the trigeminal system may be involved in the development of HFS [26, 29].

The abnormal muscle contraction has been extensively studied in human as well as in animals, and it has played an important role in studies on the pathophysiology of HFS [15, 18, 22, 26–28]. Thus, the fact that patients with HFS have several measurable signs that are related to HFS makes it possible to perform quantitative studies on the pathological signs of this disorder. Other disorders that can be cured by vascular decompression, such as trigeminal neuralgia (TN), disabling positional vertigo (DPV), and tinnitus lack such signs. The results of studies of HFS may be applicable to other disorders that are caused by vascular compression of a cranial nerve.

Symptoms and signs of hemifacial spasm

Involuntary contractions of smaller or larger portions of facial muscles, synkinesis, and the abnormal muscle response are typical signs of HFS [12]. The synkinesis is often demonstrated objectively by recording the blink reflex, but it is particularly the abnormal muscle response that has been used in studies of the pathophysiology of HFS.

The abnormal muscle response

When a branch of the facial nerve in patients with HFS is stimulated electrically, not only does the muscles that are innervated by that branch contract but also do muscles innervated by other branches [15, 22, 40, 41]. The abnormal muscle response can be elicited by electrical stimulation of the temporal branch of the facial nerve and recorded from the mentalis muscle, or it can be elicited from the marginal mandibular branch and recorded from the orbicularis oculi muscles (Fig. 1A). When elicited in either way the abnormal muscle contraction consists of an initial response with a latency of about 10 ms, thus much longer than that of the direct muscle response (M-response) from the muscles that are innervated by the branch of the facial nerve that is being stimulated electrically. This initial component of the abnormal muscle response is followed by a burst of EMG activity, the duration of which typically varies from time to time (Fig. 1B). The abnormal muscle response (also

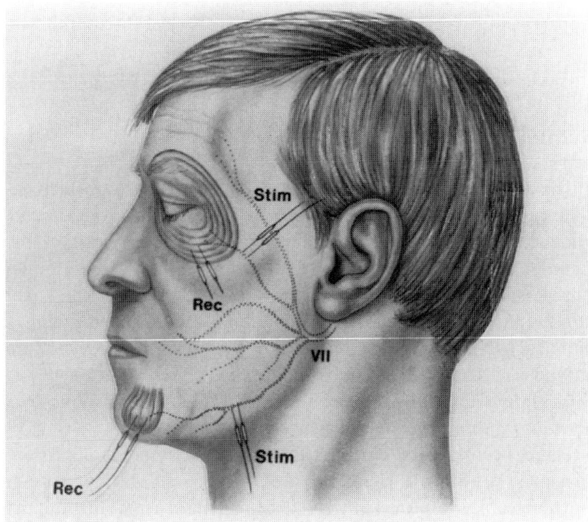

A

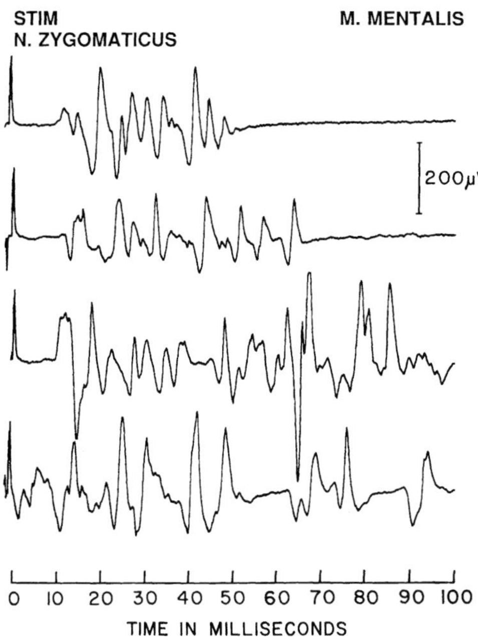

B

Fig. 1. A Illustration of how the abnormal muscle response may be elicited and recorded (from Møller and Jannetta [25]).
B Typical recordings of the abnormal muscle response in a patient with HFS who is to undergo a MVD operation (from Møller and Jannetta [24])

known as the delayed muscle response or lateral spread response) was first described by Esslen [40], and it has been used extensively in recent years in clinical studies of patients with HFS [15, 17, 18, 20], intraoperatively in MVD operations to relieve HFS [21, 22, 26, 27, 30, 36, 37], and in the development of animal models of HFS [31–35].

Although the exact physiological basis for this abnormal muscle response is not known in detail, it seems without doubt that it depends on an abnormal cross-transmission. The anatomical location of this abnormal cross-transmission has been regarded to be either in the facial nerve at the location of the vascular compression [15, 19] or in the facial motonucleus [22, 26–29, 36, 37] or a combination of both [18].

We have used the abnormal muscle contraction in intraoperative studies to determine the anatomical location of this cross-transmission in patients undergoing MVD operations to relieve HFS [22, 26, 27]. If we assume that the abnormal muscle response is a result of cross-transmission at the site of the vascular compression then the sum of the neural conduction times between 1) the stimulus site and the site of compression, and 2) between the compression site and the muscle from which the abnormal muscle response was recorded, would be equal to the latency of the abnormal muscle response. However, we found that the latency of the abnormal muscle response was about 2 ms longer than the sum of the conduction times of the nerve pathways between the stimulation site and the location of the vascular cross-compression and the pathway from the vascular compression site to the recording site [22] (Fig. 2). This indicates that the cross-transmission that causes the abnormal muscle response occurs at a more central location than that of the vascular compression. Others have presented similar results [20, 21].

This also makes it unlikely that the cross-transmission that causes the abnormal muscle response is a direct result of (ephaptic) communication between motor nerve fibers at the site of the vascular compression. This is also supported by the observation that in rare cases when the facial nerve has been manipulated extensively during MVD, an earlier component of the abnormal muscle response appears with a latency of about 8 ms, thus 2 ms shorter than the abnormal muscle contraction [28]. In the study by Møller [28], this component appeared only for a few seconds after cessation of manipulation of the facial nerve and it was

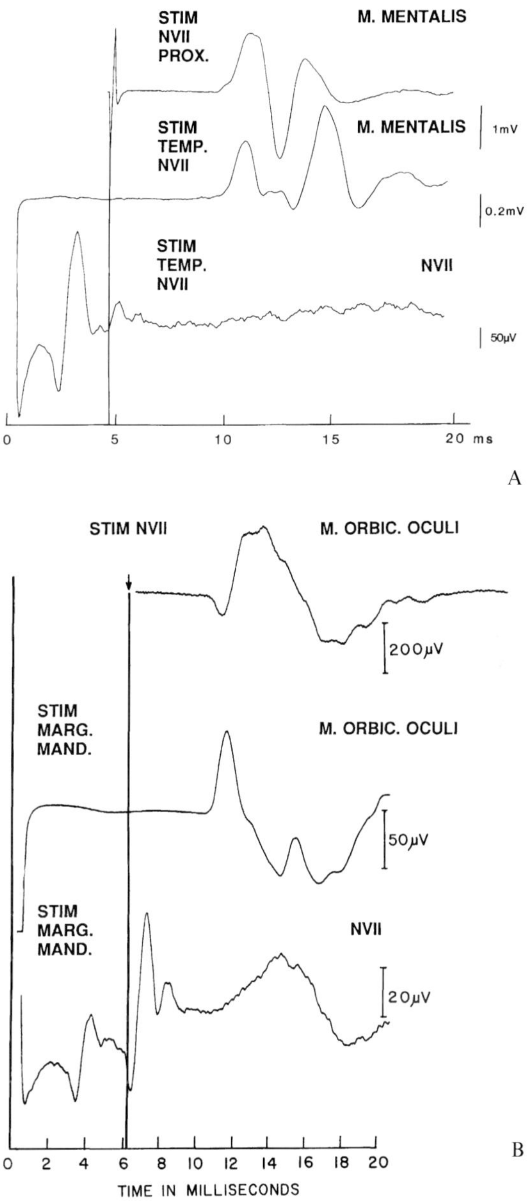

Fig. 2. Illustrations of the measurements of neural conduction times in the presumed pathway of the abnormal muscle contraction.
A The abnormal muscle response was elicited by electrical stimulation of the temporal branch of CN VII and recorded from the mentalis muscle. The response from the same muscle elicited by electrical stimulation of the intracranial portion of the facial nerve (upper tracing) was aligned in time with the abnormal muscle response. The estimated time of the occurrence of neural activity in the intracranial portion of the facial nerve that caused the abnormal muscle response is seen to be later than the CAP recorded from the facial nerve elicited by stimulation of the temporal branch of the facial nerve. (from Møller, 1993 [37])
B Graph similar to that in A, but when the abnormal muscle response was elicited by electrical stimulation of the marginal mandibular branch of the facial nerve and recorded from the orbicularis oculi muscle. Notice the second CAP in the recording from the facial nerve, the occurrence of which coincides with the presumed occurrence of the neural activity that elicited the abnormal muscle response

seen to reappear when the facial nerve was again manipulated. This early component was present in only 3 of 50 patients in this study [28], and its amplitude was 20% or less than that of the abnormal muscle response or less than 1/2% of the direct muscle response, which is consistent with the assumption that ephaptic transmission can only involve a small fraction of nerve fibers of the facial nerve. The results of this study [28] are consistent with the assumption that this early (rare) component is generated by ephaptic transmission in the intracranial portion of the facial nerve.

The generation of the abnormal muscle contraction seems to be closely related to the vascular compression of the facial nerve root. Thus it is absent after successful treatment of HFS by MVD [41, 42] and, indeed, it disappears instantaneously when the offending blood vessel is moved off the facial nerve [21, 24] (Fig. 3). Recording of the abnormal muscle response has therefore been found of practical value in MVD operations to relieve HFS, in which it is used as an indicator of which vessel is causing the signs of HFS [43, 44]. The absence of the abnormal muscle response at the end of such operations indicates the high cure rate (above 90% [43]).

The fact that the abnormal muscle response disappears instantaneously when the blood vessel is moved off the facial nerve indicates that irritation from a blood vessel is also necessary to maintain the hyperactivity of the facial motonucleus that is presumably causing the spasm and cross-transmission that cause the abnormal muscle response as well as the synkineses that are the typical signs of HFS.

There is thus considerable evidence that the facial motonucleus is the anatomical location of the physio-

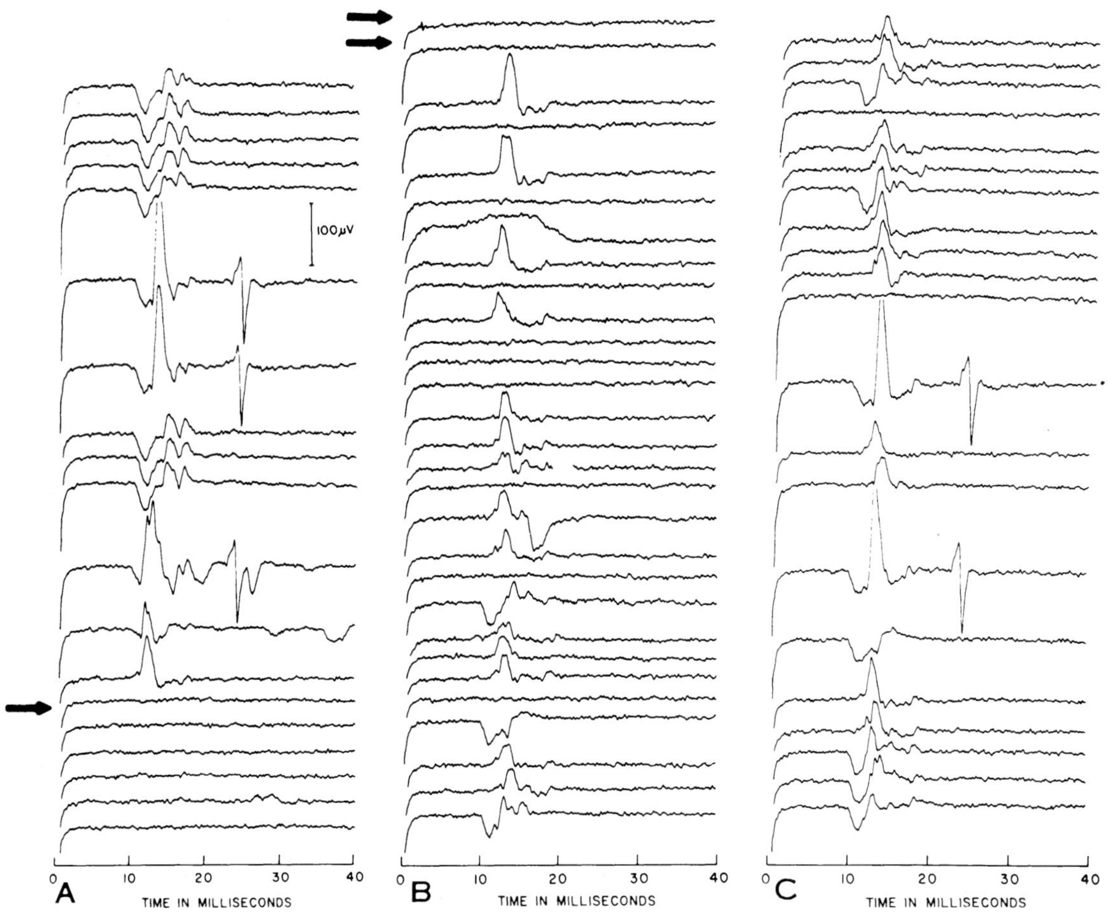

Fig. 3. Results of intraoperative recordings of the abnormal muscle response in a patient undergoing MVD operation to relieve HFS. When the offending vessel was lifted off the facial nerve (arrow) the abnormal muscle response disappeared. When the vessel was allowed to fall back onto the facial nerve (marked by two arrows) the abnormal muscle response gradually returned. The time between each stimulation was 0.2 seconds, and the graph shows consecutive recordings with a break of 10 seconds between the first and the second row (from Møller and Jannetta [24])

logical abnormality that causes both the spasm and the synkinesis that are the characteristic signs of HFS. The assumption that these abnormalities are brought about by irritation of the facial nerve from a blood vessel is strongly supported by the considerable success of MVD (cure rate above 85%) in achieving a permanent cure for patients with HFS [7, 9]. The finding that the abnormal muscle response disappears nearly instantaneously when the offending vessel is moved off the facial nerve root [24] is a further indication that vascular compression is a necessary condition to produce the symptoms and signs of HFS. The finding that patients in whom the abnormal muscle response was absent at the end of the operation had a higher probability of being free of spasm [43, 44] is a further indication that both spasm and the abnormal muscle response are related symptoms of HFS, and it makes it likely that these two signs may have the same pathophysiological basis.

The blink reflex

In patients with HFS there is a distinct EMG response from muscles of the lower face in response to electrical stimulation of the supraorbital nerve that occurs with a latency of about 10 msec. The latency of this response has a value that is similar to that of the R_1 component of the response recorded from the orbicularis oculi muscle in response to electrical stimulation of the supraorbital nerve [19]. Intraoperative studies in patients undergoing MVD operations to relieve HFS [26] show that the blink reflex elicited by electrical stimulation of the supraorbital nerve is present on the affected side, despite the effect of surgical anesthesia, which makes it impossible to elicit the blink reflex on the unaffected side. When the offending blood vessel is moved off the facial nerve, the blink reflex can no longer be elicited [26] (Fig. 4). This supports the hypotheses that the facial motonucleus is hyperactive in patients with HFS and that the close contact between the facial nerve and a blood vessel is necessary, not only to the development of the hyperactivity but also to maintaining it.

The close similarity between the latency of the abnormal muscle contraction and the R_1 component of the blink reflex could lead to the assumption that these two responses are identical, thus the abnormal muscle response could mistakenly be judged to be a result of stimulation of trigeminal sensory fibers in the face and not a result of stimulation of the facial nerve. Studies in anesthetized patients showed evidence that the response is not a result of trigeminal sensory fibers in the face being stimulated, but rather that the abnormal muscle response is indeed elicited by antidromic activ-

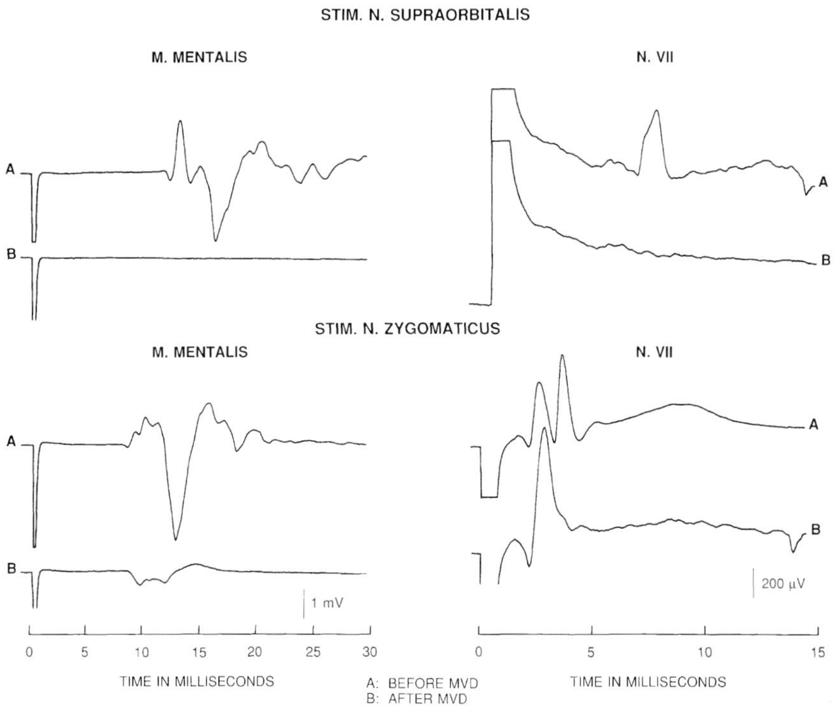

Fig. 4. Responses from the mentalis muscle to stimulation of the temporal branch of the facial nerve (abnormal muscle response) and the response from the same muscle to stimulation of the supraorbital nerve (blink reflex, synkinesis) in a patient undergoing MVD operation to relieve HFS, recorded before (A) and after MVD of the facial nerve (B). Also the response from the exposed intracranial portion of the facial nerve is shown. Notice that the second peak in the CAP from the facial nerve to stimulation of the temporal branch of the facial nerve disappears when the offending vessel is lifted off the facial nerve (from Møller and Jannetta [26])

ity in the facial motor nerve [26, 29]. Thus in the anesthetized patient, the latency of the R_1 component of the blink reflex is longer than 10 ms due to the effect of anesthesia, but the latency of the abnormal muscle response is 10 ms, as it is in unanesthetized patients. Thus, anesthesia affects the blink reflex but not the abnormal muscle response. Recordings from the exposed intracranial portions of the facial nerve also reveal evidence that the R_1 component of the blink reflex is different from the abnormal muscle response [26].

Further observations of patients with HFS

Also speaking against the hypothesis of ephaptic transmission is the fact that involuntary contractions of facial muscles seem to involve most of the facial muscles in patients who have had HFS for a long time. If the spasm was caused by such ephaptic transmission, it would require that practically all facial motor nerve fibers be in contact with each other, a situation which has no morphological evidence [17]. The fact that attacks of spasm can be evoked by emotional events also speaks against the ephaptic hypothesis as being the direct cause of the abnormal muscle response and the spasm, and, in fact, indicates a more central location of the physiological abnormality.

Basis for cross-transmission

We have suggested that dormant synapses in the facial motonucleus are opened as part of the pathophysiology of HFS [28, 37], and that the opening of such dormant synapses and the development of the hyperactivity of the motonucleus is brought about by the irritation of the facial nerve from close contact with a blood vessel. We have also suggested that the hyperactivity of the facial motonucleus that causes the signs of HFS may develop by mechanisms similar to that known as "kindling." [22]

Is contact with a blood vessel the only irritation that can maintain the abnormal muscle response?

There is evidence that other forms of irritation of the facial nerve can restore the abnormal muscle response after the facial nerve has been decompressed and the abnormal muscle response no longer able to be elicited by electrical stimulation of a branch of the facial nerve. Thus, when the cerebellopontine angle is irrigated after completion of MVD operation to relieve HFS with irrigation fluid that has a temperature below normal body temperature, general contractions of facial muscles become evident from recorded EMG activity from, for instance, the mentalis muscle (Fig. 5A). An abnormal muscle response similar to that seen before the facial nerve was decompressed will often appear in response to electrical stimulation of the temporal branch of the facial nerve during such irrigation when the recorded EMG responses are averaged (Fig. 5B). When the effect of the irrigation subsides then also this muscle response disappears.

These observations indicate that also irritations other than those caused by close contact with a blood vessel can cause an abnormal muscle response similar to that seen typically in patients with HFS before having undergone an MVD procedure.

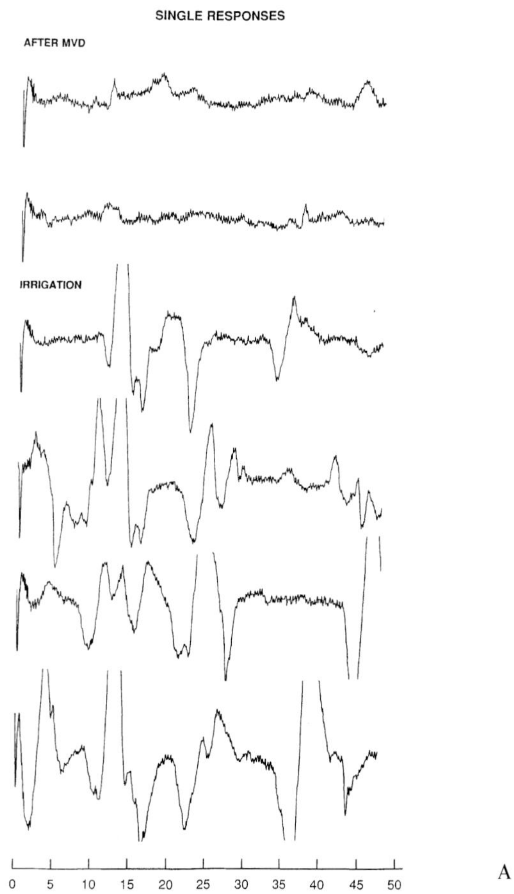

Fig. 5 (*continued*)

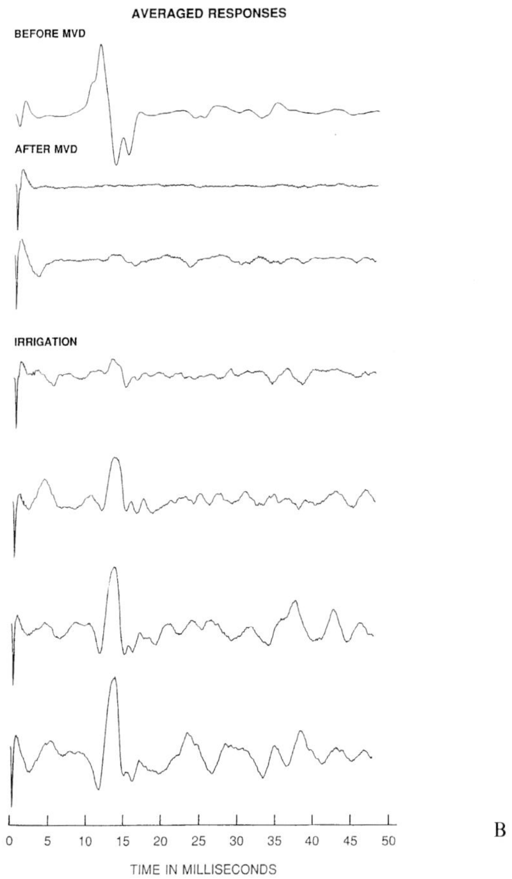

Fig. 5. A Intraoperative recordings of EMG activity from the mentalis muscle in response to electrical stimulation of the temporal branch of the facial nerve after MVD and during irrigation of the cerebellopontine angle with saline, the temperature of which was below normal body temperature. **A:** single responses. **B:** Averaged responses (25 total responses). The top tracings in B are the abnormal muscle response obtained before and after MVD

Animal models of HFS

In order to test the hypotheses that irritation of the facial nerve may over a period of time cause the development of the typical signs of HFS – an abnormal muscle response and involuntary facial movements – we performed several animal experiments [31–35]. The hypothesis that chronic irritation of the facial nerve can cause signs similar to those seen in patients with HFS is supported by several studies in animals.

In two studies it was shown that chronic electrical stimulation of the central portion of the facial nerve can result in the development of an abnormal muscle response with characteristics similar to those seen in patients with HFS [32, 33]. Recordings from the facial motonucleus in rats that showed the presence of the abnormal muscle response indicated that the abnormality that caused the abnormal muscle response was located in the facial motonucleus [31].

In subsequent and slightly different animal studies it was shown that similar signs of HFS (abnormal muscle response and spasm) may develop if a blood vessel is brought in close contact with a peripheral branch of the facial nerve [34, 35]. However, this latter study showed that a prerequisite for this to cause HFS-like signs (abnormal muscle response and spasm) is that the nerve at the location of the vascular contact is slightly injured. This study thus showed that vascular contact *alone* did not cause the development of the abnormal muscle contraction; only after a chromic suture had been placed around the facial nerve was the abnormal muscle response seen to develop.

The injury to the facial nerve in these experiments was accomplished by placing a chromic suture around the facial nerve 3 weeks before the artery was brought into contact with the facial nerve. This had been previously shown to cause a demyelination of a nerve with peripheral myelin [45–47]. The above mentioned study by Kuroki and Møller [34] also showed that a chromic suture placed around the facial nerve alone did not cause the development of an abnormal muscle response. Thus, both vascular contact and facial nerve injury are required for the abnormal muscle response to develop.

It was also shown in experiments using such HFS model rats that blocking of the neural transmission proximal to the compression site eliminated the abnormal muscle response [34]. This was taken as an indication that the anatomical location of the cross-transmission was proximal to the site of vascular compression. Other experiments in such HFS model rats using electrophysiological recordings from the facial motonucleus support the assumption that the abnormal muscle response in such rats was caused by neural activity in the facial motonucleus [35].

The results of these latter studies thus indicate that vascular irritation together with slight injury of the facial nerve may cause the development of physiological abnormalities in the facial motonucleus, whereas vascular contact alone does not cause any measureable abnormalities in the facial motor system. Thus, these results may explain why it seems only to be the root exit zone (REZ) of the facial nerve that is susceptible to the effect of close vascular contact [2, 4] because here the facial nerve is probably more vulnerable to injury, and thus vascular irritation at this location may cause HFS.

It may be that such an injury is less likely to occur at more distal locations along the intracranial course of the facial nerve.

Recent studies of patients with disabling positional vertigo (DPV) who were treated by MVD of the eighth cranial nerve (CN VIII) have shown that the vestibular nerve in such patients shows signs of injury [48], although such morphological studies cannot verify that the injury was caused by vascular compression. The injury, however, may also have occurred independent of the vascular compression; the injury may simply have been the second factor, in addition to vascular compression, necessary to cause the symptoms of DPV [36, 37].

The role of the trigeminal system in the development of HFS

There ere are several indications that the trigeminal system may be involved in the development of HFS in human. Thus most, but not all, patients with HFS report that their spasms begin in the muscles around the eye [4, 12], a region of the face where the trigeminal system has an excitatory influence on the facial motonucleus, as is evident from the fact that stimulation of the skin around the eye causes contractions of the orbicularis oculi muscles (blink reflex). It has been shown in studies of patients who are undergoing MVD to relieve HFS that electrical stimulation of the supraorbital nerve can interact with the abnormal muscle response elicited by electrical stimulation of the temporal branch of the facial nerve (Fig. 6) [29]. The results of such studies support the hypothesis that the anatomical location of the physiological abnormality that causes the abnormal muscle response is in the facial motor nucleus, but these studies also show that this interaction between the trigeminal and the facial systems is complex. It seems likely that a tonic background activity from the trigeminal sensory nucleus may influence the excitability of facial motoneurons that innervate the muscles around the eye, and that this may facilitate the development of HFS.

If the development of HFS is facilitated by the excitatory input to the facial motonucleus from the trigeminal system, it is surprising that the vascular irritation of the trigeminal nerve root that causes trigeminal neuralgia does not also cause HFS. There have been reports of a combined disorder of HFS and trigeminal neuralgia (tic convulsif [49]; for a review, see Møller [9]). However, an analysis of these published results has provided doubt as to the existence of such a combined disorder [9].

Why is hemifacial spasm so rare?

It is well known that vascular contact with cranial nerves in the cerebellopontine angle is rather common [50–52], but the occurrence of disorders that can be cured by MVD of cranial nerves such as CN VII, CN V, CN VIII and CN IX is rather rare. Thus, the incidence of HFS is less than 1 in 100,000 [53], and the incidence of trigeminal neuralgia (TN) is about 5 in 100,000 [54]. The incidences of disorders that are associated with CN VIII (DPV [55–58], and tinnitus [4, 6, 59]) and with CN IX (glossopharyngeal neuralgia [4]) are not known.

We have previously presented the hypothesis that one or more additional factors are needed for vascular compression to cause specific symptoms [36, 37, 60, 61]. Assuming that more central structures are involved in the generation of the symptoms and signs of disorders that can be cured by vascular decompression of a cranial nerve, such additional factors may be a predisposition or an acquired hyperactivity of the respective nucleus that is involved in the disease. In the case of HFS, it may be low resting membrane potentials of facial motoneurons or it may be an unusually large excitatory input from other brain areas, such as, for instance, the trigeminal system, which is known to exert excitatory influence on the facial motonucleus. Since trigeminal input from the region around the eye to the facial motonucleus is excitatory, an abnormal input from the trigeminal system to the facial motonucleus may be the additional factor that predisposes one towards the development of HFS, if vascular compression of the facial nerve is also present.

The fact that inhibitory neurons seem to disappear with increasing age at a higher rate than excitatory neurons, as evidenced from studies of other parts of the brain [62, 63] may explain why disorders caused by vascular compression of cranial nerves tend to (but not always) occur later in life.

One such additional factor could also be a weakness or slight injury of the myelin of the respective cranial nerve. This hypothesis is supported by recent neurological studies of the vestibular nerve in patients who were cured of dizziness by vascular decompression and who had exhibited pathological signs of the vestibular nerves, as seen in histopathological studies [48]. This is also supported by the results of the above

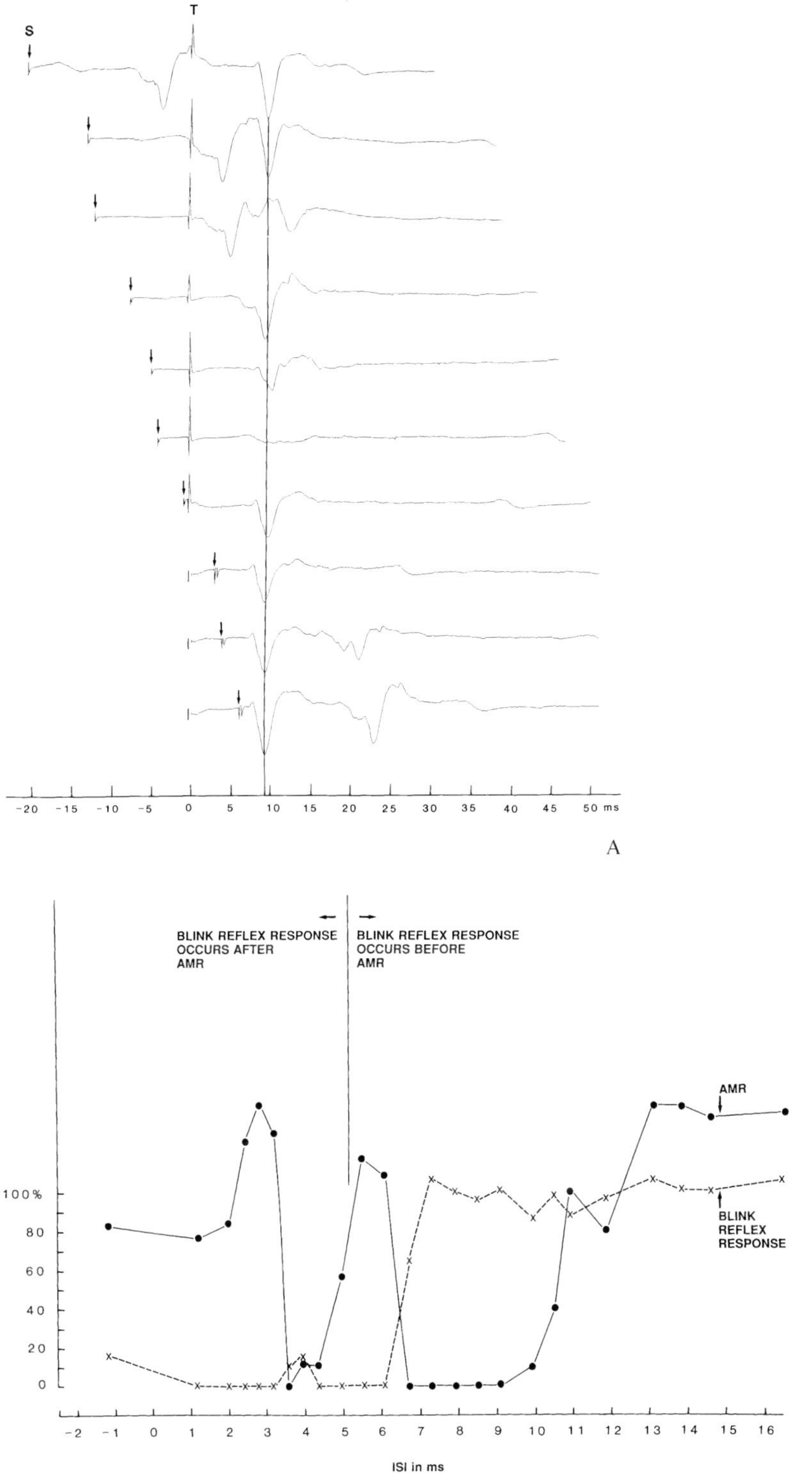

Fig. 6. Interaction between the abnormal muscle response and the response to electrical stimulation of the supraorbital nerve (blink reflex).
A Responses from the mentalis muscle to stimulation of the supraorbital nerve (*S*) and the temporal branch of the facial nerve (*T*). The different recordings show the responses obtained at different intervals between stimulation of the supraorbital nerve and that of the temporal branch of the facial nerve, with the supraorbital stimulation preceding the stimulation of the temporal branch of the facial nerve as shown in the top portion of the graph. The lower portion of the graph shows responses obtained when the stimulation of the supraorbital nerve trailed that of the facial nerve.
B The amplitude of the abnormal muscle response (*AMR*, solid line) together with that of the synkinetic response of the blink reflex recorded from the mentalis muscle (dashed line) are shown as a function of the interstimulus interval (*ISI*). (The latency of the AMR was 10 ms and that of the synkinetic response of the blink reflex – both recorded from the mentalis muscle – was 15 ms, and the difference was 5.15 ms (from Møller [29])

mentioned animal experiments that showed that both slight injury and close contact with a blood vessel is necessary to the development of HFS-like signs in rats [34].

There is thus substantial evidence that the anatomical location of the physiological abnormality that causes both the spasm and the abnormal muscle response in patients with HFS is in the facial motonucleus, but it is evident from many studies that this hyperactivity and facilitation with cross-transmission between motoneurons that innervate different parts of the face may depend on factors in addition to vascular compression.

That vascular compression of a cranial nerve may exist without any noticeable symptoms is evident from studies of hearing in patients with HFS. Thus, it has been shown that many patients with HFS have small anomalies in their pure tone audiograms (dips) that appear clearly but which do not seem to cause any symptoms [64] and therefore would go unnoticed if the person did not have an audiogram for other reasons. It was hypothesized that these anomalies are caused by vascular irritation of the auditory nerve by the same vessel that is causing HFS. Thus, the vessel that is in close contact with the facial nerve is also in close contact with the auditory nerve. These patients, however, did not have the symptoms of severe tinnitus. In other cases, the vascular compression of the cochlear nerve caused rather dramatic symptoms. Thus a large portion of patients with severe tinnitus and hypersensitivity to sound who were found to have a vascular compression of the auditory nerve could be cured of their tinnitus by MVD of the auditory nerve [6, 56–59, 65]. It has also been reported that patients with DPV often have small quiverings of the facial muscles around the eye [56] that are only apparent on close examination and that may not have been observed by the patient. This may be a sign that the vessel that is compressing the vestibular nerve and causing the symptoms of DPV is also in close contact with the facial nerve, but does not cause the symptoms of HFS, probably because the necessary additional factor(s) are not present.

These studies thus indicate that a vascular compression in itself gives only very slight signs that are not normally noticed by the patient. This contrasts sharply to the rather dramatic signs of HFS and DPV caused by anatomically similar vascular compression of respective cranial nerves. This observation supports the hypothesis that vascular compression is *not sufficient* to cause the rather noticeable symptoms and signs associated with disorders that can be cured by vascular decompression – HFS, TN, and DPV. Thus another factor seems to be necessary to create the symptoms that are typical of these disorders [36, 37, 60].

The presence of the second (or more) factor(s) alone may not cause any symptoms and a person may therefore live an entire life with such additional factors without manifesting any signs of disease or neurological abnormalities. In the same way, individuals with vascular compression, but no such additional factor, may live their entire life without manifesting any noticeable symptoms. This explains why the symptoms and signs of vascular compression disorders are so rare, although anatomical studies show such a high incidence of vascular compression of cranial nerves [50–52].

There are several unanswered questions. It is not known how vascular irritation of the facial nerve may cause the development of hyperactivity and cross-transmission in the facial motonucleus, and it is not known why it is a necessary factor for maintaining hyperactivity. Although there is evidence that the facial nerve also contains sensory afferents [66], these afferents presumably terminate in the trigeminal sensory nucleus, and it is not known if such afferents play a role in the development of HFS or in maintaining the signs of HFS.

The fact that there may be factors other than vascular compression that are necessary for the development of disorders such as HFS, TN, DPV, and tinnitus does not in any way cause doubt as to the efficacy of MVD procedures in treating such disorders. If more than one factor is *necessary* but no single one of these factors (including vascular compression) is *sufficient* in itself for the development and maintenance of the symptoms and signs of a certain disorder, then the elimination of either one of these factors obviously can cure the specific disorder. We do not know exactly what are these additional factors that are necessary for maintaining the signs of HFS and we do not know how to eliminate them.

References

1. Iwakuma T, Matsumoto A, Nakamura N (1982) Hemifacial spasm, comparison of three different operative procedures in 110 patients. J Neurosurg 57: 753–756
2. Apfelbaum RI (1988) Surgical management of disorders of the lower cranial nerves. In: Schmidek HH, Sweet WH (eds) Operative neurosurgical techniques. Indications, methods, and results, vol 2. Grune and Stratton, Orlando Florida, pp 1097–1109
3. Jannetta PJ (1970) Microsurgical exploration and decompression of the facial nerve in hemifacial spasm. Curr Top Surg Res 2: 217–220
4. Jannetta PJ (1977) Observations on the etiology of trigeminal neuralgia, hemifacial spasm, acoustic nerve dysfunction, and glossopharyngeal neuralgia. Definitive microsurgical treatment and results in 117 patients. Acta Neurochir (Wien) 20: 145–154

5. Jannetta PJ (1981) Hemifacial spasm. In: Samii M, Jannetta PJ (eds) The cranial nerves. Springer, Heidelberg, pp 484–493
6. Kondo A, Ishikawa J, Yamasaki T, Konishi T (1980) Microvascular decompression of cranial nerves, particularly of the seventh cranial nerve. Neurol Med Chir (Tokyo) 20: 739–751
7. Barker FG, Jannetta PJ, Bissonette DJ, Shields PT, Larkins MV, Jho HD (1995) Microvascular decompression for hemifacial spasm. J Neurosurg 82: 201–210
8. Gardner WJ, Sava GA (1962) Hemifacial spasm—a reversible pathophysiologic state. J Neurosurg 19: 240–247
9. Møller AR (1991) The cranial nerve vascular compression syndrome: I. A review of treatment. Acta Neurochir (Wien) 113: 18–23
10. Pollack IF, Jannetta PJ, Bissonette DJ (1988) Bilateral trigeminal neuralgia: A 14-year experience with microvascular decompression. J Neurosurg 68: 559–565
11. Burchiel KJ, Clarke H, Haglund M, Loeser JD (1988) Long term efficacy of microvascular decompression in trigeminal neuralgia. J Neurosurg 69: 35–38
12. Digre K, Corbett JJ (1988) Hemifacial spasm: Differential diagnosis mechanism and treatment. In: Tolosa E (ed) Advances in neurology, vol. 39, Facial dyskinesia. Raven Press, New York, pp 151–176
13. Gardner WJ (1962) Concerning the mechanism of trigeminal neuralgia and hemifacial spasm. J Neurosurg 19: 947–958
14. Gardner WJ (1966) Crosstalk—the paradoxical transmission of a nerve impulse. Arch Neurol 14: 149–156
15. Nielsen VK (1984) Pathophysiological aspects of hemifacial spasm. Part I. Evidence of ectopic excitation and ephaptic transmission. Neurology 34: 418–426
16. Ferguson JH (1978) Hemifacial spasm and the facial nucleus. Ann Neurol 4: 97–103
17. Esteban A, Molina-Negro P (1986) Primary hemifacial spasm: A neurophysiological study. J Neurol Neurosurg Psychiatry 49: 58–63
18. Roth G, Magistris MR, Pinelli P, Rilliet B (1990), Cryptogenic hemifacial spasm. A neurophysiological study. Electromyogr Clin Neurophysiol 30: 361–370
19. Nielsen VK (1984) Pathophysiological aspects of hemifacial spasm. Part II. Lateral spread of the supraorbital nerve reflex. Neurology 34: 427–431
20. Itagaki S, Saito S, Nakai O (1989) Electrophysiological study on hemifacial spasm-usefulness in etiological diagnosis and pathophysiological mechanism. Brain Nerve (Tokyo) 41: 1005–1011
21. Saito S, Itagaki S, Nakai O (1990) Neurophysiological study on hemifacial spasm—the abnormality and origin of the electromyographic response to stimulation of the facial nerve. Brain Nerve (Tokyo) 42: 621–627
22. Møller AR, Jannetta PJ (1984) On the origin of synkinesis in hemifacial spasm: Results of intracranial recordings. J Neurosurg 61: 569–576
23. Møller AR, Jannetta PJ (1985) Hemifacial spasm: Results of electrophysiologic recording during microvascular decompression operations. Neurology 35: 969–974
24. Møller AR, Jannetta PJ (1985) Microvascular decompression in hemifacial spasm: Intraoperative electrophysiological observations. Neurosurgery 16: 612–618
25. Møller AR, Jannetta PJ (1985) Synkinesis in hemifacial spasm: Results of recording intracranially from the facial nerve. Experientia 41: 415–417
26. Møller AR, Jannetta PJ (1986) Blink reflex in patients with hemifacial spasm: Observations during microvascular decompression operations. J Neurol Sci 72: 171–182
27. Møller AR, Jannetta PJ (1986) Physiological abnormalities in hemifacial spasm studied during microvascular decompression operations. Exp Neurol 93: 584–600
28. Møller AR (1987) Hemifacial spasm: Ephaptic transmission or hyperexcitability of the facial motor nucleus? Exp Neurol 98: 110–119
29. Møller AR (1991) Interaction between the blink reflex and the abnormal muscle response in patients with hemifacial spasm: Results of intraoperative recordings. J Neurol Sci 101: 114–123
30. Itagaki S, Saito S, Nakai O (1988) Intraoperative recording of evoked EMG in patients with hemifacial spasm-possible physiological mechanism. Facial N Res Jpn 8: 143–146
31. Møller AR, Sen CN (1990) Recordings from the facial nucleus in the rat: Signs of abnormal facial muscle response. Exp Brain Res 91: 18–24
32. Sen CN, Møller AR (1987) Signs of hemifacial spasm created by chronic periodic stimulation of the facial nerve in the rat. Exp Neurol 98: 336–349
33. Saito S, Møller AR (1993) Chronic electrical stimulation of the facial nerve causes signs of facial nucleus hyperactivity. Neurol Res 15: 225–231
34. Kuroki A, Møller AR (1994) Facial nerve demyelination and vascular compression are both needed to induce facial hyperactivity: A study in rats. Acta Neurochir (Wien) 126: 149–157
35. Kuroki A, Møller AR, Saito S (1994) Recordings from the facial motonucleus in rats with signs of hemifacial spasm. Neurol Res 16: 389–392
36. Møller AR (1991) The cranial nerve vascular compression syndrome: II. A review of pathophysiology. Acta Neurochir (Wien) 113: 24–30
37. Møller AR (1993) Cranial nerve dysfunction syndromes: Pathophysiology of microvascular compression. In: Barrow DL (ed) Neurosurgical Topics Book 13. Surgery of Cranial Nerves of the Posterior Fossa, Chapter 2. American Association of Neurological Surgeons, Park Ridge, Illinois, pp 105–129
38. Goddard GV (1964) Amygdaloid stimulation and learning in the rat. J Comp Physiol Psychol 58: 23–30
39. Wada JA (1981) Kindling 2. Raven Press, New York
40. Esslen E (1957) Der Spasmus facialis eine Parabiosserscheinung: Elektrophysiologische Untersuchungen zum Entstehungsmechanismus des Facialisspasmus. Dtsch Z Nervenheil 176: 149–172
41. Auger RG (1979) Hemifacial spasm: Clinical and electrophysiological observations. Neurology (NY) 29: 1261–1272
42. Auger RG, Piepgras DG, Laws ER Jr, Miller RH (1981) Microvascular decompression of the facial nerve for hemi-facial spasm: Clinical and electrophysiologic observations. Neurology 31: 346–350
43. Møller AR, Jannetta PJ (1987) Monitoring facial EMG responses during microvascular decompression operations for hemifacial spasm. J Neurosurg 66: 681–685
44. Haines SJ, Torres F (1991) Intraoperative monitoring of the facial nerve during decompressive surgery for hemifacial spasm. J Neurosurg 74: 254–257
45. Howe JF, Calvin WH, Loeser JD (1976) Impulses reflected from dorsal root ganglia and from focal nerve injuries. Brain Res 116: 129–144
46. Howe JF, Loeser JD, Calvin WH (1977) Mechanosensitivity of dorsal root ganglia and chronically injured axons: A physiological basis for the radicular pains of root compression. Pain 3: 25–41

47. Lehman HJ, Ule G (1964) Electrophysiological findings and structural changes in circumscript inflammation of peripheral nerves. Prog Brain Res 6: 169–173
48. Colletti V, Carner M, Fiorino FG, Sbarbati A (1994) The vestibular nerve in Meniere's disease: Ultrastructural findings. (Submitted)
49. Cushing H (1920) The major trigeminal neuralgias and their surgical treatment based on experience with 332 Gasserian operations. The varieties of facial neuralgia. Am J Med Sci 160: 157–184
50. Matsushima T, Inoue T, Fukui M (1990) Arteries in contact with the cisternal portion of the facial nerve in autopsy cases: Microsurgical anatomy for neurovascular decompression surgery of hemifacial spasm. Surg Neurol 34: 87–93
51. Sunderland S (1948) Microvascular relations and anomalies at the base of the brain. J Neurol Neurosurg Psychiatry 11: 243–257
52. Ouaknine GE (1981) Microsurgical anatomy of the arterial loops in the ponto-cerebellar angle and the internal acoustic meatus. In: Samii M, Jannetta PJ (eds) The cranial nerves. Springer, Heidelberg, pp 378–390
53. Auger RG, Whisnant JP (1990) Hemifacial spasm in Rochester and Olmsted County, Minnesota, 1960 to 1984. Arch Neurol 47: 1233–1234
54. Katusic S, Beardd CM, Bergstralh E, Kurland LT (1990) Incidence and clinical features of trigeminal neuralgia, Rochester, Minnesota 1945–1984. Ann Neurol 27: 89–95
55. Jannetta PJ, Møller MB, Møller AR (1984) Disabling positional vertigo. N Engl J Med 310: 1700–1705
56. Møller MB, Møller AR, Jannetta PJ, Sekhar LN (1986) Diagnosis and surgical treatment of disabling positional vertigo. J Neurosurg 64: 21–28
57. Møller MB, Møller AR, Jannetta PJ, Jho HD, Sekhar LN (1993) Microvascular decompression of the eighth nerve in patients with disabling positional vertigo: Selection criteria and operative results in 207 patients. Acta Neurochir (Wien) 125: 75–82
58. Møller MB, Møller AR, Jannetta PJ, Jho HD (1993) Vascular decompression surgery for severe tinnitus: Selection criteria and results. Laryngoscope 103: 421–427
59. Jannetta PJ (1987) Microvascular decompression of the cochlear nerve as treatment of tinnitus. In: Feldmann H (ed) Proceedings of the Third International Tinnitus Seminar (held in Munster, 'West Germany, June 11–13, 1987). Harsch, Karlsruhe, pp 348–352
60. Møller AR (1989) Letter to the Editor, Views on microvascular decompression: Comments on article by Adams CBT. "Microvascular compression: An alternative view and hypothesis" (published in J Neurosurg 1989; 57: 1–12.) J Neurosurg 71: 459–460
61. Møller AR (1989) Possible mechanisms of tinnitus. In: Mahon WJ (ed) Tinnitus 1989. The Hearing Journal 42: 65–67
62. Caspary DM, Raza A, Lawhorn Armour BA, Pippin J, Arneric SP (1990) Immunocytochemical and neurochemical evidence of age-related loss of GABA in the inferior colliculus: Implications for neural presbycusis. J Neurosci 10: 2363–2372
63. Raza A, Milbrant JC, Armeric SP, Caspary DM (1994) Age-related changes in brainstem auditory neurotransmitters: Measures of GABA and acetylcholine function. Hear Res 77: 221–230
64. Møller MB, Møller AR (1985) Audiometric abnormalities in hemifacial spasm. Audiology 24: 396–405
65. Møller MB (1987) Vascular compression of the eighth nerve as cause of tinnitus. In: Feldmann H (ed) Proc. III International Tinnitus Seminar (held in Munster, West Germany, June 11–13, 1987). Harsch, Karlsruhe, pp 340–347
66. Radpour S, Gacek RR (1985) Anatomical organization of the cat facial nerve. Otolaryngol Head Neck Surg 93: 591–596

Correspondence: Aage R. Møller, Ph.D., Department of Neurological Surgery, Suite B-400 Presbyterian-University Hospital, 200 Lothrop Street, Pittsburgh, Pennsylvania 15213, U.S.A.

Magnetic resonance imaging in hemifacial spasm

J.-C. Froment and **M. LeDelliou**

Hopital Neurologique Pierre Wertheimer, University Claude Bernard, Lyon, France

Summary

Twenty-two patients with hemifacial spasm (HFS) underwent magnetic resonance imaging (MRI). Seventeen patients had contrast injection of Gadolinium. Six patients underwent microvascular decompression of the seventh cranial nerve (CN VII). Two patients underwent controlled MRI after surgery. Transverse 3-D Gradient Echo (GE) and transverse 3-D magnetic resonance angiography (MRA) were the most adequate sequences to individualize both nerves and arteries. Contract injection did not improve the visualization of small vessels. The examination showed a neurovascular conflict in 21 patients; it was always ipsilateral to the HFS; and there was no abnormal vessel on the contralateral side. Surgery confirmed the preoperative diagnosis of neurovascular conflict for the 6 patients who underwent operation. Postoperative control MRIs did not show any clear differences from the preoperative examination. MRI should be considered as the screening procedure of choice in patients with HFS. MRA appears to be the best sequence, as it offers both projectional and native thin sections. 3-D GE or CISS sequences are to be used in addition in order to get a better delineation of CN VII.

Key words: Hemifacial spasm, magnetic resonance imaging, magnetic resonance angiography, vertebral arteries, basilar arteries.

Introduction

The main purpose of performing imaging studies in patients with hemifacial spasm (HFS) is to search for a compression of the facial nerve at its root exit zone (REZ) by a vascular loop [8]. The use of conventional or digital subtraction angiography (DSA) [3] has been discontinued because of its inability to show neural structure and because it is an invasive technique. Computerized tomography (CT-scan) can be effective in diagnosing large dolicho arteries [9], but it is inadequate for showing the relationship between the facial nerve and nearby smaller vessels. Both of these tests have been replaced by magnetic resonance imaging (MRI) for examining patients with HFS. MRI appears to be the present technique of choice, as it allows one to obtain images of both nerves and arteries with optimal contrast and good resolution. MRI makes it possible to diagnose with precision the relationship between the facial nerve and vessels in the area of the REZ, and furthermore it can provide an angiogram of the vertebro-basilar system.

Patients and methods

Between September, 1993 and May, 1994, 22 patients with HFS underwent magnetic resonance imaging (MRI) in our Department. This study group comprised 10 men and 12 women, 23 to 73 years old (mean age, 52 years old). Examinations were performed with a Siemens Magnetom 63 SP 1.5 T unit. All patients had sagittal FLASH 2-D (TR = 120 ms, TE = 10 ms, flip angle = 10 degrees, slice number = 5, thickness = 7 mm, field of view = 250 mm, matrix size = 200 × 256, number of acquisitions = 2, measure time = 50 seconds), transverse 3-D Gradient Echo (GE) FLASH (TR = 30 ms, TE = 6 ms, flip angle = 35 degrees, slab number = 1, thickness = 64 mm, field of view = 256 mm, matrix size = 256 × 256, number of acquisition = 1, number of 1-mm thick 3-D partitions = 64, measure time = 8 mn 14 sec), and transverse FISP 3-D magnetic resonance angiography (MRA) (TR = 43 ms, TE = 8 ms, flip angle = 20 degrees, slab number = 1, thickness = 52 mm, field of view = 200 mm, matrix size = 256 × 512, number of acquisition = 1, number of 0.812-mm thick 3-D partitions = 64, parallel saturation slab above the 3-D volume, measure time = 11 mn 47 sec). Projectional angiography was obtained by postprocessing the MRA data using coronal-to-sagittal maximum intensity projection (MIP) algorithms after segmentation of the vertebrobasilar system to erase the carotid arteries. Seventeen patients in our study group had previous contrast injection of Gadolinium; the other 5 patients did not have any contrast injection. Two patients had comparative pre- and postcontrast transverse FLASH 3-D acquisition, and 1 patient had comparative pre-operative postcontrast and postoperative noncontrast MRA. Additionally, T2 weighted 2-D Turbo Spin Echo (TSE) was performed in 9 patients. A transverse 3-D CISS acquisition (TR = 14.65 ms, TE = 21 ms, flip angle = 65 degrees, slab number = 1, thickness = 22.4 mm, field of view = 170 mm, matrix size = 256 × 256, number of acquisition = 1, number of 0.7-mm thick 3-D partitions = 32, measure time = 2.02 mn × 2 was performed in 2 patients.

Six patients in this series underwent microvascular decompression (MVD) of the seventh cranial nerve (CN VII) (surgery performed by M. Sindou). Two patients underwent controlled MRI, one 7 days after surgery and the other 7 months after surgery.

Results

1) Transverse 3-D GE and transverse 3-D MRA (Figs. 1–13) were the *most adequate sequences to individualize both nerves and arteries.* Projectional angiography was necessary to show the vascular pathway of the incriminated vessels and to identify them. Contrast injection did not improve the visualization of small vessels, neither when using transverse 3-D nor 3-D MRA. A comparison between post-contrast and non-

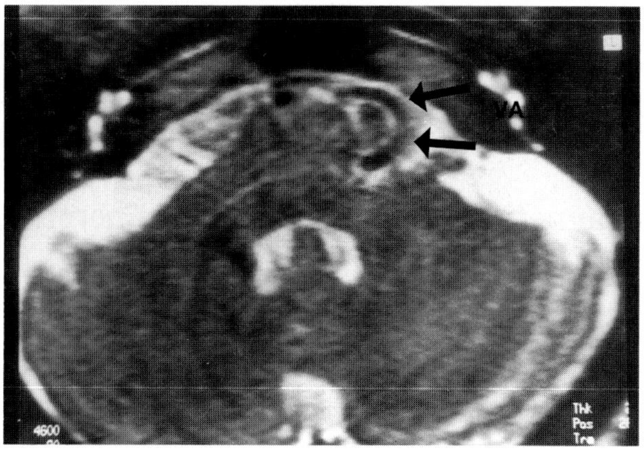

Fig. 2

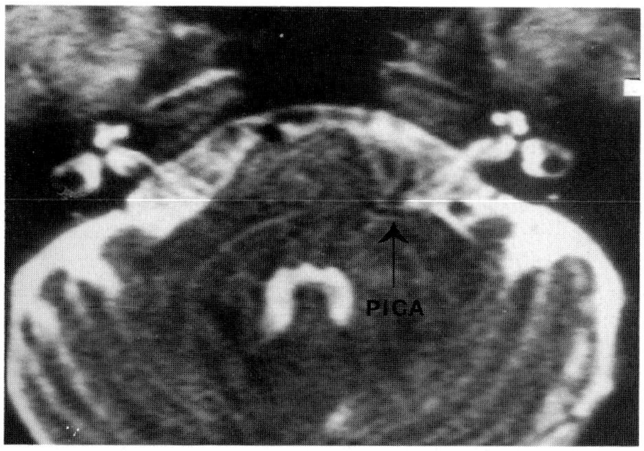

Fig. 3

Figs. 2, 3. Axial T2-weighted TSE images (Flip angle: 90, TR: 4600, TE: 90, 3 acquisitions, Acquisition time: 9mn 23): there is, close to the REZ, a signal void curved vascular structure (left *VA*), and just above it a signal void transversal structure (PICA)

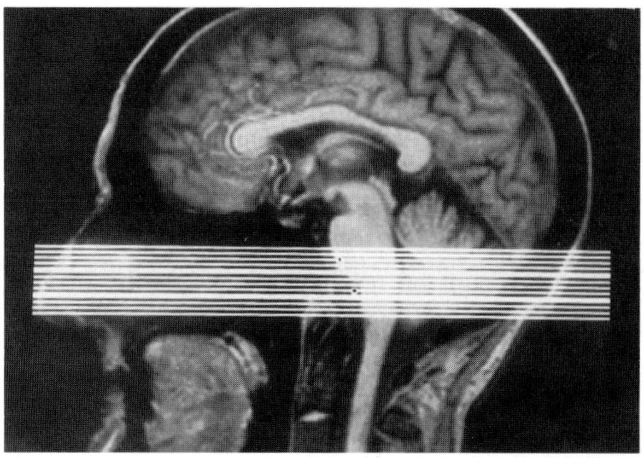

Case 19: 57-year-old female with HFS on the left side for 1 year. (Figs. 1–13)

Fig. 1. Sagittal T1-weighted localizer image: eleven, 2 mm thick, axial, T2-weighted TSE sections have been selected on the ponto-medullary junction

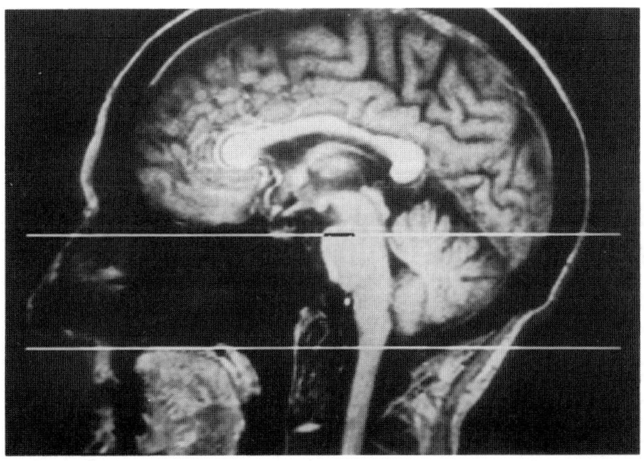

Fig. 4. Sagittal T1-weighted localizer image: the two lines represent the area of coverage of the axial 3-D GE acquisition, which is centered on the junction between the pons and the medulla oblongata

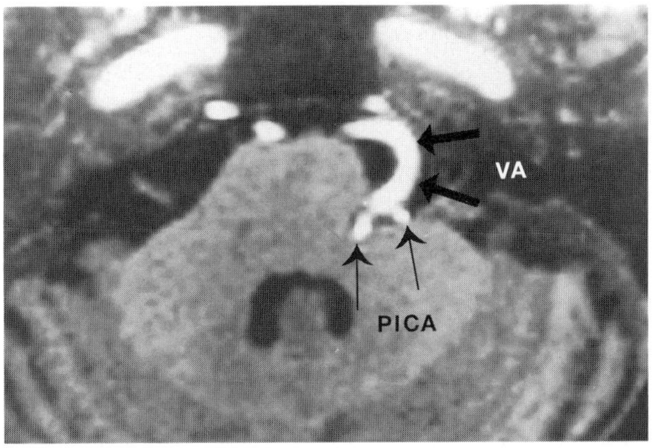

Fig. 5

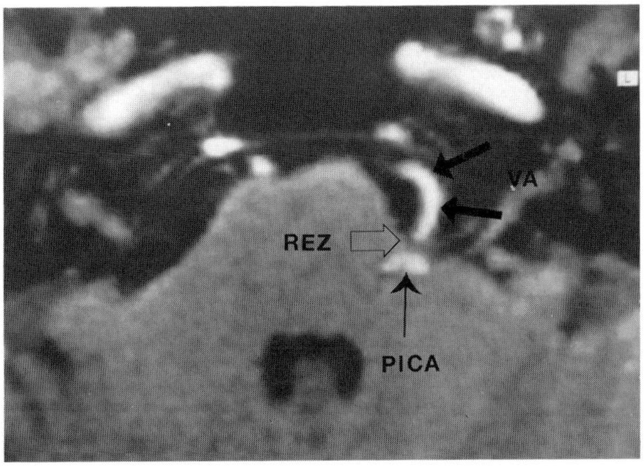

Fig. 6

Figs. 5, 6. Axial 3-D GE 1.3 mm thick sections (Flip angle: 40, TR: 30, TE: 6, 2 acquisitions, acquisition time: 8mn 14): compression of the *REZ* by *PICA* and left *VA*

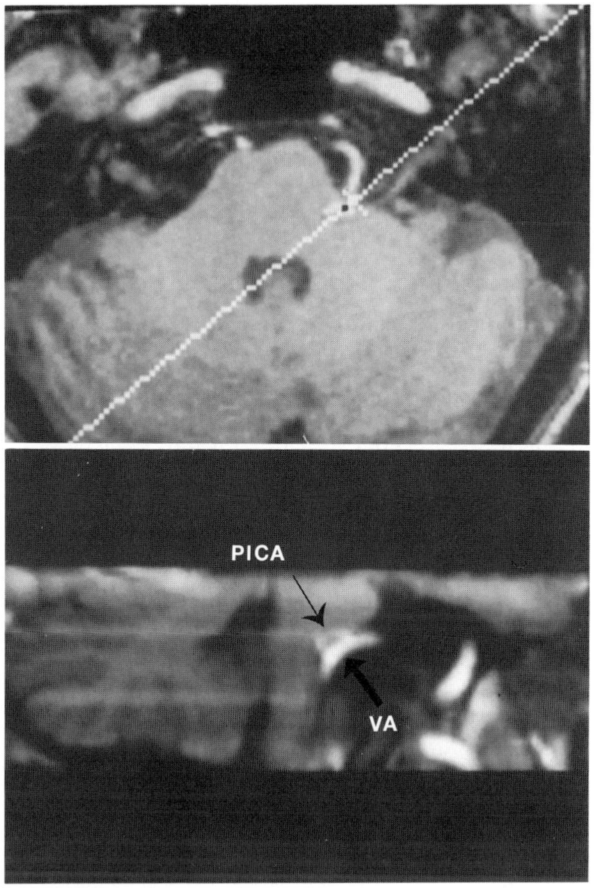

Fig. 7. 3-D GE coronal oblique multiplanar reconstruction along the long axis of the nerve

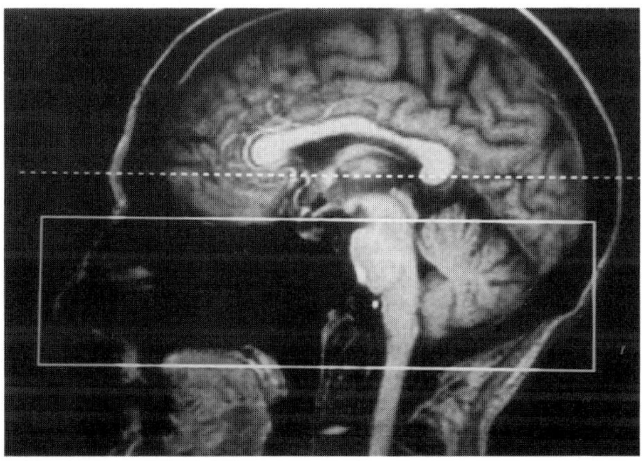

Fig. 8. Sagittal T1-weighted localizer image: the two lines represent the area of coverage of the MRA acquisition, and the dotted line delimits a presaturation volume to exclude veins on the angiogram

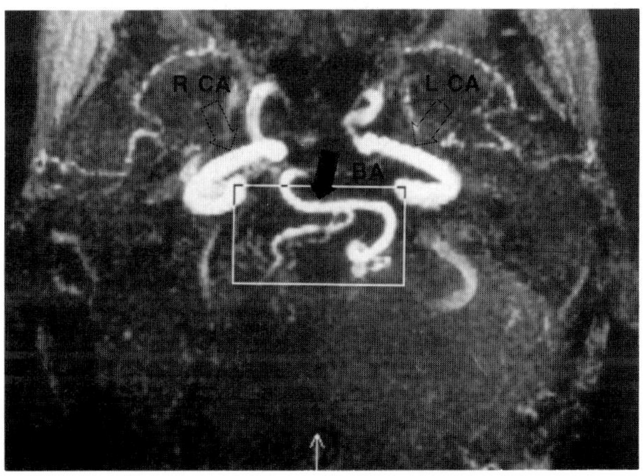

Fig. 9. Selection of a box to exclude the carotid arteries

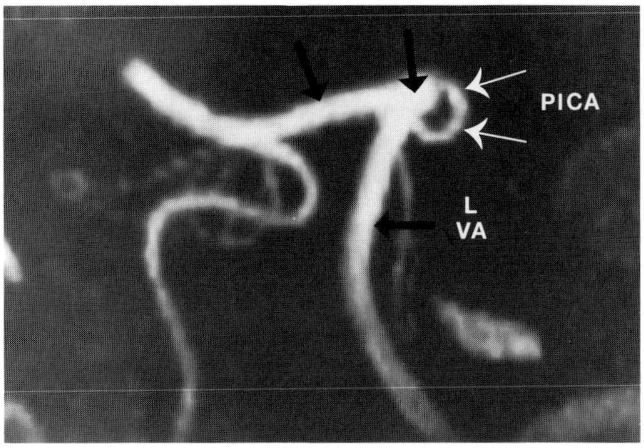

Fig. 10. Projectional MRA (frontal view): dolicho vertebral arteries with a loop of the *PICA* emerging at the convexity of the left *VA*; compression of CN VII is not visualized

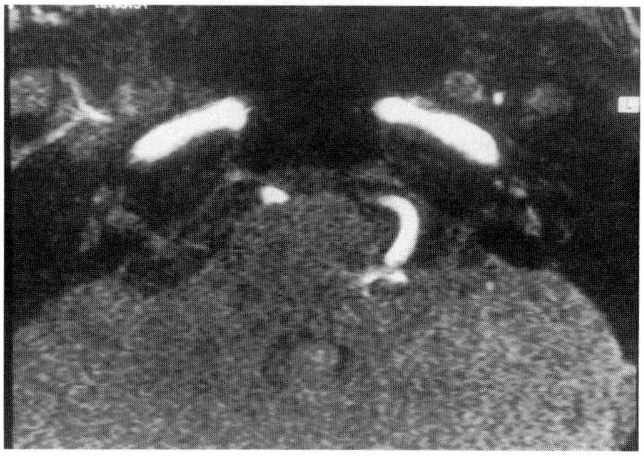

Fig. 11

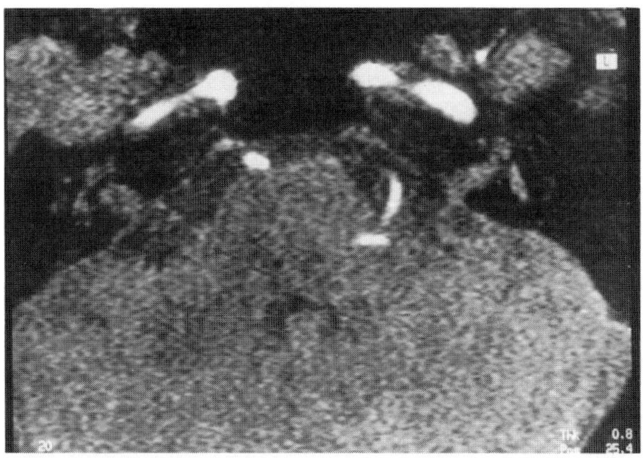

Fig. 12

Figs. 11, 12. Individual native angiographic 0.8-mm thick sections (Flip angle: 20, TR: 43, TE: 8, 1 acquisition, acquisition time: 11 mn 47): same aspect as Figs. 5 and 6

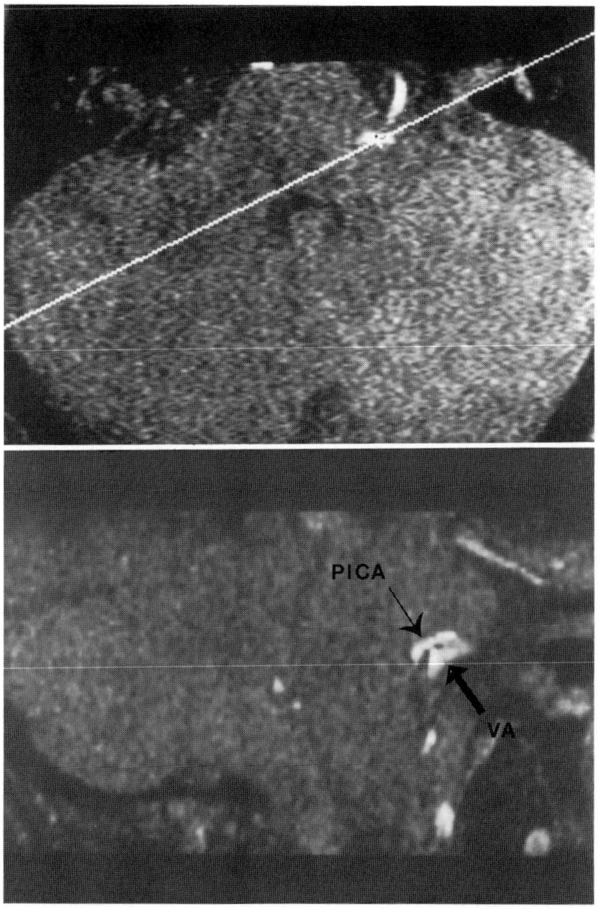

Fig. 13. MRA coronal oblique multiplanar reconstruction along the long axis of the affected nerve: *VA* and *PICA* are well depicted at the REZ of the nerve

contrast MRA (Figs. 14–19) indicated that noncontrast angiography is preferable, since it did not have any venous artifacts. 2-D TSE did not add any significant information to the information that was provided by transverse 3-D and 3-D MRA. 3-D CISS acquisition did not give enough information because of signal void artifacts due to the pulsations of cerebrospinal fluid (CSF).

2) *The examination showed a neurovascular conflict* in nearly all 21 patients (Table 1). There was a vascular contact with the REZ of CN VII in 21 patients (95%), and contact with a deformity of the REZ in 11 patients (50%). The abnormalities were ipsilateral to HFS in all patients (21 out of 21 cases), and there was no abnormal vessel on the contralateral side. In only one case was the vascular contact with the REZ questionable.

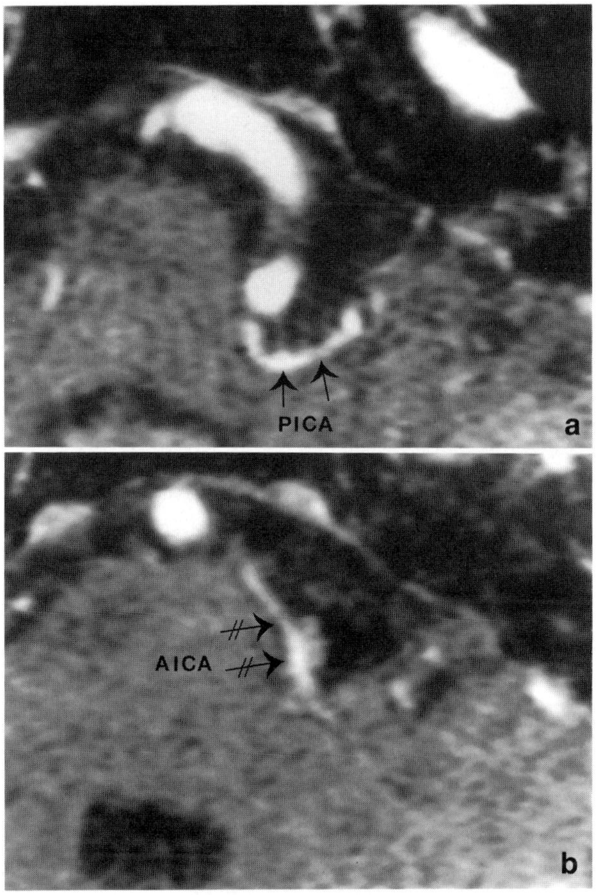

Fig. 14

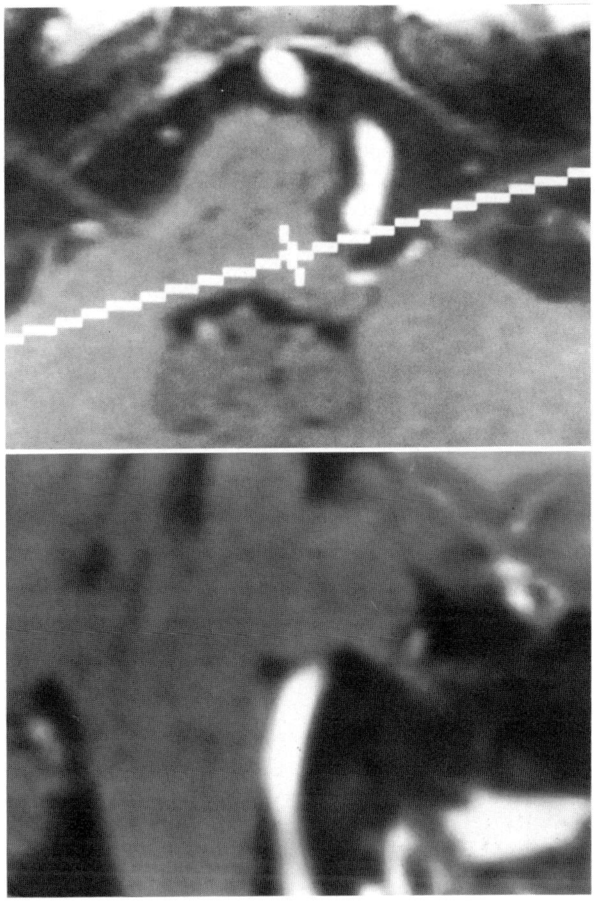

Fig. 15

Case 7: 43-year-old female with HFS on the left side for 2 years. (Figs. 14–19)

Fig. 14. 3-D GE FLASH section: **a** loop of the *PICA* emerging from a dolicho *VA* at the REZ of the facial nerve. **b** contribution of the *AICA* to the neurovascular conflict

Fig. 15. 3-D GE FLASH oblique coronal reformatted section: deformity of the REZ due to the *VA*

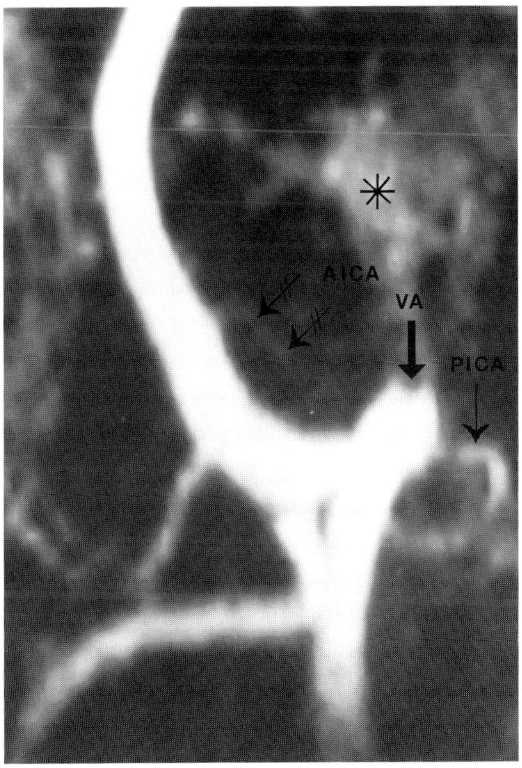

Fig. 16. Post-contrast projectional MRA (frontal view): the three arteries contributing to the conflict (*VA*, *PICA*, and *AICA*) are well seen; note the venous artifacts due to the injection of contrast medium

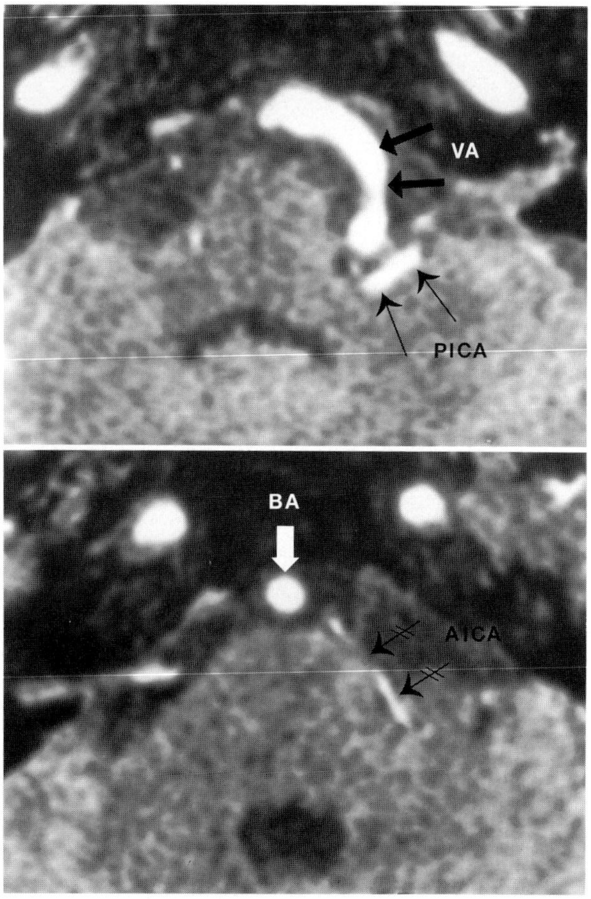

Fig. 17. 3-D GE postoperative control examination: same aspect as Fig. 14

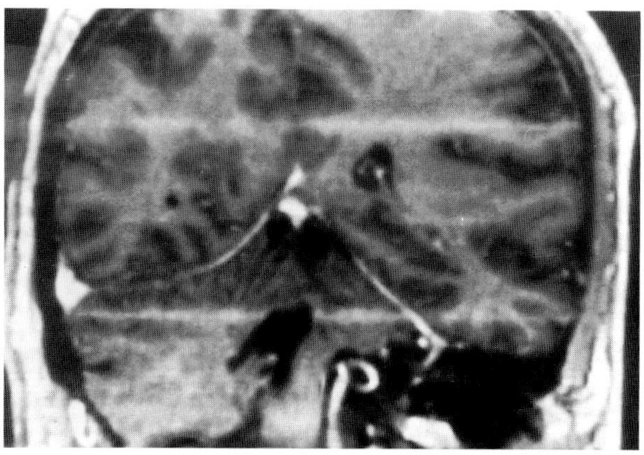

Fig. 18. 3-D GE postoperative oblique coronal reformatted section: deformity of the REZ due to the loop of the PICA

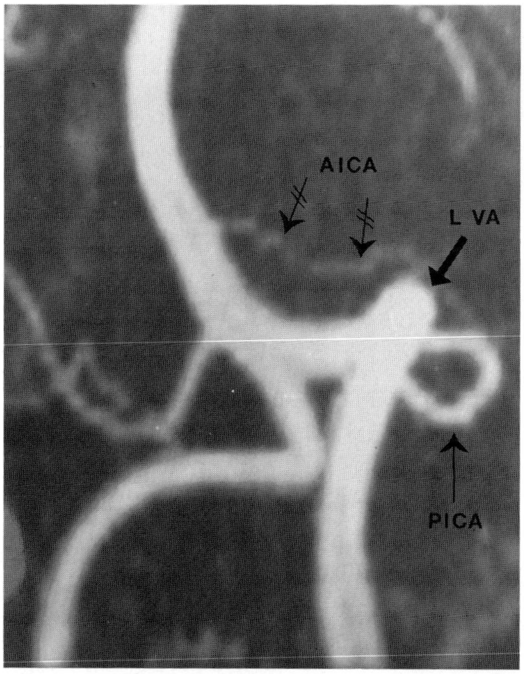

Fig. 19. Projectional postoperative MRA (frontal view): same aspect as on Fig. 16; no venous artifact (the patient had no contrast injection)

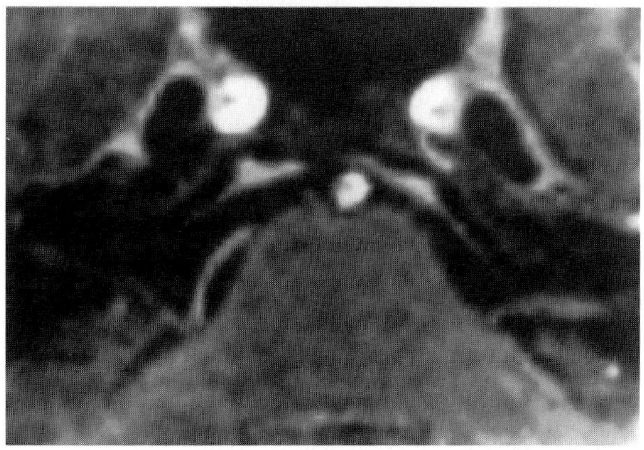

Case 16: 34-year-old female with HFS on the right side for 2 years. (Figs. 20–22)

Fig. 20. 3-D FLASH GE 1 mm thick section: contact between the nerve and a vascular branch originating at the right VA/BA junction (PICA?)

3) In 8 patients the *vessels responsible for the conflict* were the vertebral artery (VA) and the posterior inferior artery (PICA) (Figs. 20–22), in 6 patients it was the anterior inferior artery (AICA) alone, in 2 patients it was the PICA alone, in 2 patients it was the VA, PICA and AICA, in 1 patient it was the VA and AICA, in 1 patient it was both the basilar artery (BA) and the

Table 1. MRI and surgical findings in 22 patients with essential hemifacial spasm

Case N°/patient name	Age sex	HFS side	MR Finding					Surgical findings NVC/REZ
			Dolicho arteries	Contact	Compression	NVC/REZ	NVC side	
1. CHA	73 M	L	+	+	+	VA, PICA, AICA	L	
2. VID	26 F	L	–	+	–	AICA	L	AICA
3. COS	64 M	L	+	+	+	VA, PICA	L	
4. AMA	41 F	R	–	+	–	AICA	R	
5. VAS	58 M	L	+	+	+	VA	L	
6. BAR	46 F	L	+	+	–	VA, PICA	L	
7. SAU	43 M	L	+	+	+	VA, PICA, AICA	L	AICA, PICA, VA
8. EMO	55 F	L	–	+	–	PICA	L	
9. LAL	23 F	R	–	?	–	?	?	
10. CHA	60 M	L	+	+	+	VA, PICA	L	
11. LER	38 F	R	–	+	–	AICA	R	
12. BAT	69 F	L	+	+	+	VA, PICA	L	
13. OMR	51 F	L	+	+	–	VA, AICA	L	
14. BOI	58 M	L	+	+	+	AICA	L	
15. MEN	59 F	L	+	+	–	AICA	L	
16. OLI	34 F	R	+	+	+	VA, PICA	R	PICA (+dolicho VA)
17. CIC	64 M	R	+	+	–	AICA	R	
18. GRA	62 M	L	+	+	+	VA, PICA	L	
19. SCH	57 F	L	+	+	+	VA, PICA	L	PICA (+dolicho VA)
20. PEY	32 M	L	–	+	–	PICA	L	
21. PIG	70 M	L	+	+	+	BA, AICA	L	PICA (+ dolicho BA)
22. LIN	66 F	L	+	+	–	VA, PICA	L	PICA (+dolicho VA)
* PER	44 F	L				Neurinoma	L	Neurinoma

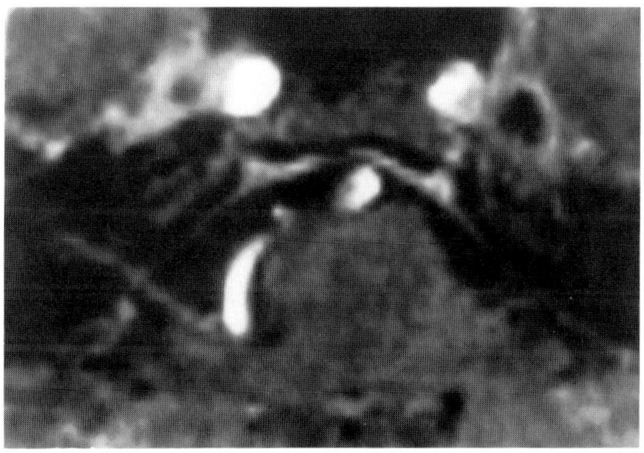

Fig. 21. 3-D FLASH GE 1 mm thick section: contact between the right facial nerve and a dolicho VA

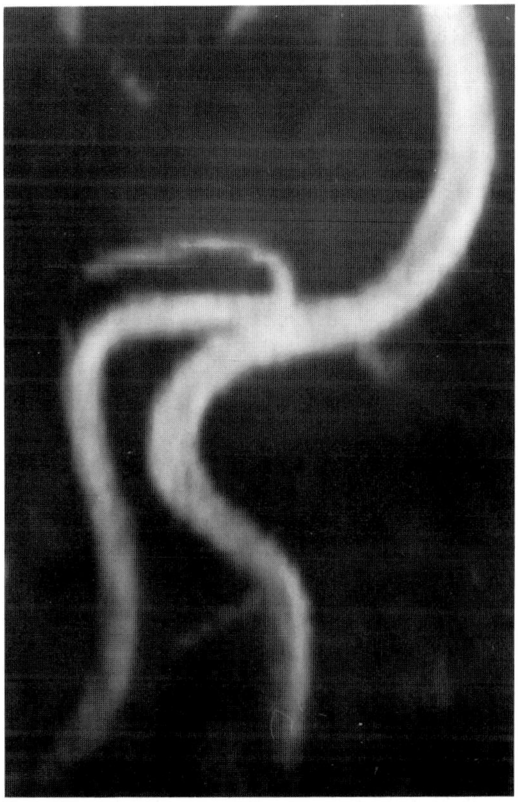

Fig. 22. Projectional MRA: dolicho, convex toward the symptomatic size, vertebral arteries, and vascular branch (right PICA?) contributing to the compression of the nerve

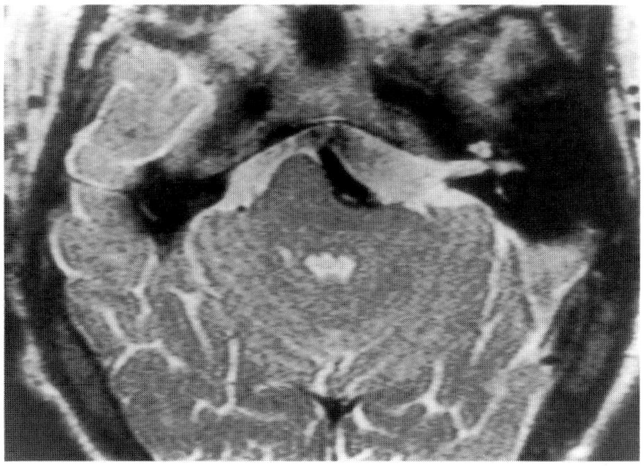

Case 21: 70-year-old male with HFS on the left side. (Figs. 23, 24)

Fig. 23. Axial T2-weighted 2 mm thick TSE section: compression of the REZ by a vascular loop

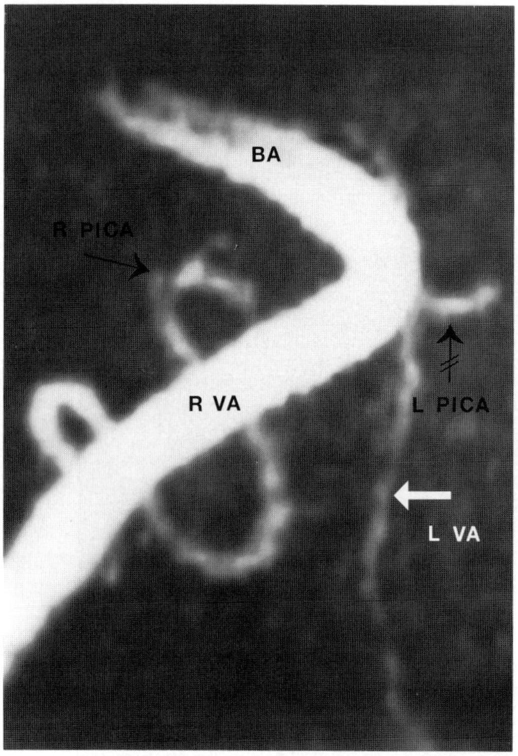

Fig. 24. Projectional MRA: large dolicho right vertebrobasilar artery, hypotrophic left *VA*; loop of the left *PICA*

PICA (Figs. 23–24), and in 1 patient it was the VA alone.

Surgery confirmed the magnetic resonance preoperative diagnosis of neurovascular conflict for the 6 patients who underwent operation. In one case (patient 21), MRI indicated the incriminated arteries to be the AICA and the BA, but during surgery the incriminating artery was seen to be the PICA and a dolicho BA.

4) *Postoperative control MRIs* did not show any clear differences from the preoperative examination (Figs. 14–19).

Discussion

1. MRI procedures

The area of interest to search for a neurovascular contact or compression is the cerebellopontine angle, whose level on an MR sagittal scout view (Figs. 1, 4, and 8) is the junction between the pons and the medulla oblongata. For this purpose, there is a wide range of techniques available, such as T1- or T2-weighted images (T1WI, T2WI) using 2-D or 3-D acquisitions, and MR angiography.

Routinely applied two-dimensional, spin-echo, MR techniques (2D-SE) provide sections that are 3 to 5 mm thick. Vascular structures appear dark, due to time-of-flight effects, which limits the differentiation of small vessels from cerebrospinal fluid on T1-weighted images. With high-resolution fast spin-echo (or turbo-spin-echo) sequences (FSE), 2-mm thick T2-weighted sections can be obtained (Figs. 2, 3, and 23). Better spatial resolution and high signal intensity of CSF improves the differentiation of small vessels from CSF as well as the delineation of the nerves.

Three-dimensional GE FLASH MR studies allow one to obtain 1-mm contiguous sections, on which CSF has a hypointense signal and arteries have a hyperintense signal (Figs. 5, 6, 20, and 21). Nerves have an isointense signal. The data can be postprocessed using multiplanar reconstruction (MPR) algorithms to reconstruct images along specific orientations (coronal, oblique coronal along the axis of the facial nerve, or perpendicular to it) (Figs. 7, 15, and 18).

MRA uses saturation pulses that suppress the signal arising from the brain tissue so that the blood vessels that have a fast flow appear as areas of higher signal intensity. A vertebrobasilar angiogram can be obtained without any superposition of the carotid arteries by creating a box in which only the area of interest is included (Figs. 9 and 10) and then by postprocessing the data using MIP algorithms. Projectional angiography allows one to visualize the entire vertebrobasilar system from different viewing angles, with the vessels being rotated either along a head-feet axis (Figs. 10, 16,

19, 22, and 24) or along a right-left axis. Projectional angiography is very helpful to understand the complex architecture of the vertebrobasilar system, but it does not show neural structures at all. To cancel this disadvantage, Tien and Wilkins [11] suggested that a projectional MR angiogram be superimposed on a T1-weighted image that shows the REZ of CN VII. Contiguous 0.8-mm thick individual native angiographic sections (Figs. 11–12, 14, and 17) are very important to consider; by adjusting the window width and level on the MR console, the relationship between the arteries and the cranial nerves and brain tissue can be demonstrated. Axially-acquired native angiographic sections can be reformatted into coronal or coronal oblique MR images [1, 2] (Fig. 13).

The CISS (Constructive Interference in Steady State) sequence [4, 7] is a special three-dimensional sequence that provides 1-mm thick sections with a hyperintense signal from the CSF. It has to be optimized to avoid signal voids due to CSF pulsations, and thus it would be then the best sequence to delineate CN VII and CN VIII. MPR algorithms can be used to reconstruct any incidence.

Which strategy has to be applied to perform the examination?

Most authors (Table 2) utilize transverse acquisitions, except Tien [11], who prefers to acquire 2-D sections and 3-D MRA volume by orientating them parallel to the clivus.

3-D GE and MRA acquisitions are the best sequences, since they provide millimetric sections that can be postprocessed to obtain reformatted sections in any orientation. Such data postprocessing is unfortunately time consuming. MRA is of particular interest because it offers both projectional angiography, which like DSA shows the entire vertebrobasilar system, and individual native angiographic sections, which are more informative to delineate small vessels in relation to the facial nerve.

Contrast medium injection does not add any information to the non-contrast MRI data [1] when used in patients with HFS. We prefer to perform projectional MRA without any injection to avoid venous artifacts (Figs. 16 and 19).

The study protocol that we recommend includes:

- Fast 2-D sagittal Gradient Echo sequence to place the area of interest on the cerebellopontine angle (pons/medulla oblongata junction),
- Transverse 3-D MRA acquisition,
- and additional transverse 3-D GE or optimized CISS sequence.

No contrast injection is required.

2. *Neurovascular conflict*

The relationship between the REZ of CN VII and the vertebrobasilar system can be divided into three categories [10]:

Table 2. HFS: MRI findings (literature review)

	Patients NB	Sequences	MR Findings		Surgery
Tash-1991 (10)	HFS = 13	Axial T1 WI	Vascular structure at the REZ 13		1
	Control = 70	Coronal T1 WI	Contact	30 (21%)	
	(140 VII nerves)		Contact and deformity	2 (1%)	
			Ipsilateral compression	24 (64,9%)	
Adler-1992 (1)	HFS = 37	Axial T1 WI	Controlateral compression	3	
		T2 WI	Negative	10 (27%)	
	Control = 16	3D MRA	Compression	1 (6,3%)	
Felber-1992 (5)	HSF = 14	Axial T2 WI	Ipsilateral contact	12	
	Control = 20	3D MRA	Contact	4	
			Compression	5	6
Furuya-1992 (6)	HSF = 6	Axial 3D Flash	Prothesis compressing the VIIth	1	(Second surgery in one case)
Girard-1993 (7)	HSF = 24	Axial 3D CISS 3D Turboflash	Compression	20	10
Tien-1993 (11)	HSF = 1 Control = 5	Coronal 3D MRA T1 WI	Compression	1	1

1) no contact;
2) contact with the REZ. The vascular structure is adjacent to the REZ of CN VII without deformity of the nerve;
3) deformity of the REZ when there is a neurovascular contact and a deformity of the REZ or a clear deformation of the adjacent pons by the vascular structure.

In most cases the offending vessels are the PICA, AICA, VA, or associations of two or more vessels.

The PICA can be recognized easily because it originates from the VA and makes a loop. The association of a dolicho VA extending into the cerebellopontine angle with a loop of the PICA compressing the brain stem and the REZ of the facial nerve gives a typical aspect.

The AICA originates from the basilar artery (BA) and has an antero-posterior course; it can be the only causative vessel, or it can be associated with a PICA, with a VA, or with both a PICA and a VA (Figs. 14–16).

Naming the exact vessel which is in contact with the REZ is not always easy (Figs. 20–22 and 24), but knowing this has no practical importance.

Sometimes it can be difficult to determine whether or not there are more than one compression site in a patient.

In most cases MRI cannot easily distinguish between CN VII and CN VIII. This could be avoided by using the CISS sequence.

The most important point is that it is not easy to differentiate a real cross-compression, a mere contact, or a vicinity relationship between the nerve and the arterial loop: Mere contact is not a specific aspect of a neurovascular conflict, because there is a high rate of occurrence of contact at the REZ in the asymptomatic individual—21% according to Tash et al. [10], 20% according to Felber et al. [5]. For this reason it is difficult to be sure that the offending vessel is really responsible for the patient's symptoms. It is, however, of great diagnostic value to detect vascular abnormalities at the REZ ipsilateral to the HFS side, with a comparative contralateral normal aspect. Deformity of the REZ is more specific than isolated contact. According to Tash and co-workers [10], it has been found in only 1% of asymptomatic individuals.

The definitive diagnosis will be based on the anatomical findings reported by the surgeon, who has a direct real 3-D vision of the neurovascular conflict. The purpose of MRI is to provide a preoperative evaluation of the vascular topography and to precisely indicate any vascular loop at the REZ of the facial nerve on the affected side. Sometimes MRI can also be useful to the surgeon because it can identify the offending vessel when it is difficult to identify due to a very narrow operative field of view that is rendered by the "keyhole" approaches that are now routinely used.

Postoperative MRI of patients who have had a good outcome is similar to the preoperative MRI, since the material (Teflon or Dacron) that is interposed between the vessel(s) and CN VII is too thin to be seen on a MRI scan. In patients with postoperative complications, MRI can indicate a compression of CN VII by, for example, a prosthesis [6].

In conclusion, we find that MRI adequately depicts in a single, noninvasive examination the relationship of the REZ of CN VII to the vertebrobasilar system. Therefore, MRI should be considered as the screening procedure of choice in patients with HFS, and it should be recognized that there is no need to perform computerized tomography (CT-scan) or digital subtraction angiography.

MRA appears to be the best sequence as it offers both projectional angiography and native thin sections that can be reformatted. 3-D GE or CISS sequences are to be used in addition in order to get a better delineation of CN VII.

References

1. Adler CH, Zimmerman RA, Savino PJ, Bernardi B, Bostley TM, Sergott RC (1992) Hemifacial spasm: Evaluation by magnetic resonance imaging and magnetic resonance tomographic angiography. Ann Neurol 32: 502–506
2. Bernardi B, Zimmerman RA, Savino PJ, Adler C (1993) Magnetic resonance tomographic angiography in the investigation of hemifacial spasm. Neuroradiology 35: 606–611
3. Carlos R, Fukui M, Hasuo K, Uchino A, Matsushima T (1986) Radiological analysis of hemifacial spasm with special reference to angiographic manifestations. Neuroradiology 28: 288–295
4. Casselman JW, Kuhweide R, Deimling M, Ampe W, Dehaene I, Meeus L (1993) Constructive interference in steady state-3-D FT MR imaging of the inner ear and cerebellopontine angle. AJNR 14: 47–57
5. Felber S, Birbamer G, Aichner F, Poewe W, Kampfl A (1992) Magnetic resonance imaging and angiography in hemifacial spasm. Neuroradiology 34: 413–416
6. Furuya Y, Ryu H, Uemura K, Sugiyama K, Isoda H, Hasegawa S, Takahashi M, Kaneko M (1992) MRI of intracranial neurovascular compression. J Comput Assist Tomogr 16: 503–505

7. Girard N, Poncet M, Raybaud Ch, Chays A, Magnan J (1993) 3-D FT MR (Turbo-Flash and CISS sequence) of neurovascular relationships in case of arterial compression of the facial or trigeminal nerves, with surgical correlations. Neuroradiology 35: S59
8. Jannetta PJ, Abbasy M, Maroon JC, Ramos FM, Albin MS (1977) Etiology and definitive microsurgical treatment of hemifacial spasm. Operative techniques and results in 47 patients. J Neurosurg 47: 321–328
9. Pamir MN, Ozer AF, Keles GE, Erzen C, Gurmen N (1992) The aid of computerized tomography in hemifacial spasm. J Neuroradiol 19: 293–300
10. Tash R, DeMerritt J, Sze G, Leslie D (1991) Hemifacial spasm: MR imaging features. AJNR 12: 839–842
11. Tien RD, Wilkins RH (1993) MRA delineation of the vertebral-basilar system in patients with hemifacial spasm and trigeminal neuralgia. AJNR 14: 34–36

Correspondence: Prof. J. C. Froment, Hopital Neurologique et Neuro-Chirurgical Pierre Wertheimer, 59 boulevard Pinel, F-69003 Lyon Cedex 03, France.

Electrophysiological investigations of peripheral and central changes in hemifacial spasm

G. Lamas[2], N. Danziger[1], I. Fligny[2], S. Poignonec[2], J. Soudant[2], H. Lacombe[3], Y. Kéravel[3], M. Vidailhet[1], and J. C. Willer[1]

[1]Laboratory of Clinical Neurophysiology, and [2]Department of E.N.T., Hôpital Pitié-Salpétrière, Paris, France
[3]Department of Neurosurgery, Hôpital Henri Mondor, Créteil, France

Summary

A short review of the literature and of some personal data that deals with the electrophysiological observations that can be made in patients with hemifacial spasm and that allow one to discuss the two hypotheses that are proposed as possible mechanisms for the pathophysiology of hemifacial spasm is presented. The first part of the paper summarizes the technological and methodological aspects used for investigations. The second part presents data that support the peripheral nerve hypothesis. Although the peripheral nerve hypothesis has been prominent for a long time, recent data in the literature as well as the authors personal findings, as reported in the third section, favour the central or 'nucleus' hypothesis, which seems actually the most probable to explain as a whole the clinical and electrophysiological characteristics of HFS.

Key words: Hemifacial spasm, electrophysiology, blink reflex, facial nucleus, hyperexcitability.

Introduction

Classically, the syndrome of idiopathic hemifacial spasm (HFS) is characterized by spontaneous clonic and tonic contractions of facial muscles localized on one side of the face and associated with synkinesia of variable intensity and topography. This syndrome occurs most of the time as a consequence of a compressive process (usually by blood vessels) of the facial nerve at its root entry zone (REZ). It must be emphasized that between the brainstem and the internal auditory meatus, the intracranial portion of the facial nerve exhibits some characteristics that must be considered in an explanation of its vulnerability to a compressive process: a) this intracranial segment represents a section of transition between the central (oligodendroglial) and the peripheral (Schwann cells) myelination of the nerve fibres; and b) there is no interfascicular connective tissue separating the fibres traveling to the different peripheral branches [13, 26]. Thus, the anatomy of the facial nerve causes it to be very sensitive to any, even mild, pressure in the cerebellopontine angle (see the chapter by H. Lacombe in this volume). Even a minor compression may cause an increase in interstitial pressure and result in the generation of ephaptic synapses.

There are two hypotheses on the pathophysiology of HFS: the peripheral nerve hypothesis and the central or "nucleus" hypothesis. The *peripheral nerve hypothesis* states that the clinical features of HFS are due to ectopic excitation and ephaptic transmission at the site where the nerve is injured by the compression [2, 3, 35, 36]. The *central or "nucleus" hypothesis* states that compression of the facial nerve induces a synaptic reorganization of the functional connection within the facial nucleus that is associated with a general hyperexcitability of the whole motoneuronal pool of this nucleus. This would in turn result in spontaneous contractions and in synkinetic spasms of facial muscles [4, 12, 14–20, 27, 29].

The present paper is a review of the literature and summarizes some personal electrophysiological observations that provide evidence that both central and peripheral nerve hypotheses can be valid in explaining the mechanisms of HFS.

Subjects and methods

Thirty-eight patients were examined using electrophysiological methods, 25 women and 13 men with typical HFS, the onset of which began between 2 and 8 years prior to examination. Their ages ranged from 43 to 71 years, with a median age of 53 years. In 20 of the patients the right side was affected and in 18 the left side was affected. None had any history or clinical sign of facial nerve palsy. In all patients, examinations were carried out on both normal and affected sides. Six normal subjects (members of the medical staff: 3 women and 3 men) served as a matched control group.

During electrophysiological recording all subjects were comfortably reclined in a bed with a headrest in order to obtain good general muscle relaxation.

Electrophysiological methods

These examinations [32] did not differ much from those reported in the literature [4, 11]. The facial nerve was stimulated with a couple of surface electrodes (placed 1 cm apart) applied to the skin after the skin had been cleaned with a mixture of ether-acetone. The stimulus was a single rectangular shock of 0.2 ms duration delivered at the frequency 0.5 Hz. For all patients, the stimulus intensity was adjusted to be clearly supramaximal (usually between 30 and 50 mA).

For studying the blink reflex, the supraorbital (V_1) nerve was stimulated with a single rectangular shock of 0.1 ms duration at the frequency 0.2 Hz while the stimulus intensity was adjusted to 1.5 times the threshold of the R_1 component, usually between 8 and 12 mA. For all stimulations (of the facial or supraorbital nerves), a constant-current stimulator (maximal impedance of 5 kOhm) was used, and thus the skin was cleaned before placement of the electrode to ensure an adequate impedance of the stimulating circuit.

Since the central pathway of the R_1 response is known to be oligosynaptic (2 or 3 synapses) and completely intrapontine [8, 9, 10], we decided to explore the facial motorneurons to detect any excitability as evidenced in the R_1 reflex response in order to quantify the hyperexcitability of the facial nucleus. For this purpose, we used the classic double-shock technique that has been described elsewhere in detail [32]. Briefly, the test stimulus (used to stimulate the ipsilateral supraorbital nerve) was adjusted to elicit stable R_1 and R_2 reflex responses, and the conditioning stimulus (used to stimulate the contralateral supraorbital nerve) was adjusted so as to be just infraliminar to any reflex response. The R_1 reflex response was integrated and qualitified within a time window of 15 ms beginning 10 ms after the onset of the test stimulus. Under these conditions, after a 5–10 minute control period, during which only the test stimulus was delivered, both stimuli were applied together with an interstimulus interval that varied between 0 and 600 ms. Since previous studies have shown that similar data are obtained when using random time intervals as when using increasing time intervals [33, 34], we used the latter technique on the three muscular groups (orbicularis oculi, orbicularis oris, and chin) on both the normal and affected sides of patients and in control subjects. EMG signals were full-wave rectified, integrated, and on-line quantified by a computerized system. Numerical values of the R_1 response were then converted into percent in order to allow intra- and inter-individual comparison. For each muscle, the 100% value represented the mean of 40 responses obtained during the control period preceding each conditioning procedure.

According to need, the recordings were made with either needle or surface electrodes. When studying the electrophysiological features of the motor units at rest and during voluntary contractions from frontalis, inferior orbicularis oculi, orbicularis labii, and mentalis muscles, recordings were obtained with the use of concentric monopolar needle electrodes (0.25 mm in diameter) inserted near the endplate zone of the muscle in question. However, when studying evoked motor responses elicited either by stimulation of the facial or the trigeminal nerves, recordings were obtained with surface electrodes (0.5 cm in diameter) placed 1 cm apart on the cleansed skin above each concerned muscle.

General procedure

In general, the nerves were stimulated only when no spontaneous electrical activity was detected in the facial muscles in order to avoid any artifactual response, which could occur during a spasm.

For studying direct motor responses, the facial nerve was stimulated at its stylomastoidian pathway, with the cathode placed in front of the earlobe. On both sides of patients as well as normals the distance between the stimulation site and the recorded muscle was about 10 cm for the orbicularis orculi muscles and 12.5 cm for the mental muscles. For studying ephaptic reponses, the zygomatic and mandibular branches of the facial nerve were alternatively stimulated according to a procedure described in detail by Nielsen [21].

After studying the direct motor and ephaptic responses, the blink reflex responses were studied on both sides, elicited alternatively by ipsi-and contralateral stimulations of the supraorbital nerve.

Special attention was paid to the characteristics of the R_1 component, since its simple oligosynaptic central pathway [9] makes it a reliable index for central integration of afferent trigeminal messages as well as intracranial conduction of the seventh nerve. In all cases (direct motor, ephaptic, and blink reflex responses), the threshold was defined (in mA) as the minimal stimulus intensity giving rise to a probability of 80% of responses. Then a supramaximal stimulus was given (direct motor and ephaptic responses) to allow the latency (in ms) to be measured from the stimulus onset to the first deflexion of the baseline, and the peak-to-peak amplitude was measured to the nearest 0.1 mV. A similar procedure was applied to the blink reflex response elicited by a stimulus 1.5 times the threshold for R_1 component.

Electrophysiological data supporting the peripheral nerve hypothesis

This chapter describes some clinical and electrophysiological observations that show that the trunk of the facial nerve is clearly involved in some clinical and electrophysiological features of HFS: *ectopic focus of spontaneous firing, autoexcitation, and ephaptic transmission*, as described by Nielsen [21–24].

An *ectopic focus* of spontaneous firing can be observed either clinically or electromyographically during a spontaneous spasm, since several facial muscles are involved in the synkinetic contraction. It is also possible to trigger a spontaneous spasm by asking a patient to hyperventilate for several (usually 2–3) minutes, thereby inducing a respiratory alkalosis and a decrease of the Ca^{++} level. By contrast, it is also possible to completely block the spasm during apnea. *Autoexcitation*, also termed as late activity [21, 23], is characterized by either tonic activity of single, double, or multiple spikes that appear spontaneously infraclinically or that appear as an after-discharge following a voluntary contraction of facial muscles or that appear after electrical stimulation of the trigeminal and facial nerves. It is actually difficult to speculate on a precise pathophysiological mechanism that could explain these observations. However, attention should be placed on the role of Na^+ channels in the mechanisms of both ectopic excitation and autoexcitation, since the initiation of trains of action potentials mainly depends of the voltage-sensitive Na^+ channel [7]. Such Na^+ channel immunolocalization has been recently observed in peripheral mammalian axons after nerve injury and neuroma formation [5], suggesting that this accumulation of voltage is likely a precursor to hyperexcitability in injured nerves. It is thus tempting to suggest that a similar mechanism can be responsible for ongoing activity, autoexcitation, and ectopic neural excitation observed in patients with HFS or in patients with other nerve injury [1].

Ephaptic transmission and hyperexcitable fibres are classical observations in many models of nerve injury in which are commonly seen a reduction in the surrounding extra-axonal space, resulting in a focal demyelinization with a slowing of the conduction velocity at the site of the lesion [1, 6, 21, 22].

In patients with HFS, stimulation of the mandibular or of the zygomatic branches of the seventh nerve on the affected side elicits a delayed 'ephaptic' response in the orbicularis oculi or in the mentalis muscles, respectively, whereas on the unaffected side such is not the case nor is it the case in normal subjects [12, 25]. Interestingly, in our patients the threshold for the ephaptic response was often slightly higher than that for the direct orthodromic motor response, and the latency of the ephaptic response ranged from 6 to 10 ms, depending on the muscle recorded, and its amplitude was always lower than that of the direct orthodromic motor response. As previously demonstrated by Nielsen [21–24], these responses imply that antidromic impulses run upstream in a branch of the stimulated facial nerve, cross over through an ephaptic synapse somewhere in the facial nerve trunk, and travel down through another branch of the facial nerve to activate a remote and distant muscle. From these data, it is difficult to locate the exact site of cross-transmission based on the latency of the ephaptic response, since the conduction velocity along facial nerve fibres is not homogeneous. This may be, at least in part, due to the slowed conduction velocity of these fibres produced by the focal demyelination, which can be observed at the root entry zone. In conclusion, it is clear that peripheral (extracranial) ectopic excitation and ephaptic transmission within facial nerve fibres represent important mechanisms in the pathophysiology of hemifacial spasm.

Observations supporting the central (or "Nucleus") hypothesis

This hypothesis was presented due to the possibility that ectopic and abnormal peripheral nervous activity induces an increased excitability in the facial motonucleus by creating a permanent antidromic neuronal excitation. In support of this hypothesis it has been observed that when the peripheral irritated facial nerve focus was removed by decompression of the nerve, the facial motonucleus was no longer subjected to the abnormal antidromic impulses and thus behaved normally [17]. Another argument that supports this hypothesis is the perseverance of the R_1 component on the affected side during anaesthesia whereas it is abolished on the normal side [14, 15, 19, 20].

With the use of qualitative and quantitative electrophysiological methods (see Methods section), we provide data that substantiates this latter hypothesis that a central hyperexcitability exists in the facial motoneurons of patients with hemifacial spasm (HFS).

In a first set of experiments described in this chapter, we studied trigemino-facial reflexes elicited by electrical stimulation of supraorbital nerves on both the affected and unaffected sides of patients with HFS as well as in 8 matched control subjects using the classic conventional techniques described previously [2, 11, 32].

Crossing of the R_1 blink reflex component

In control subjects, supraorbital nerve stimulation elicited the well-known blink reflex pattern of responses, i.e., R_1 and R_2 on the ipsilateral orbicularis oculi muscles and R_2 on the contralateral orbicularis oculi muscles. When such stimulation was applied on the patient's unaffected side, a crossed oligosynaptic blink response of the R_1 type was observed on the contralateral (HFS) side in addition to the normal crossed R_2 component. This crossed R_1 response was observed separately in the orbicularis oculi muscles in 29 patients, in the orbicularis oris muscles in 3 patients, in the mentalis muscles in 5 patients, and in 1 patient, surprisingly, in the platysma muscles, whereas it was not observed in normal subjects under similar experimental conditions. By contrast, such a crossed R_1 response could be elicited in normal subjects in whom hyperexcitability was produced into the facial motoneurons in two situations: a) during a slight voluntary contraction of the eyelids and b) when infraliminar conditioning stimuli were delivered to the contralateral trigeminal afferents (V^1–V^2 or V^3) using paired stimuli delivered at variable interstimulus intervals, usually between 30 and 40 ms [33, 34]. The appearance or absence of this crossed R^1 response clearly depends on the existence or absence of background activity in the facial motoneurons. It is thus tempting to suggest that such a finding in HFS patients is a good argument in support of the existence of a critical state of depolarization in some facial motoneurons. Furthermore, in these patients the observation of a crossed R_1 blink reflex response in one muscle but not in others provides a good argument in support of hyperactivity of the facial motonucleus as being the pathophysiology of HFS.

When supraorbital nerve stimulation was delivered on the side with spasm, the R_1–R_2 blink reflex responses were also recorded in the other facial muscles on the affected side, mainly the orbicularis oris and the mental muscles. Such blink reflex responses were not observed in homologous muscles of these patients' normal side nor was it observed in control subjects, at least during this specific experimental procedure, which required as much relaxation as possible. These data suggest that there could exist a state of hyperexcitability in the facial motoneurons involved in the blink reflex as well as a widespread hyperexcitability of the entire facial motoneuronal pool, which would be in agreement with numerous other findings already described in the literature [see 16].

This facial motoneuronal excitability exhibited in the R_1 reflex response was investigated using quantitative methods in order to quantify the hyperexcitability of the facial nucleus. Thus we used a classic double-shock technique described above in the Methods section.

In all of the patients in this study, and only on the affected side, the infraliminar conditioning stimulus induced an important facilitation of the R_1 reflex response that was elicited by the test stimulus delivered to all of the facial muscles whose reflexes were tested. In the orbicularis oculi muscles, the onset of the facilitatory effect occurred within a shorter interstimulus interval ($Dt = 0$ ms) than that which was observed in recordings from the patients' normal side and from control subjects ($Dt = 30$ ms). The maximum facilitatory effect was significantly higher (+330%) on the affected side than on the normal side (+220%) and it remained significantly higher for longer interstimulus intervals (+50% for $Dt = 100$ ms) on the affected side than on the normal side (+2% for $Dt = 100$ ms). In the orbicularis oris and chin muscles a similar pattern in the R_1 excitability curve was observed on the affected side whereas, as already mentioned above, no reflex response was elicited in homologous muscles on the normal side or in control subjects. Furthermore, in these latter cases, the conditioning stimuli were ineffective in producing any reflex activity. These data clearly shows that the central hyperexcitability of facial motoneurons that has been observed in patients with HFS can be quantified accurately with the use of paired stimuli. Furthermore, since the onset of facilitation observed in the R_1 reflex response occurred early in the excitability curve, i.e. when both conditioning and test stimuli were delivered simultaneously ($Dt = 0$ ms), one can suggest that the facial motoneurons involved in the R_1 reflex response receive convergent afferent messages through a similar oligosynaptic pathway from both conditioning (contralateral) and test (ipsilateral) stimuli. This idea is supported by the fact that a crossed R_1 response can be recorded in the orbicularis oculi muscle on the affected side when the contralateral supraorbital nerve is excited, thus indicating the existence of a crossed disynaptic or trisynaptic afferent pathway projecting to the same motoneuronal pool as when the ipsilateral supraorbital nerve is excited.

Although direct anatomical connections between the trigeminal sensory nucleus and the contralateral facial nucleus have been described [28], most investigators agree on the strictly ipsilateral distribution of the R_1 component. Consequently, our present data raises the question of whether these crossed oligosynaptic excitatory effects as well as the ectopic R_1 responses are produced by abnormal synaptic connections or by existing synapses that are normally unresponsive to contralateral supraorbital nerve stimulation.

Thus, experiments were carried out on normal subjects to explore the possibility of eliciting these "abnormal" facial reflexes during constant slight and specific voluntary contractions of the eyelids, of the mouth, and of the chin, respectively, and when any reflex response was observed, we tested the excitability of the R_1 response using paired stimuli as described above. In all normal subject's, during voluntary closure of the eyelids, crossed R_1 responses appeared in the contralateral orbicularis oculi muscle (in response to supraorbital nerve stimulation) and the amplitude of the R_2 component increased. When we were able to extract the blink components from the tonic EMG activity, the crossed R_1 response became larger and larger, indicating the strength of the eyelids' contractions. Similarly, two components of the reflex responses (R_1 and R_2) were recorded in the orbicularis oris and chin muscles, respectively, when a specific voluntary contraction was maintained in these muscles, whose reflexes are not normally activated by supraorbital nerve stimulation. Under this condition, which simulates pathological HFS, the facial motoneurons involved in the R_1 reflex response were subjected to central hyperexcitability brought about by the pyramidal messages (the descending controls of voluntary contraction), as revealed by the excitability curves of the R_1 response for each muscle under study. It is thus tempting to conclude that both the crossed R_1 response and the "ectopic" or so-called "abnormal trigeminofacial reflex" responses recorded from all of the facial muscles exist potentially in normal subjects but cannot be elicited when trigemino-facial reflexes are obtained using the classic methods previously described in the literature [11], i.e., using unilateral supraorbital nerve stimulation in relaxed subjects with the "eyes gently closed." Consequently, the appearance of these ectopic reflexes would depend on the existence of background activity in the facial motoneurons. This idea is supported by observations in animal experiments (monkeys) in which both the crossed R^1 blink reflex responses and the trigemino-naso-labial reflexes, normally elicited by supraorbital nerve stimulations and often associated with tonic EMG activities in facial muscles, showed a physiological hyperexcitability in the monkeys' facial motoneurons [30, 31].

In conclusion, it now seems quite clear that both peripheral and central mechanisms are involved in the pathophysiology of hemifacial spasm. Although the peripheral hypothesis has been prominent for a long time, recent data reported in the literature as well as our own personal findings favor the central hypothesis.

Acknowledgements

This work was supported by INSERM (Contrat de Recherche Externe), Assistance Publique-Hopitaux de Paris (Contrat de Recherche Clinique), and by la Fondation pour la Recherche Médicale. We thank Professor A. Møller and his staff for English corrections and suggestions in the preparation of this manuscript.

References

1. Amir R, Devor M (1993) Ongoing activity in neuroma afferents bearing retrograde sprouts. Brain Res 630: 283–288
2. Auger RG (1979) Hemifacial spasm: Clinical and electrophysiological observations. Neurology 29: 1261–1272
3. Auger RG, Piepgras DG, Laws ER, Miller RH (1981) Microvascular decompression of the facial nerve for hemifacial spasm: Clinical and electrophysiological observations. Neurology 31: 346–350

4. Bratzlavsky M, Eecken H van der (1977) Altered synaptic organization in facial nucleus following facial nerve regeneration: an electrophysiological study in man. Ann Neurol 2: 71–73
5. Devor M, Govrin-Lipmann R, Angelides K (1993) Na^+ channel immunolocalization in peripheral mammalian axons and changes following nerve injury and neuroma formation. J Neurosci 13: 1976–1992
6. Gardner WJ (1966) Crosstalk- The paradoxical transmission of a nerve impulse. Arch Neurol 14: 149–156
7. Hille B (1984) Ionic channels of excitable membranes. Sinauer, Sunderland, Maine, pp 1–426
8. Hiraoka M, Shimamura M (1977) Neural mechanisms of the corneal blinking reflex in cats. Brain Res 125: 265–275
9. Holstege G (1990) Neuronal organization of the blink reflex. In: Paxinos G (ed) The human nervous system. Academic Press, New York, pp 287–296
10. Iwata N, Kitai ST, Olsen S (1972) Afferent component of the facial nerve: Its relation to the spinal trigeminal and facial nucleus. Brain Res 43: 662–667
11. Kugelberg E (1952) Facial reflexes. Brain 75: 385–396
12. Lamas G, Poignonec S, Fligny I, Soudant J, Willer JC (1994) Recovery of normal excitability of the facial nerve motor nucleus following facial nerve decompression in hemifacial spasm. Eur Arch Otorhinolaryngol [Suppl]: 555–556
13. Martin MR, Lodges D (1977) Morphology of the facial nucleus of the rat. Brain Res 123: 1–12
14. Møller AR (1987) Hemifacial spasm: Ephaptic transmission or hyperexcitability of the facial motor nucleus? Exp Neurol 98: 110–119
15. Møller AR (1991) Interaction between the blink reflex and the abnormal muscle response in patients with hemifacial spasm: Results of intraoperative recordings. J Neurol Sci 101: 114–123
16. Møller AR (1993) Cranial nerve dysfunction syndromes: Pathophysiology of microvascular decompression. In: Barrow DL (ed) Neurosurgical Topics Book 13, Surgery of Cranial Nerves of the Posterior Fossa, Chapter 2. American Association of Neurological Surgeons, Park Ridge, Illinois, pp 105–129
17. Møller AR, Jannetta PJ (1984) On the origin of synkinesis in hemifacial spasm: results of intracranial recordings. J Neurosurg 61: 569–576
18. Møller AR, Jannetta PJ (1985) Hemifacial spasm: results of electrophysiologic recordings during microvascular decompression operations. Neurology 35: 969–974
19. Møller AR, Jannetta PJ (1986) Blink reflex in patients with hemifacial spasm: Observations during microvascular decompression operations. J Neurol Sci 72: 171–182
20. Møller AR, Jannetta PJ (1986) Physiological abnormalities in hemifacial spasm studied during microvascular decompression operations. Exp Neurol 93: 584–600
21. Nielsen VK (1984) Pathophysiology of hemifacial spasm: I. Ephaptic transmission and ectopic excitation. Neurology 34: 418–426
22. Nielsen VK (1984) Pathophysiology of hemifacial spasm: II. Lateral spread of the supraorbital nerve reflex. Neurology 34: 427–431
23. Nielsen VK (1985) Electrophysiology of the facial nerve in hemifacial spasm: Ectopic/ephaptic excitation. Muscle Nerve 8: 545–555
24. Nielsen VK, Jannetta PJ (1984) Pathophysiology of hemifacial spasm: III. Effects of facial nerve decompression. Neurology 34: 891–897
25. Poignonec S, Vidailhet M, Lamas G, Fligny I, Soudant J, Jedynak P, Willer JC (1994) Electrophysiological evidence for central hyperexcitability of facial motoneurons in hemifacial spasm. Eur Arch Otorhinolaryngol S 216–217
26. Radpour S (1977) Organization of the facial nucleus in the cat. Laryngoscope 87: 557–574
27. Roth G, Magistris MR, Pinelli P, Rilliet B (1990) Cryptogenic hemifacial spasm. A neurophysiological study. Electromyogr Clin Neurophysiol 30: 361–370
28. Ramon Y, Cajal SR (1909) Histologie du Systéme Nerveux de L'homme et des Vertébrés. Maloine, Paris, pp 859–888
29. Sen CN, Møller AR (1987) Signs of hemifacial spasm created by chronic periodic stimulation of the facial nerve in the rat. Exp Neurol 98: 336–349
30. Willer JC, Lamour Y (1975) Analyse électrophysiologique d'un réflexe facial chez le singe: Le réflexe trigémino-naso- labial. CR Soc Biol 169: 1177–1185
31. Willer JC, Lamour Y (1975) Etude électrophysiologique du réflexe de clignement chez le macaque (macacus cynomolgus). CR Acad Sci (Paris) 281: 563–566
32. Willer JC, Lamour Y (1977) Electrophysiological evidence for a facio-facial reflex in the facial muscles in man. Brain Res 119: 459–464
33. Willer JC, Roby A, Boulu P, Albe-Fessard D (1982) Depressive effect of high frequency peripheral conditioning stimulation upon the nociceptive component of the human blink reflex. Lack of naloxone effect. Brain Res 239: 322–326
34. Willer JC, Boulu P, Bratzlavsky M (1984) Electrophysiological evidence for crossed oligosynaptic trigemino-facial connections in normal man. J Neurol Neurosurg Psychiatry 47: 87–90
35. Williams HL, Lambert EH, Woltman HW (1952) The problem of synkinesis and contracture in case of hemifacial spasm and Bell's palsy. Ann Otol Rhinol Laryngol 61: 850–872
36. Woltman HW, Williams HL, Lambert EH (1951) An attempt to relieve hemifacial spasm by neurolysis of the facial nerve: A report on two cases of hemifacial spasm with reflection on the nature of the spasm, the contracture and mass movements. Proc Staff Meet Mayo Clin 26: 236–240

Correspondence: Jean Claude Willer, Laboratory of Clinical Neurophysiology, Hôpital Pitié-Salpétrière, 91, Boulevard de L'Hôpital, F-75013 Paris, France.

Surgical treatment of hemifacial spasm by microvascular decompression

G. L. Rosseau[1] and **P. J. Jannetta**[2]

[1]Chicago Institute of Neurosurgery and Neuroresearch, Chicago, Illinois, U.S.A.
[2]Department of Neurological Surgery, University of Pittsburgh School of Medicine, Pittsburgh, Pennsylvania, U.S.A.

Summary

An outline of the clinical syndromes of hemifacial spasm (HFS), the history of surgical treatments for this condition and a detailed description of the authors' preferred form of operative treatment is provided. Operative findings, results, and complications in HFS patients treated at the University of Pittsburgh, Presbyterian-University Hospital during the period between 1972 and 1993 is reviewed. It is concluded at this time that a retromastoid craniotomy and microvascular decompression (MVD), in experienced hands, is a safe and highly effective procedure to treat both forms of HFS.

Key words: Microvascular decompression, surgical techniques.

History of surgical treatment for hemifacial spasm

The descriptive term, hemifacial spasm (HFS), was originally suggested by Gowers in 1888 [9]. However, even earlier, in 1875, Shultze [38] described a case in which postmortem examination had revealed aneurysmal compression of the facial nerve in the cerebellopontine angle. Despite these two reports suggesting a vascular etiology for the condition, HFS was for many years thought to be epileptiform and, therefore, its cause was considered to be localized in the supratentorial space. In the late 1940's, Campbell and Keedy [3] and Laine and Nayrac [24] described ectatic basilar arteries in patients with HFS. During this same period, Revilla described several patients in whom hemifacial spasm was attributed to tumors in the cerebellopontine angle [36, 37].

In 1962, Gardner [7] described the similarities in the etiologies of HFS and trigeminal neuralgia. In that same year Gardner and Sava [8] described "abnormal" blood vessels close to the facial nerve in 6 of 19 patients. Gardner's hypothesis [7] was excellent. His observations and therapy, however, were inadequate because of the inadequate technology that was available of the time. In 1966, Jannetta performed the first microvascular decompression (MVD) of the facial nerve to treat HFS [21].

In the past, surgical trauma to the facial nerve, either peripherally or centrally, was used to treat patients with HFS [6]. The introduction of the operating microscope, however, provided the recognition and clarification of the vascular etiology of HFS, and now MVD of the facial nerve is the accepted surgical treatment for this condition [1, 2, 12–16, 19, 21, 22, 39, 40].

To date, no medication has been shown to have a therapeutic effect on HFS.

Clinical presentation

Jannetta et al. [22] was the first to clarify the two varieties of HFS and to correlate each with a separate clinical pathology.

The two varieties of HFS are *typical HFS and atypical HFS*. *Typical HFS* begins as irregular, intermittent, and spasmodic contractions of one of the orbicularis oculi muscles [4, 13]. Typically, the spasm in this form of HFS is uniformly progressive, but may progress either slowly (over years) or rapidly (over weeks or months). The syndrome is more common in women than in men, and is more common on the left side than on the right. It most often occurs during the fifth and sixth decades of life.

From the one orbicularis oculi muscle, the spasm progresses to involve the other muscles of the face on the same side, often including the platysma. The rostral-to-caudal progression of the spasm is the hallmark of typical HFS. Involvement of the frontalis muscle is uncommon in typical HFS. The spasm is usually exacerbated by the use of the face muscles as well as by emotional tension and fatigue. In some patients, changes in the position of the head may exacerbate or lessen the spasm. The most common position that is reported to ease the spasm is the contralateral-decubitus position. The spasm may occur during sleep and, on rare occasions, may even awake the patient. Patients with typical HFS may complain of tinnitus and, occasionally, they describe a clicking noise, which is caused by spasm of the stapedius muscle [23].

Over time, the spasm increases in frequency and severity, and may be such to render the patient socially, economically and/or psychologically disabled. It is generally at this point that a patient seeks medical attention. Eventually, a "tonus phenomenon" may occur. This phenomenon is a forced and sustained contraction of all the involved muscles that causes severe grimacing, a drawing up of the corner of the mouth, and eye closure, which may be complete. Although the tonus phenomenon may be brought on by the use of face muscles, it frequently occurs spontaneously. In tandem with the development of the tonus phenomenon is the development of mild peripheral facial weakness. This facial weakness may be seen alone without observing the tonus phenomenon, but is almost always noticeable when the tonus phenomenon is present. The earliest sign of facial weakness is the inability to bury the eyelashes on the ipsilateral side during forced eye closure shortly thereafter followed by an inability to draw up the ipsilateral corner of the mouth. Although pain is not a prominent symptom of HFS, patients with the tonus phenomenon may develop an aching discomfort in the face.

Eight percent of the patients referred to us with HFS have what we refer to as "*atypical hemifacial spasm*" [22]. In these patients, the typical rostral-to-caudal progression of spasm that is seen in typical HFS is reversed, and the first spasms occur in the buccal or orbicularis oris muscles and the progression of the symptom is upward over the face, and often with considerable involvement of the frontalis muscle. All other symptoms of atypical HFS are the same as for typical HFS. The differences in presentation and progression are important to clarify, however, as patients with atypical HFS are surgically observed to have a different relationship between the offending vessel and the facial nerve than what is usually the case for patients with typical HFS (see detailed observations below) [12, 17, 18, 20].

Preoperative evaluation

The diagnosis of HFS is a clinical one. Electromyography (EMG) may be useful in verifying the diagnosis and for clarifying that it is not a general orofacial movement disorder, myokymia, or a functional disorder. Audiologic tests are performed, including pure tone audiogram and speech discrimination scores, as well as recording brainstem auditory evoked potentials (BAEP). An ipsilateral mild hearing loss is observed in approximately 17% of HFS patients [34], many of whom have often not subjectively noted this deficit.

Computerized tomography (CT-scan) or magnetic resonance imaging (MRI) with and without contrast enhancement is performed to rule out tumors in the cerebellopontine angle, aneurysms, arteriovenous malformations, or the presence of ectatic posterior circulation arteries, all of which may infrequently cause HFS. A benign extra-axial tumor in the cerebellopontine angle may cause HFS by causing vascular compression of the facial nerve.

Operation using a retromastoid craniectomy and MVD is indicated for otherwise healthy patients of virtually any age who are disabled by HFS.

Surgical technique for microvascular decompression

The surgeon's goal in performing MVD procedure to relieve HFS is threefold: 1) to identify the offending vessel that is compressing the facial nerve, 2) to move this vessel away from the nerve without causing nerve injury, and 3) to keep the vessel away from the nerve in the future. More than one blood vessel may be contributing to the HFS, and even extremely small arterioles and venules may be responsible [16]. The neurovascular compression may be subtle and require careful observation on the part of the surgeon. In particular, the surgeon must fully explore the facial nerve at and proximal to its root exit zone as well as its non-fascicular portion, as this is the site where vascular compression causes HFS [13]. The surgeon should diligently search for and treat *all* offending vessels in this area, regardless of size, until the intraoperative EMG demonstrates that the abnormal muscle response (lateral spread] [5, 29] has disappeared [11, 33].

Preoperative considerations

Preoperatively, the patient is given perioperative antibiotics using a modification of Malis' regimen [25]. The patient is anesthetized and intubated with muscle endplate blocking agents, succinylcholine and 3 mg tubocurarine, with no additional muscle relaxants used after intubation. Although it is extremely rare to see a venous air embolism during procedures in which a patient has been placed in the lateral decubitus position [15], we place a central venous pressure catheter and a Doppler ultrasound monitor over the sternum before beginning the operation. An arterial line is preferred, but if placing this line presents much difficulty the operation may proceed without it. An indwelling urethral catheter is not required.

Positioning the patient

The operating table is positioned so that the patient's head is at the foot of the table, allowing knee room for the seated surgeon. The patient's head is placed in a three-point headholder and the patient is then rolled into a contralateral-lateral-decubitus position. An axillary roll is used to protect the opposite (down-side) brachial plexus. The neck is moderately stretched, minimally flexed, and the head slightly rotated toward the ipsilateral side. (If necessary, the head may be contralaterally flexed downward toward the floor a few degrees in order to expose the occipital bone maximally). The headholder is then secured in this position. The ipsilateral shoulder is taped caudally and anteriorly. Padding is placed between the knees, and the body is secured to the table with straps and adhesive tape so that lateral tilting of the table may be permitted during exposure of the cerebellopontine angle. We prefer the contralateral-lateral-decubitus position because it reduces intraoperative cardiovascular stress and decreases the risk of venous emboli, and results in less postoperative headache. Disadvantages of this position include a minimally increased risk of venous bleeding into the operative field, which would require suctioning to be done in the cerebellopontine angle, as well as alterations in the relationship between the facial nerve and nearby blood vessels due to a differential movement of the brainstem and these blood vessels that could occur while the patient is in this position. Long hair is combed and held out of the way by adhesive tape, and the hair in the ipsilateral occipital region is shaved. The skin is prepped and draped.

Operative technique

One fingerbreadth posterior to the mastoid eminence, a skin incision 3–6 cm wide is made parallel and posterior to the hairline. This incision is shorter in Asians as well as slender, long-necked people, but it must be longer in heavily muscled, short-necked people who are dolichocephalic. The incision is extended down to the occipital bone by means of electrocauterization. Soft tissues are separated from the occipital bone using a large periosteal elevator and electrocauterization as needed. In particular, the medial and posterior aspects of the mastoid eminence must be cleared of soft tissue. The transverse occipital artery may be seen in the lower reaches of a longer incision. In such cases, this artery is ligated or coagulated and divided. An inferior-lateral emissary vein is sometimes found, which must also be coagulated and divided. An angulated or straight Weitlaner retractor is put into place.

A 2.5 × 3.0 cm, roughly triangular, craniectomy is then fashioned. It should extend laterally to the sigmoid sinus and caudally to the floor of the posterior fossa. It is important that this craniectomy be low and laterally placed, and that its most rostral extent be located at or just below the junction of the lateral and sigmoid sinuses. Particularly in dolichocephalic patients it may be necessary to remove mastoid air cells that may have extended across the sigmoid sinus. If any mastoid air cells that need not be removed is entered, they must be meticulously filled with bone wax at opening and again at time of closure.

The dura mater is opened obliquely from the superolateral to the inferomedial corner of the craniectomy. A "T" incision is made into the inferiolateral corner. Alternatively, a curvilinear incision may be used in a brachycephalic patient. Inferiolateral exposure is particularly important in cases of typical HFS. The dural flaps are held out of the way with retention sutures. An experienced surgeon may choose to do a smaller craniectomy.

A microsurgical self-retaining retractor with a long narrow blade that is protected with a rubber dam (fashioned from a rubber glove) and a cottonoid is placed low over the cerebellum. It is important that the blade be bent proximally 20–30 degrees, but it should not be curved. A surgical binocular microscope with a 250-mm objective is swung into place and used for the remainder of the intradural portion of the procedure. The cerebellum is gently elevated rather than retracted.

Following modest cerebellar elevation, the subarachnoid cisterns over the ninth and tenth cranial nerves (CN IX and CN X) are opened by sharp dissection. The resulting spontaneous drainage of cerebrospinal fluid (CSF) causes the cerebellum to fall away by gravity alone. Patience is important at this point of the procedure. With adequate CSF drainage and gentle aspiration, gravity and time will provide most of the needed exposure.

In patients with typical HFS the approach to the site of the pathology is from the caudal side. This approach is over CN IX and CN X and under CN VIII. After sharply dividing the pia-arachnoidal bands between the cerebellum and CN IX and CN X, the flocculus can be elevated. The choroid plexus of the lateral recess of the fourth ventricle then comes into view. The retractor tip is placed over the choroid plexus. Occasionally, it may be necessary to use bipolar coagulation to shrink redundant portions of the choroid plexus to facilitate better visualization of the lower pons and the proximal facial nerve.

The offending blood vessel may be the posterior inferior cerebellar artery (PICA), the vertebral artery (VA), the anterior inferior cerebellar artery (AICA), or a vein. If it is the PICA or the VA, the mobilization may proceed laterally and caudally from the inferior aspect of the facial nerve. Perforating arteries from the PICA or from the VA perfuse the medulla, elongate into a looping configuration, and move rostrally with the major vessels. The situation is different, however, for perforating branches of arteries from the AICA, where the perforating vessels are located in the lower pons. Preserving these latter vessels is vital, despite the fact that they may restrict mobilization of the AICA. All blood vessels, regardless of size, encountered at or proximal to the root exit zone should be mobilized away from the nerve and treated. Veins and venules are coagulated and divided. Preservation of blood flow during and after mobilization of arterioles and perforating branches of arteries is essential, as these are frequently physiologic end-arteries, and obstruction of blood flow in these vessels could lead to stroke.

In patients with atypical HFS the site of the vascular-neural conflict may be found on the rostral side of CN VII, posterior to and between CN VII and CN VIII. Occasionally, an AICA branch may be detected running vertically between these cranial nerves and causing atypical HFS. The AICA, or a major branch thereof, frequently gives off one or more important perforating branches to the pons that restrict the mobilization of the vessel that is necessary in order to perform vascular decompression. In such cases, the artery must be carefully mobilized off the pons by placing small soft implants around the artery, rostrally as well as caudally, taking care to avoid injuring any perforating branches of the AICA. Occasionally, both a rostral and a caudal vessel may be observed lying in a "scissors-like" configuration, causing the atypical syndrome. In such cases, both vessels must be treated. Finally, any veins located in this region should be coagulated and divided, carefully avoiding the spread of heat or current to adjacent nerves. Intraoperative EMG monitoring is most important to assure that the MVD has been as complete as possible before ending the operation [11, 33].

Implant material

Many different implant materials have been advocated for use in MVD, including muscle, fat, Ivalon sponge (Unipoint Company, NC), and silicone sponge. The implant materials used in the present series of 648 patients [2] was predominantly shredded Teflon (477 patients), but in the earlier stages of this study muscle (76 patients) and Ivalon sponge (63 patients) were used. In a few of the first patients in this study silicone and gelatin sponge were used (19 and 6 cases, respectively). In two cases the implant material was not recorded. At present, the preferred implant material is shredded Teflon felt (C.R. Bard Co., Bard Implants Division, Billerica, MA). This material comes in the shape of a flat square and it is used by cardiovascular surgeons to support cardiac and aortic sutures. The implants are formed by shredding the flat-shaped material with toothed forceps and rolling it into American football or cigar shapes of various sizes. It has the physical characteristic of absorbent cotton. The advantages of this material are that it remains in place, is not eroded by arteries over time, and causes only modest tissue reaction.

Intraoperative monitoring

Monitoring of brainstem auditory evoked potentials (BAEP) is done throughout the procedure [10, 26, 27, 35]. Compound action potentials are also frequently recorded via an electrode placed directly on CN VIII as soon as it is identified in the cerebellopontine angle [26–28]. The advantage of this technique is that it gives immediate feedback to the surgeon, and thereby minimizes the risk of ipsilateral hearing loss. With the use of these techniques, the rate of ipsilateral hearing loss has dropped to less than 1.5% [35].

Intraoperative recording of the abnormal muscle response (lateral spread) is valuable in assuring complete microvascular decompression [11, 33], because this response seems to remain until the last vessel that is causing the HFS is removed [30–32]. This immediate disappearance of the lateral spread response is a reliable sign that the facial nerve has been adequately decompressed [11, 33].

Wound closure

Multiple Valsalva maneuvers are performed to assure the adequacy of hemostasis. The Valsalva maneuver is also performed as an attempt to ensure that the relationships of the prosthesis to the artery, nerves, and brainstem will persist. The self-retaining retractor, rubber dam, and cottonoid are removed slowly while maintaining constant visualization of the pertinent relationships as the retraction is being released. The cerebellopontine angle is gently filled with a balanced salt solution. The dura mater is closed in a watertight fashion. A pledget of Gelfoam[R] (Upjohn Company, Kalamazoo, MI) is placed over the craniectomy defect. In recent years, we have covered the bony defect by performing a cranioplasty, which has dramatically decreased the incidence of postoperative headache. The soft tissues are closed in layers.

Postoperative care

The patient is monitored in the Neurosurgical Intensive Care Unit overnight and returned to his or her room the following day. Most patients are ambulatory the morning after the operation and resume a normal diet that same day. Fluid intake is not restricted during the postoperative period. The only medications that are necessary are mild narcotic analgesics and antiemetics, as needed. If a severe headache is reported within 48 hours after the operation, a CT-scan is performed. If the CT-scan is normal, a therapeutic lumbar puncture usually resolves the headache. CSF pressure may be moderately elevated. White blood cells and some red cells are usually observed. Gram stains and cultures are performed. Infection is rare.

Results

This series includes 703 patients (705 sides and 782 MVD operations) who underwent MVD operation to relieve hemifacial spasm between the years 1972 and 1993 at the University of Pittsburgh Presbyterian-University Hospital [2]. Of these 703 patients, 648 patients had not undergone prior intracranial procedures to treat their HFS; 65% were female; the mean age was 52 years; and the mean preoperation duration of the symptoms of HFS was 7 years. Onset was typical in 92% and atypical in 8% [2]. Using Kaplan-Meier statistics, the results of the MVD procedure were found to be excellent in 79%, and in 5% there was partial success 10 years postoperatively [2]. In this series of patients, vascular compression by PICA was the predominant cause of HFS (see Table 1) in 442 patients. A vein in combination with an artery was the cause of HFS in 132 patients. A compressing vein alone caused the HFS in 19 patients.

Table 1. Operative findings in 648 consecutive first operations for hemifacial spasm

Compressing Vessel	No. of Patients	Percent of Total
PICA*	442	68.2
AICA	229	35.3
Vertebral artery	155	23.9
Labyrinthine artery	19	2.9
SCA	4	0.6
Basilar artery	2	0.3
Unnamed small artery	71	11.0
Vein	132	20.4
Vein only	19	2.9
Unnamed small artery or vein only	38	5.9

*PICA = Posterior inferior cerebellar artery; AICA = Anterior inferior cerebellar artery; SCA = superior cerebellar artery. (From Barker et al., 1995)

Many patients still had some degree of HFS at the time of their discharge from the hospital. The general trend is toward improvement over time. Of the 15 patients in this series who had no immediate relief, 13 underwent at least one additional re-exploration. This included those patients who had no response to the initial procedure, as well as those who had a delayed recurrence of HFS following an initial good response. When necessary, an early re-operation is preferred, as late operation is more difficult because of scar formation in the cerebellopontine angle.

Complications

The complications experienced by the 648 patients with typical HFS in this series who underwent MVD for the first time are indicated in Table 2. There were no operative deaths. One patient suffered persistent neurological deficits (0.2%). The postoperative complications were facial weakness and (ipsilateral) hearing loss.

Table 2. Operative complications*

Complication	First Operation in 648 Patients		782 Operations in 703 Patients	
	No.	%	No.	%
Operative death	0	0	1	0.1
Brainstem infarct	1	0.2	2†	0.3
Cerebellar hematoma	2†	0.3	4	0.5
Facial weakness				
transient	25	3.9	25	3.2
mild permanent	12	1.9	14	1.8
moderate permanent	4	0.6	7	0.9
severe permanent	6	0.9	12	1.5
Hearing loss				
mild permanent	1	0.2	1	0.1
moderate permanent	3	0.5	3	0.4
deaf ear	17	2.6	21	2.7
Cerebrospinal fluid leak	16	2.5	19	2.4
Wound infection	7	1.1	9	1.2
Wound hematoma	1	0.2	1	0.1
Pseudomeningocele	2	0.3	4	0.5
Bacterial meningitis	4	0.6	4	0.5

*Other complications included: transient hoarseness or dysphagia (11), transient sixth nerve palsy (2), permanent fourth nerve palsy (1), exacerbation of multiple sclerosis with transient quadriparesis (1), postoperative Guillain Barre syndrome with persistent neurological deficit (1), pneumonia (1), sepsis (1), and gastrointestinal hemorrhage (1).

†One cerebellar hematoma after first microvascular depression and one brainstem infarction after reoperation resulted in permanent neurological deficit. (From Barker et al., 1995)

Complications were not more common in re-operations, although in this group one death occurred on the fourth postoperative day—a woman with a Chiari malformation who died from respiratory failure.

Conclusions

The intraoperative observations and results of MVD in this large series support the hypothesis that HFS is due to vascular cross-compression of the nerve at or before the root exit zone. With experience, thorough understanding of the principles involved and thoughtful use of electrophysiologic monitoring, MVD can be performed with minimal morbidity and rare mortality. The operative procedure as described above is the only non-destructive technique currently available to treat this debilitating condition effectively.

References

1. Apfelbaum RI (1988) Surgical management of disorders of the lower cranial nerves. In: Schmidek HH, Sweet WH (eds) Operative neurosurgical techniques. Indications, methods, and results, vol. 2, Grune and Stratton, Orlando Florida, pp 1097–1109
2. Barker FG, Jannetta PJ, Bissonette DJ, Shields PT, Larkins MV, Jho HD (1995) Microvascular decompression for hemifacial spasm. J Neurosurg 82: 201–210
3. Campbell E, Keedy C (1947) HFS: A note on the etiology in two cases. J Neurosurg 4: 342–347
4. Digre K, Corbett JJ (1988) Hemifacial spasm: Differential diagnosis mechanism and treatment. In: Tolosa E (ed) Advances in neurology, vol. 39, Facial dyskinesia. Raven Press, New York, pp 151–176
5. Esslen E (1957) Der Spasmus facialis eine Parabiosserscheinung: Elektrophysiologische Untersuchungen zum Entstehungsmechanismus des Facialisspasmus. Dtsch Z Nervenheil 176: 149–172
6. Fisch U, Esslen E (1972) The surgical treatment of facial hyperkinesia. Arch Otolaryngol 95: 400–405
7. Gardner WJ (1962) Concerning the mechanism of trigeminal neuralgia and hemifacial spasm. J Neurosurg 19: 947–957
8. Gardner WJ, Sava GA (1962) Hemifacial spasm – A reversible pathophysiologic state. J Neurosurg 19: 240–247
9. Gowers R (1988) Manual of diseases of the nervous system. JA Churchill, London
10. Grundy BL (1983) Intraoperative monitoring of sensory evoked potentials. Anesthesiology 58: 72–87
11. Haines SJ, Torres F (1991) Intraoperative monitoring of the facial nerve during decompressive surgery for hemifacial spasm. J Neurosurg 74: 254–257
12. Jannetta PJ (1970) Microsurgical exploration and decompression of the facial nerve in hemifacial spasm. Curr Top Surg Res 2: 217–220
13. Jannetta PJ (1977) Observations on the etiology of trigeminal neuralgia, hemifacial spasm, acoustic nerve dysfunction, and glossopharyngeal neuralgia. Definitive microsurgical treatment and results in 117 patients. Acta Neurochir (Wien) 20: 145–154
14. Jannetta PJ (1980) Neurovascular compression in cranial nerve and systemic disease. Ann Surg 192: 518–525
15. Jannetta PJ (1981) Hemifacial spasm. In: Samii M, Jannetta PJ (eds) The cranial nerves. Springer, Heidelberg, pp 484–493
16. Jannetta PJ (1984) Hemifacial spasm caused by a venule: Case report. Neurosurgery 14: 89–92
17. Jannetta PJ (1985) Neurovascular contact in hemifacial spasm. In: Portmann M (ed) Facial nerve. Masson, Paris, pp 45–48
18. Jannetta PJ (1987) Hemifacial spasm: Etiology and treatment. In: English G (ed) Otolaryngology, vol. 1, LL Lippincott, Philadelphia, pp 1–10
19. Jannetta PJ (1990) Cranial rhizopathies. In: Youmans JR (ed) Neurological surgery. W. B. Saunders, Philadelphia, pp 4169–4182
20. Jannetta PJ (1992) Microvascular decompression of the facial nerve for hemifacial spasm. In: Wilson CB (ed) Neurosurgical procedures: personal approaches to classic operations. Williams and Wilkins, Baltimore, pp 154–162
21. Jannetta PJ, Hackett E, Ruby JR (1970) Electromyographic and electronmicroscopic correlates in hemifacial spasm treated by microsurgical relief of neurovascular compression. Surg Forum 21: 449–451
22. Jannetta PJ, Abbasy M, Maroon JC, Ramos FM, Albin MS (1977) Etiology and definite microsurgical treatment of hemifacial spasm: Operative technique and results in 47 patients. J Neurosurg 47: 321–328
23. Kim P, Fukushima T (1984) Observations on synkinesis in patients with hemifacial spasm. J Neurosurg 60: 821–827

24. Laine E, Nayrac C (1948) Hemispasme facial gueri par intervention sur la fosse posterieure. Rev Neurol 80: 38–40
25. Malis LI (1967) Petrous ridge compression and its surgical correction. J Neurosurg 26: 163–167
26. Møller AR (1988) Evoked potentials in intraoperative monitoring. Williams and Wilkins, Baltimore
27. Møller AR (1995) Intraoperative neurophysiologic monitoring. Gordon and Breach, Langhorne Pennsylvania (In press)
28. Møller AR, Jannetta PJ (1983) Monitoring auditory functions during cranial nerve microvascular decompression operations by direct recording from the eighth nerve. J Neurosurg 59: 493–499
29. Møller AR, Jannetta PJ (1984) On the origin of synkinesis in hemifacial spasm: Results of intracranial recordings. J Neurosurg 61: 569–576
30. Møller AR, Jannetta PJ (1985) Hemifacial spasm: Results of electrophysiologic recording during microvascular decompression operations. Neurology 35: 969–974
31. Møller AR, Jannetta PJ (1985) Microvascular decompression in hemifacial spasm: Intraoperative electrophysiological observations. Neurosurgery 16: 612–618
32. Møller AR, Jannetta PJ (1985) Synkinesis in hemifacial spasm: Results of recording intracranially from the facial nerve. Experientia 41: 415–417
33. Møller AR, Jannetta PJ (1987) Monitoring facial EMG responses during microvascular decompression operations for hemifacial spasm. J Neurosurg 66: 681–685
34. Møller MB, Møller AR (1985) Audiometric abnormalities in hemifacial spasm. Audiology 24: 396–405
35. Møller AR, Møller MB (1989) Does intraoperative monitoring of auditory evoked potentials reduce incidence of hearing loss as a complication of microvascular decompression of cranial nerves? Neurosurgery 24: 257–263
36. Revilla AG (1947) Neurinomas of cerebellopontine recess. A clinical study of one hundred and sixty cases including operative mortality and end results. Johns Hopkins Hosp Bull 80: 254–296
37. Revilla AG (1948) Differential diagnosis of tumors at the cerebellopontine recess. Johns Hopkins Hosp Bull 33: 187–212
38. Schultze F (1875) Linksseitiger Facialiskrampf in Folge eines Aneurysma der Arteria vertebralis sinistra. Virchows Arch 65: 385–391
39. Wilkins RH (1991) Hemifacial spasm: A review. Surg Neurol 36: 251–277
40. Wilkins RH (1993) Cranial nerve dysfunction syndromes: Evidence for microvascular compression. In: Barrow DL (ed), Neurosurgical Topics Book 13, Surgery of Cranial Nerves of the Posterior Fossa, Chapter 4. American Association of Neurological Surgeons, Park Ridge, Illinois, pp 155–163

Correspondence: Peter J. Jannetta, M.D., Department of Neurological Surgery, University of Pittsburgh, School of Medicine, Presbyterian-University Hospital, Suite B-400, 200 Lothrop Street, Pittsburgh, Pennsylvania 15213, U.S.A.

Surgical treatment of hemifacial spasm by microvascular decompression: a forty-patient series study

G. Broggi, A. Franzini, S. Giombini, and **F. Pluchino**

Department of Neurosurgery, Istituto Nazionale Neurologico "C. Besta", Milano, Italy

Summary

Between 1980 and 1993 at the Istituto Nazionale Neurologico "C. Besta" in Milan, Italy, 40 patients with hemifacial spasm underwent microvascular decompression of the facial nerve in the posterior fossa. The role of preoperative neuroradiological and neurophysiological examinations is discussed, with particular attention to the presence of small meningiomas or schwannomas provoking the hemifacial spasm. The nature of arterial or venous neurovascular contact is discussed and the results of long-term follow-ups are presented.

Key words: Hemifacial spasm, microvascular decompression, meningioma, schwannoma.

Introduction

Hemifacial spasm (HFS) is a rare socially disabling condition which in Italy affects about 70 individuals per year. A considerably higher incidence is reported in Asiatic people and particularly in populations where congenital vascular abnormalities are prevalent [8].

The etiology of this condition fulfills epidemiological considerations; in fact, since the early published report by Gardner [6], the cause of HFS is now accepted worldwide as being a blood-vessel that is compressing the facial nerve at its entry zone (REZ) into the brainstem [6, 10]. As in other "hyperactive" cranial and peripheral nerve dysfunction syndromes [4], the motor symptoms are always unilateral. The spasms may affect localized parts of the face or the entire face on one side to different degrees.

The neurophysiological mechanisms underlying the disease are still debated, but the hypothesis that the antidromic activity is a result of ephaptic transmission at the site of the neurovascular contact has recently been disputed on the basis of neurophysiologic intraoperative monitoring in affected patients [11]. Since the 1970 report by Jannetta on his series of HFS patients [9], microvascular decompression of the nerve where it emerges from the brainstem has been the most common surgical procedure chosen to treat this condition [5], and other palliative treatments [7] were quickly discontinued, although Scott et al. [13] and Elston [3] attempted to create selective facial muscle palsy with injections of botulinum toxins.

In the present study, the results of microvascular decompression in 40 consecutive patients are discussed.

Patients and methods

Between 1980 and 1993, at the Istituto Nazionale Neurologico "C. Besta" of Milano, 40 patients between 10 and 67 years of age (mean age 47 years) with HFS underwent microvascular decompression of the facial nerve in the posterior fossa. The time between the manifestation of the first symptoms and the operation varied between 2 and 15 years. Preoperative neuroradiological examinations included contrast-enhanced computer tomography (CT-scan) and, since 1986, magnetic resonance imagery (MRI) (32 patients); since 1991, paramagnetic contrast-enhanced MRI has been used routinely. In only a few cases was an unequivocal neurovascular cross-compression of the facial nerve indicated preoperatively, as characterized by a "mega-dolicho-basilar" artery [2] and grossly tortuous vessels within the cerebellopontine region. The character and severity of the clinical symptomatology led to surgery on these patients, but also the patients who had no neuroradiological evidence of a neurovascular contact underwent surgery. Preoperative otoneurovestibular examinations failed to provide clear evidence of a compression in the acoustico-facial nerve complex.

Twenty-nine patients were operated on in the sitting position. The remaining 11 patients were operated on in the lateral decubitus position, as this position has been preferred since 1986 due to fewer associated anesthesio-logic problems. Intraoperative neurophysiological monitoring of the auditory nerve and of facial nerve function was performed by recording brainstem auditory evoked potentials (BAEP) and facial electromyography [12]. A small (1.5 cm diameter) craniectomy was performed, with its cranial boundary at the transverse sinus and its anterior boundary at the sigmoid sinus, thereby avoiding a wide exposition of these structures in most cases. After gentle retraction of the cerebellar hemisphere, which allowed the release of a considerable amount of cerebrospinal fluid (CSF), the acoustico-facial nerve complex was exposed and dissected from arterial and venous blood vessels as well as from arachnoid fibrous bundles. The vessel that was primarily compressing the facial nerve was then identified by higher magnification directed at its origin from the brainstem. In 20 patients the identified neurovascular contact was relieved by placing pieces of muscle or adipose tissue fragments between the nerve and the offending vessel. In the remaining 20 patients Teflon bundles or Teflon squares were placed between the nerve and the offending vessel.

In patients with evidence of venous conflict the vessels were coagulated and cut. The mastoid cells were filled with wax and fibrin glue. Tight closure of the dura was always reinforced by fibrin glue and then a round-shaped heterologous collagen lamina was forced into and sealed within the burr hole. CSF was drained via lumbar puncture repeatedly performed within the first 2–3 postoperative days.

In all cases the neurovascular cross-compression was due to arterial vessels belonging to the PICA system, and in only two cases was a considerable venous compression found in addition to the arterial conflict. A compression of the facial nerve by veins alone has never been detected in any patient, whereas venous compression occurred in 10% of 200 patients operated on to relieve trigeminal neuralgia in our Institution since 1986. In 2 of the HFS patients in the present study small vestibular schwannomas (5 to 6 mm diameter) were found, and in 1 patient a meningioma that originated in the tentorial-petrous sinus region was detected (see Table 1). Preoperative MRI was not performed in this patient with a meningioma because of the patient's phobic fears, but a CT-scan that was done was negative.

Table 1. Summary of HFS patients who underwent surgery, with particular attention to the position for surgery and etiology of the disease

N. Cases: 40 (27 F and 13 M)	Mean Age: 12–67*	
Sitting Position	29	
Prone Position	11	
Intraoperative monitoring	since 1986	
Neurovascular conflict	Arterious	37
	also venous	3
Tumoral conflict	VIII Neurinoma	2
	Petrous bone meningioma	1*

*MRI not performed because of claustrophobia; CT read as negative

Results

Hemifacial spasm (HFS) disappeared within a few days or immediately after surgery in 38 of the 40 patients in the present study without evidence of a recurrence on follow-up, which occurred between 1 and 13 years (mean, 6 years) after the surgery. In the 2 remaining patients HFS recurred within the first 2 months after surgery: 1 of these patients underwent a reoperation that was successful; the other patient refused to undergo reoperation.

In our series, there was no operative mortality (see Table 2), and the morbidity included transient impairment of the facial nerve in 7 patients and transient vestibular syndrome in 16 patients, which completely disappeared within 24–48 hours. Permanent morbidity consisted of hearing loss in 3 patients (2 of whom

Table 2. Side effects of surgery on the HFS patients

Complications		
Facial nerve deficit	transitory	7 cases (17,5%)
– sitting position	permanent	nil
– prone position	transitory	2 cases (5%)
	permanent	nil
Hearing deficit:		
– sitting position	transitory	9 cases (22,5%)
	permanent	2 cases (5%)
– prone position	transitory	3 cases (7,5%)
	permanent	1 case (2,5%)
Ataxia		nil
Dysphagia		nil
CSF Fistula	transitory	4 cases (10%)

were operated on in the sitting position). CSF wound fistula or rhino-liquorrhea occurred in 4 patients and was successfully treated by lumbar CSF drainage in all but 1 of these patients, who underwent surgical revision of the mastoid cells and dural tear.

Discussion

Definitive long-term results and morbidity in this small series are similar to those reported by Fukushima [5] and by Sindou (this volume). The peculiarity of our series is the high incidence of small benign tumors (7.5%) found on operation and missed by both preoperative neurophysiological assessment and contrast-enhanced CT examination. Paramagnetic contrast-enhanced MRI seems mandatory for HFS patients, particularly so those HFS patients who are candidates for treatment with botulinum toxin, which provokes definitive damage of neuromuscular end-plates [1].

In conclusion, we recommend the surgical approach as the first choice of treatment for HFS, when an accurate preoperative clinical, neurophysiological, and neuroradiological assessment is performed, whereas treatment with botulinum toxin, in our opinion, must be confined to atypical cases of HFS and to patients with idiopathic bilateral blepharospasm [11].

References

1. Alderson K, Holds JB, Anderson RL (1991) Botulinum-induced alteration of nerve-muscle interactions in the human orbicularis oculi following treatment for blepharospasm. Neurology 41: 1800-1805
2. Boeri R, Passerini A (1964) The megadolichobasilar anomaly. J Neurol Sci 1: 475–484
3. Elston JS (1986) Botulinum toxin treatment of hemifacial spasm. J Neurol Neurosurg Psychiatry 49: 827–829
4. Franzini A, Scaioli V, Leocata F, Palazzini E, Broggi G (1995) Pain syndrome and focal myokymia due to anterior interosseous neurovascular relationships: Report of a case and neurophysiological considerations. J Neurosurg 82: 578–580
5. Fukushima T (1984) Results of posterior fossa microvascular decompression in the management of hemifacial spasm. Facial N Res Jpn 4: 9–14
6. Gardner JW (1962) Concerning the mechanism of trigeminal neuralgia and hemifacial spasm. J Neurosurg 19: 947–958
7. Hori T, Fukushima T, Terao H, Takakura K, Sano K (1981) Percutaneous radiofrequency facial nerve coagulation in the management of facial spasm. J Neurosurg 54: 655–658
8. Iwakuma T, Matsumoto A, Nakamura N (1982) Hemifacial spasm: comparison of three different operative procedures in 110 patients. J Neurosurg 57: 753–756
9. Jannetta PJ (1970) Microsurgical exploration and decompression of the facial nerve in hemifacial spasm. Curr Top Surg Res 2: 217–220
10. Lillie HI, Craig WM (1936) Anomalous vascular lesion in cerebellopontine angle. Severe neuralgic pain in the ear and profound nervous disturbance: Operation and recovery. Arch Otolaryngol Head Neck Surg 23: 642–645
11. Møller AR (1987) Hemifacial spasm: Ephaptic transmission or hyperexcitability of the facial motor nucleus? Exp Neurol 98: 110–119
12. Møller AR, Jannetta PJ (1987) Monitoring facial EMG responses during microvascular decompression operations for hemifacial spasm. J Neurosurg 66: 681–685
13. Scott AB, Kennedy RA, Stubbs HA (1985) Botulinum A toxin injection as a treatment for blepharospasm. Arch Ophthalmol 103: 347–350

Correspondence: Giovanni Broggi, M.D., Department of Neurosurgery, Istituto Nazionale Neurologico "C. Besta", Via Celoria N. 11, I-20133 Milano, Italy.

Microsurgical vascular decompression for hemifacial spasm: a retrospective study of a 65-patient series

M. Sindou[1], Y. Keravel[3], C. Fischer[2], S. Derraz[1], and S. Palfi[3]

[1] Department of Neurosurgery, and [2] Department of Clinical Neurophysiology, Hopital Neurologique Pierre Wertheimer, Lyon, France
[3] Department of Neurosurgery, Hôpital Henri Mondor, University of Creteil, Paris, France

Summary

The results of a series of 65 consecutive patients operated on to relieve hemifacial spasm (HFS) at Pierre Wertheimer Hospital in Lyon and at the Henri Mondor Hospital in Creteil using the same microvascular decompression (MVD) method are reported.

MVD was performed through a retromastoid keyhole approach. A neurovascular conflict (NVC) was found in 62 cases (i.e., 95.4%). The conflicting vessel was the posterior inferior cerebellar artery (PICA) in 23 cases (35.4%), the anterior inferior cerebellar artery (AICA) in 22 cases (33.8%), the vertebro-basilar artery (VBA) with PICA and/or AICA in 13 cases (20%), and the VBA alone in 4 cases (3.1%). The conflicting artery was maintained apart from the REZ of VII nerve by interposing a ball made of Teflon fibers and/or a plaque of Dacron.

Forty-five patients (69.2%) were totally cured, 16 patients (24.6%) had only a partial (i.e., more than 50%) improvement, and in 4 patients (6.2%) surgery failed. Follow-up ranged from 1 month to 13 years (mean: 4 years and 8 months). It is important that in 9 patients, total relief of spasm occurred only secundarily with a delay sometimes as long as one year.

Postoperative complications were dominated by: 1) facial deficits in 16 cases (24.6%), of which 14 were transient and 2 were permanent; 2) hearing decrease in 10 cases (15.4%), of which 5 were transient and 5 were permanent. These complications were encountered at the beginning of the surgery and at a time when monitoring of intraoperative brainstem auditory evoked potentials (BAEP) was not routinely done.

A comparison of our data with that published in the literature is concordant.

Key words: Hemifacial spasm, microvascular decompression, neurovascular conflict.

Introduction

Over the last 20 years, especially through the extensive and outstanding work achieved by P. J. Jannetta and A. R. Møller at the Presbyterian-University Hospital of the University of Pittsburgh, microvascular decompression (MVD) has become a popular conservative treatment for hemifacial spasm (HFS). This chapter is a report of our brief personal experience and a concise review of the surgical literature concerning this treatment.

Material

Sixty-five patients underwent MVD to relieve HFS from 1982 to 1994 in our institutions: 40 females (61.5%) and 25 males (38.5%) ranging in age from 23 to 78 years (50 years mean average) (Fig. 1). In 40 cases (61.5%) the HFS was on the left side, predominantly so in the males (72%) compared to the females (55%) (see Table 1). In all cases the spasm was typical, as it always began at the level of the orbicularis oculi muscle. Not one patient in our series had atypical HFS, i.e., that which begins in the lower facial territory.

In 4.6% of our cases, the onset of the disease coincided with a severe psychological trauma. In 52.3% of our cases, psychological disturbances played a role in intensifying the disease.

Ipsilateral symptoms—tinnitus, lachrymation, and a decrease in hearing—were associated with the HFS in 26.2% (17 patients) (see Table 2). Systemic hypertension was present in 18% (12 patients).

The duration of HFS in our series of patients prior to surgery varied from 10 months to 20 years (mean: 4 years, 6 months). All of our patients were initially treated with various medications, e.g., carbamazepine, clonazepam, baclofen, which failed to control the spasms, and in 16 of the patients repeated botulinic toxin injections had become ineffective.

Preoperatively, all patients had a "standard" computer topography (CT) scan and/or a magnetic resonance image (MRI) test to exclude symptomatic HFS resulting from a tumor, aneurysm, arterio-venous malformation, etc.

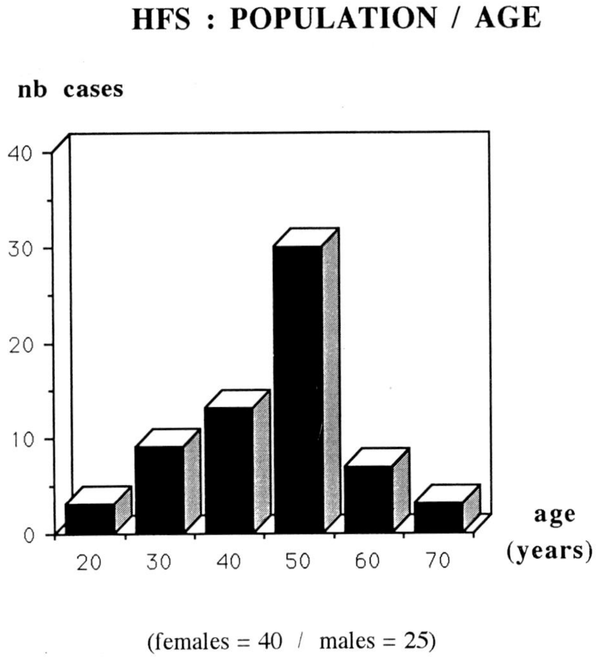

Fig. 1. Distribution of population of patients with HFS according to age

Table 1. Distribution of incidence of HFS between sides according to sex

Side / Sex	Right	Left	Total
Male	7 (28%)	18 (72%)	25 (100%)
Female	18 (45%)	22 (55%)	40 (100%)

Table 2. Clinical symptoms associated with HFS

Ipsilateral Symptoms	NB
Tinnitus	8
Lacrimation	6
Trigeminal Neuralgia	1
Otalgia	1
Corneal Hypoesthesia	1
Total	17 (out of 65)

In the last 4 cases of our series, a fine special MRI examination of the Root Exit Zone (REZ) of the facial nerve was done (see Chapter by Froment and Ledelliou in this book). In all 4, the Neuro-Vascular Conflict (NVC) was demonstrated and its type recognized; in 3 patients the NVC involved an anterior inferior cerebellar artery (AICA) (Fig. 2) and in 1 patient it involved a posterior inferior cerebellar artery (PICA) and a megadolichobasilar artery (Fig. 3).

A pure tone and speech audiogram was performed preoperatively in 47 patients: in 30, it was normal, in 14 it showed a bilateral sensorineural hearing loss of the presbycusis type, in 2 a conductive hearing loss, and in only 1 a sensorineural hearing loss ipsilateral to the HFS. Brainstem auditory evoked potentials (BAEP) were recorded preoperatively in 40 patients: in 34, BAEP were normal, in 2 BAEP evidenced cochlear disturbances, and in only 1 there was an increase in the latency of wave III; in 2 patients BAEP were not interpretable.

A facial electromyogram (EMG) was obtained preoperatively in 13 patients: in 8 it showed synkinesis, in 3 neurogenic atrophy, 2 of whom had botulinic toxin injections previously. The response of the blink reflex was recorded in 14 patients: in 11 it was normal, and in 3 abnormal responses were seen.

Methods

The first 10 patients were operated on in the sitting position. The remaining 55 patients were placed in the lateral decubitus position. We consider the latter position to be better [2] because it: 1) avoids the risk of an air embolism (which occurred in one of our patients, who had systemic hypotension while in sitting position), 2) causes less cerebrospinal fluid loss during surgery and, consequently, less collapse of the cerebrum, 3) allows easier access to the inferior aspect of the REZ of the seventh nerve, which is usually the site of the vascular compression.

The head of the patient is fixated in a three-pin headholder and is slightly flexed with a contralateral incline of 15 degrees. After the patient has been prepared for BAEP monitoring, the retromastoid region is shaved within a limited area, sterilized, and draped.

Operative procedure

The surgical approach involved a 4-cm long skin and muscle incision, followed by a low lateral retromastoid craniectomy (Fig. 4). The bone opening was semilunar-shaped (2 cm × 1.5 cm) and posterior to the sigmoid sinus, the edge of which was exposed to make the approach as lateral as possible. In almost all cases, the

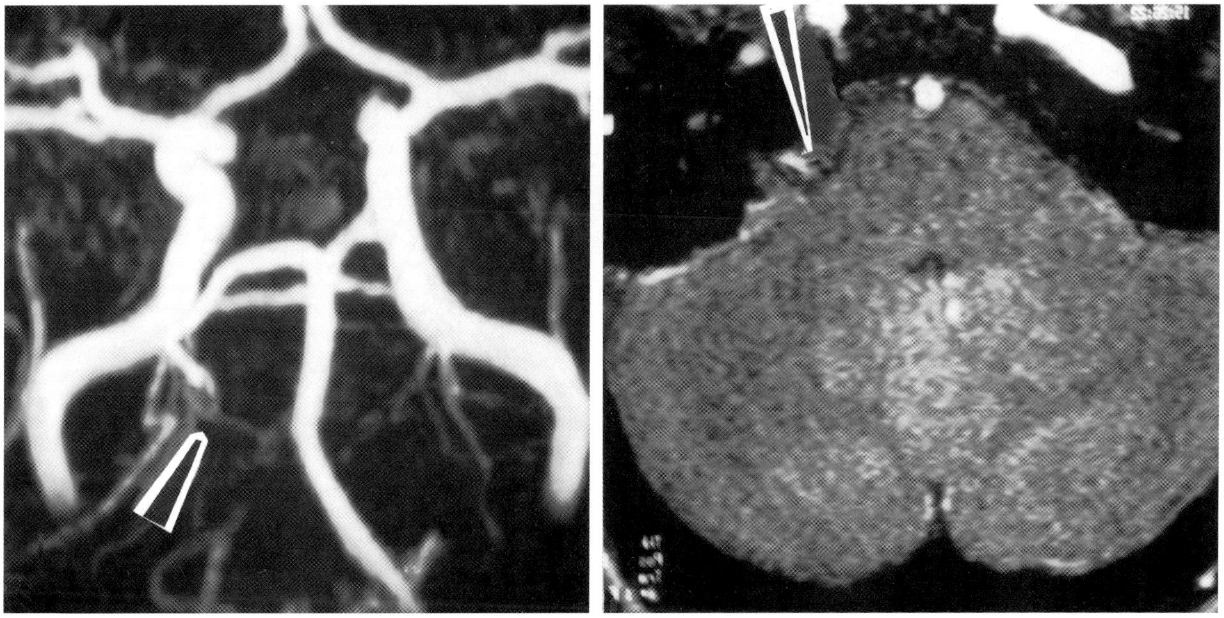

Fig. 2. HFS on right side, due to vascular compression of the facial root entry zone (REZ) and anterior-inferior cerebellar artery (AICA). *Left*: Angio-MR (A-P view); *Right*: MRI (transverse section). The arrow shows the offending AICA loop compressing the facial REZ

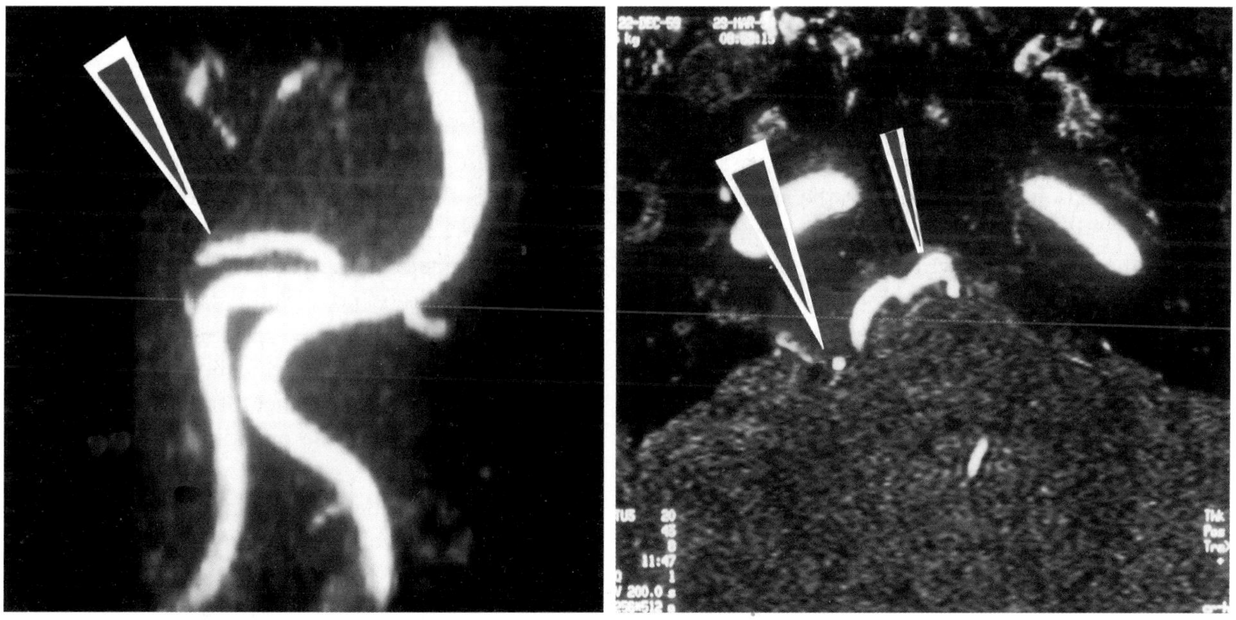

Fig. 3. HFS on right side due to vascular compression of the REZ of the facial nerve and the posterior-inferior cerebellar artery (PICA). *Left*: Angio-MR (A-P view); *Right*: MRI (transverse section). The small arrow shows the megadolichovertebral- artery, and the large arrow shows the offending PICA loop compressing the facial REZ

mastoid cells were opened and occluded by packing with small pieces of muscle and bone wax. A curved dural incision was made and the small dural flap was reflected and retracted on the sigmoid sinus.

A narrow self-retaining retractor (2 mm wide at the tip) was placed over a protective piece of rubber and a cottonoid on the inferior-lateral aspect of the cerebellar hemisphere, as far down as the arachnoid mem-

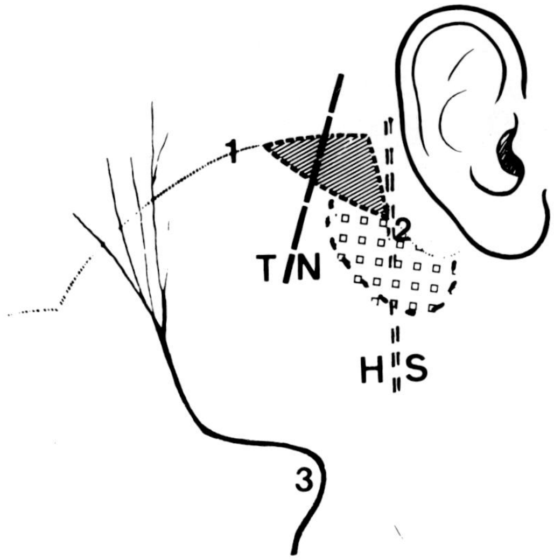

Fig. 4. Retromastoid approach (on right side) in the lateral position. Superior nuchal line (*1*) and mastoid process (*2*). Skin incision (dotted line) for the trigeminal (*TN*) and the facial (*HS*) approaches. Triangular craniotomy (hatched area) for the trigeminal nerve, and ovoid craniotomy (dotted area) for the facial nerve. Skin incisions avoid injury to the great occipital nerve (*3*)

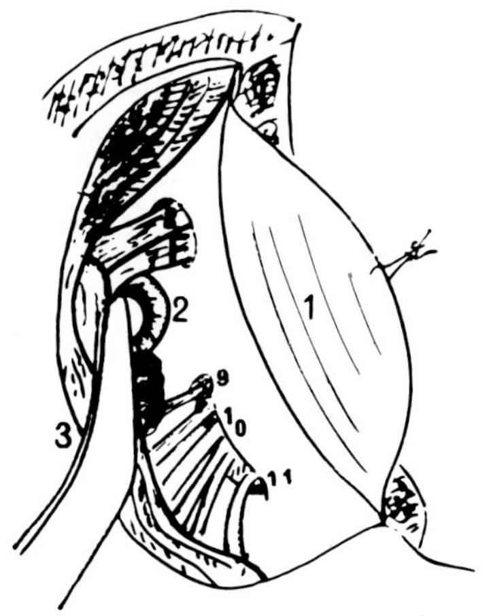

Fig. 5. Lower part: right inferolateral cerebellar approach (*3*), posterior to the mastoid tip (*1*), along the nerves of jugular foramen (*9*, *10*, *11*). The retractor tip is located between the flocculus (above) and the choroid plexus of the Luschka of foramen (below). Anterior-inferior cerebellar artery (*2*) contact with the facial nerve (*7F*)

brane covering the ninth and tenth cranial nerves and the choroid plexus that emerges from the lateral recess though the foramen of Luschka. Care must be taken not to tear bridging veins going from the cerebellar surface to their dural drainage points. The arachnoid membrane was incised from over the ninth cranial nerve to over the flocculus and the eighth cranial nerve.

Then the tip of the retractor was gently placed on the flocculus. Excessive traction, before detaching the flocculus from the eighth cranial nerve, must be avoided because this could result in stretching the nerve and consequently postoperative hearing loss. Therefore, as soon as this stage begins, it is very important to begin monitoring BAEP. When separating the flocculus from the eighth nerve, attention must be paid to not compromising the tiny vasculature of the nerve and to injuring the bridging nutrient vessels going from the surface of the cerebellum to the eighth nerve. Transfer of heat to the nerve from bipolar coagulation (if needed) must absolutely be prevented. After the flocculus was elevated from the brain stem and the pia-arachnoidal filaments of the cistern were divided, the pontomedullary sulcus was reached, with the REZ of the eighth nerve posterior and the inferior aspect of the REZ of the seventh nerve anterior (Fig. 5).

Because the offending artery(ies) is(are) almost always coming from the ventrocaudal side through the cerebello-medullary cistern, the REZ must be approached from below, i.e., from the ninth nerve and at the level of the choroid plexus up to the seventh nerve. The conflicting artery(ies), which is(are) the AICA, PICA, and/or VBA (see the "Operative Findings" section in this Chapter), has(have) to be identified and then transposed laterally with extreme care not to damage their perforating branches (Figs. 6 and 7).

Since the artery(ies) is(are) frequently atherosclerotic, mobilization may be dangerous, especially when there is a large megadolichobasilar artery involved in the vascular conflict. Stretched perforating collateral arising from the offending loop(s) also implies operative risks.

Transposition of the vessels can be difficult to maintain. To secure vessels in place, we routinely:

- use traction on the loop with teflon tape passed around the artery (the strips of tape are 4 cm in length × 3 mm in width and are made from fibers of Teflon cardiac felt);
- and/or place Teflon ball(s) (approximately 5 mm in diameter) in between the compressing vessel and the REZ of the seventh nerve, which are also made from fibers of Teflon felt;
- and, if necessary (which is frequent), place a piece of a semi-rigid plaque of Dacron (a square approxi-

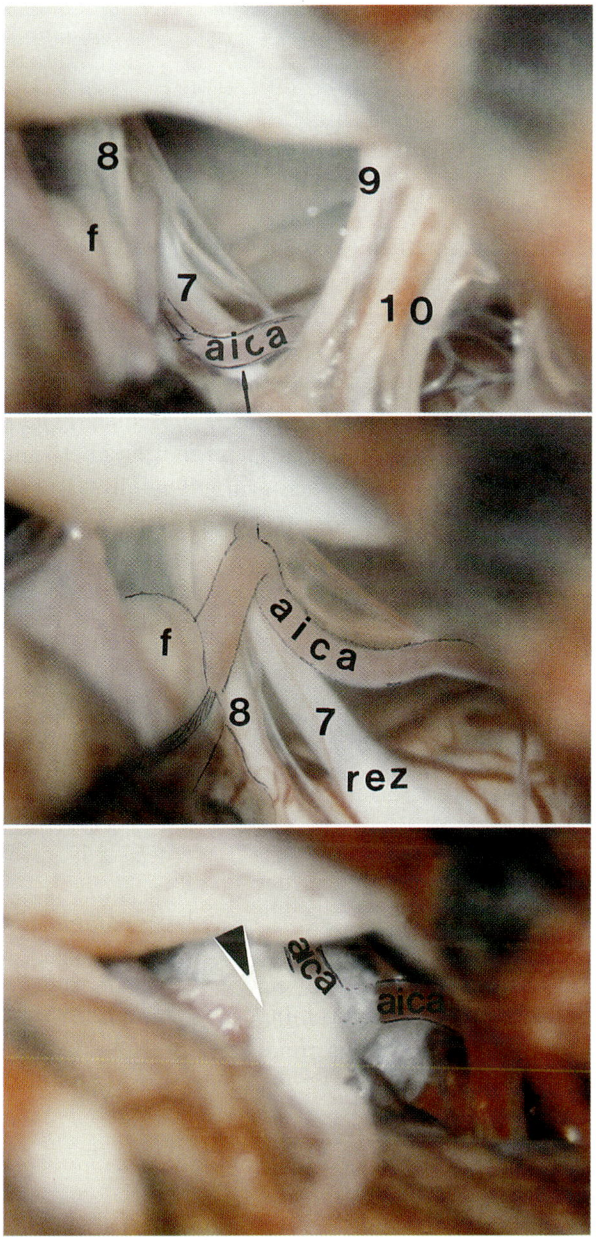

Fig. 6. HFS on right side due to vascular compression of the facial nerve by the AICA. Top: right inferolateral cerebellar route, passing along the ninth and tenth nerves, to approach the seventh nerve REZ (arrow) at its inferior aspect where the offending AICA loop is located. Middle: Magnified view (with a different view angle) of the seventh nerve REZ. The retractor is on the flocculus (*f*), which allows one to see the eighth nerve REZ. The AICA loop is well visible. Bottom: Postoperative view. The offending AICA loop has been pulled apart from the REZ by Teflon-fiber tape, and was kept apart with a Teflon-fiber absorber ball (arrow)

mately 1 cm^2) between the arterial loop and the nerve.

After completion of the decompression, it is important to check that the arteries are not kinked and/or

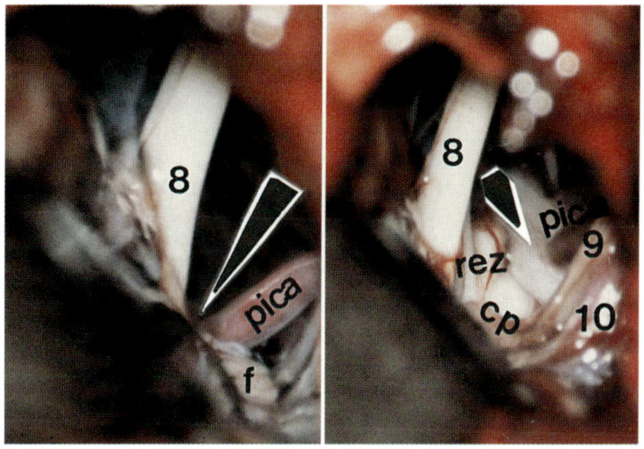

Fig. 7. HFS on right side due to vascular compression of the facial nerve from PICA. Left: The retractor is on the flocculus (*f*), which makes visible the offending PICA loop (arrow). The seventh nerve is hidden by the eighth nerve. Right: Postoperative view. The offending PICA loop has been pushed away from the seventh nerve REZ and is kept apart by Teflon-fiber tape (arrow) by pulling the loop downward. The choroid plexus (*CP*) emerging from the lateral recess of the fourth ventricle though the foramen of Luschka, as well as the ninth and tenth nerves, are visible

constricted. Careful hemostasis is achieved with several Valsalva maneuvers. Cisterns are irrigated with papaverine in saline to suppress eventual mechanical vasospasm due to manipulation of the arteries.

Finally, the dura is closed by single stitches and is made watertight by extradural apposition of a small piece of fat harvested from the retromastoid subcutaneous tissue. The muscular, subcutaneous, and cutaneous layers are closed by interrupted sutures. Then a compressive protective draping is applied on the operated area.

Intraoperative BAEP monitoring

BAEPs were recorded in 40 patients. Intraoperative changes were graded according to the classification we have described in previous reports [5, 34, 35], which was a modification of that described by Grundy et al. [12] (see Table 3). The technique [9] and the detailed results are reported by Fischer et al. in another chapter in this book.

Operative findings (Table 4)

No obvious responsible vessel could be found in 4.6% (3 cases) of the patients in this series. In the other

Table 3. Categories of intraoperative BAEP changes

Categories	Changes
1	Minimal changes
2	Increase in latency returning to normal before end of Surgery
2a	Increase in latency without normalization before end of Surgery
3	Abolition or partial decrease of responses returning to normal before end of Surgery
3a	Abolition or partial decrease of responses without complete normalization before end of Surgery
4	Total loss of responses lasting through entire procedure

Table 4. Types of vascular compression: *AICA* antero-inferior cerebellar artery; *PICA* postero-inferior cerebellar artery; *VBA* vertebro-basilar artery

HFS: Conflicting vessels	NB
Postero-Inferior Cerebellar A.	23
Antero-Inferior Cerebellar A.	22
VBA + PICA	5
VBA + AICA + PICA	4
PICA + AICA	2
Vertebro-Basilar Artery	2
Labyrinthine Artery	2
AICA + Labyrinthine A.	1
Vein	1
Non Identified vessel	3

95.4% (62 cases), the conflicting vessel varied: in 35.4% (23 patients) it was the postero-inferior cerebellar artery (PICA), in 33.8% (22 patients) it was the antero-inferior cerebellar artery (AICA), in 20% (13 patients) it was the vertebro-basilar artery (VBA) and PICA and/or AICA, in 3.1% (2 patients) it was the VBA alone, in 3.1% (2 patients) it was the labyrinthine A, and in 1.5% (1 patient) it was a vein.

Results

On hemifacial spasm

Immediate results and evolution (Table 5)

Table 5. Postoperative evolution of 65 HFS

Immediate outcome (D1)	Long-term outcome
No spasm 45 cases (69,2%)	Total cure: 36 Partial cure: 7 Recurrence: 2
Spasm 20 cases (30,8%)	Total cure: 9 Partial cure: 9 Failure: 2

Table 6. Long-term results of MVD operations for HFS (65 cases)

Total cure	Partial cure	Failure
45 (69.2%)	16 (24.6%)	4 (6.2%)

Forty-five patients (69.2%) had total relief on awakening from anesthesia; but 7 of them subsequently experienced a partial recurrence and 2 of them a complete recurrence.

Of the 20 patients who did not have an immediate postoperative total relief of HFS, 9 subsequently had total relief and 9 acquired partial relief (delays between 6 and 12 months). In 2 patients surgery totally failed—HFS remained the same postoperatively as it was preoperatively.

Overall late results (Table 6)

The results after follow-ups ranging from 6 months to 13 years (4 years and 7 months on average) were as follows: 45 patients (69.2%) were totally cured, 16 (24.6%) had a partial but beneficial (i.e, more than 50%) relief, and for 4 (6.2%) the surgery proved to be a total failure.

Complications

There were no mortalities in this series. Postoperative complications are detailed in Table 7. They were dominated by:

Facial weakness

A slight facial deficit was noticed immediately after surgery in 16 patients (24.6%). In 14 of these (21.5%), it subsided within a few months, but in 2 (3.1%) the weakness remained permanent.

Hearing loss

A decrease in hearing occurred in 10 patients (15.4%). In 5 of these (7.7%) it was transient within a few weeks, but in the 5 others (7.7%) the deficit was permanent.

These complications were encountered at the beginning of our study, at a time when intraoperative BAEP monitoring was not being routinely used (see Fig. 8).

Table 7. Postoperative complications of HFS

HFS Complications		Nb	Description
Meningitis		2	Successfully treated by antibiotherapy
Rhinorrhea		6	Requiring CSF depletion by Lumbar punctures in 4 and Lumbar drainage in 2.
Meningocoela		2	Requiring CSF depletion by Lumbar punct.
Delayed Healing and/or Infection		8	Requiring surgical repair in 2.
Neuralgia of Occipital N.		2	Mild; not requiring any medication
Facial paralysis	Transient	14	Within 2 months
	Permanent	2	Lower territory
Hearing Loss	Transient	5	Within 1 months
	Permanent	5	
Vago-Glosso-Pharyngeal paresis (transient)		3	Within 1 week
Trigeminal hypoesth. (transient)		2	Within 2 weeks
Phlebitis		2	Successfully treated by Heparin
Mortality		none	

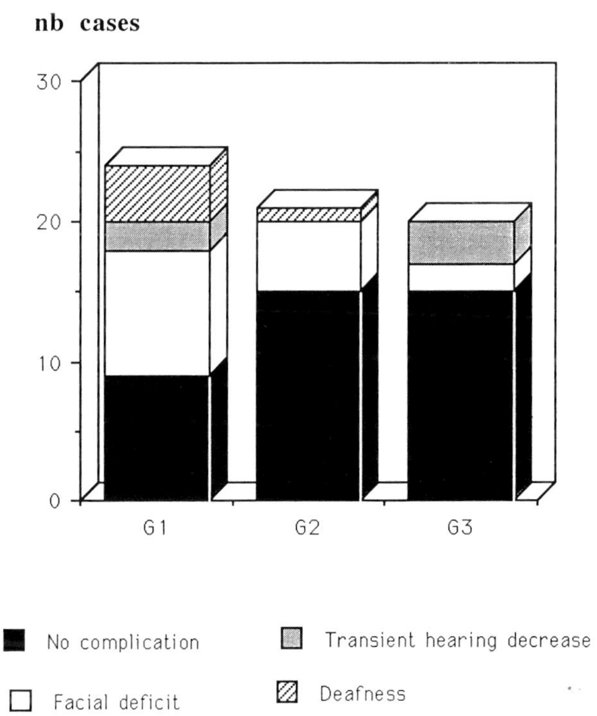

Fig. 8. Postoperative complications before and after BAEP monitoring. G1: Group operated on before BAEP monitoring; G2: Group operated on at the begining experience of BAEP monitoring; G3: Group operated on during the last experience of BAEP monitoring

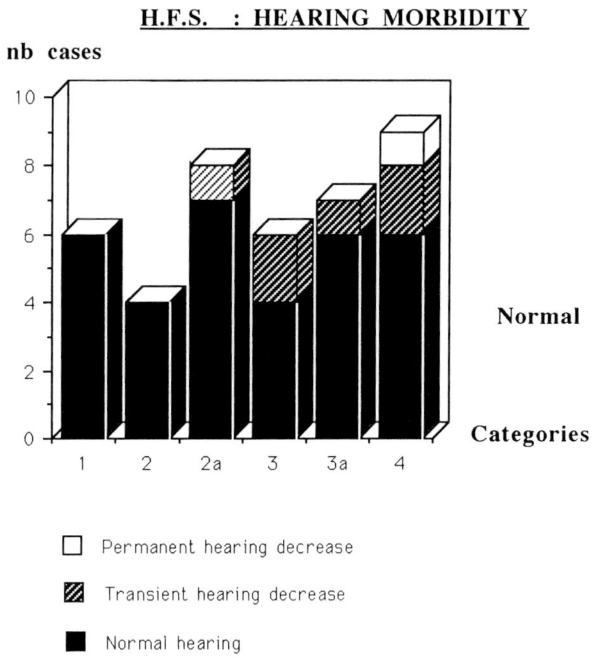

Fig. 9. Postoperative morbidity in patients with HFS as function of intraoperative BAEP modifications (see Table 3 for classification)

Data from intraoperative BAEP monitoring

Intraoperative changes in BAEP occurred in all of the patients in our series who had recordings (40 patients; see Fig. 9). In 6 patients these changes (see Table 3 for classification) were minimal, in 12 they consisted of an increase in latency, in 13 there was a decrease in amplitude, and in 9 there was a total abolition of waves that lasted for the remainder of the operation.

Figure 9 clearly shows that there was a good correlation between the severity of intraoperative changes in BAEP and the postoperative morbidity. In fact, 6 of the 7 patients who had a postoperative hearing decrease had significant changes in their intraoperative BAEP (see categories 3, 3a, and 4 in Fig. 9), as did the patient who suffered a permanent postoperative hearing loss (see category 4 in Fig. 9).

EMG data

Because EMG examination was not included in our protocol, only 4 patients had pre- and postoperative EMG recordings. The results are summarized in Table 8. In addition to these 4, 11 patients had a postoperative EMG only. These data are detailed in Table 9.

Table 8. Pre- and postoperative EMG data in patients with HFS

Case No.	Pre-operative EMG	Post-operative EMG	Post-oper. clinical data
1	– Involuntary potentials – Synkinesis – Normal Blink Reflex	– Nerve atrophy act. – Mild involuntary potentials – Increase of R_1 latency	Partial remission
2	– Nerve atrophy act. – Synkinesis – Involuntary potentials – Increase R_1 and R_2 latencies	– Nerve atrophy act. – Decrease R_1 and R_2 latencies without normalization	Total cure
3	– Synkinesis – Normal Blink Reflex	– Without changes	Total cure
4	– Normal Blink Reflex	– Normal Blink Reflex	Total cure

According to all this (fragmentary) information, there is no evidence that a curing of HFS could be correlated to lesioning of the nerve during the operation by excessive manipulation, surgical injury, and/or neocompression with interposed prosthesis.

Discussion

Strong similarities can be seen when comparing the data in our present series of patients with those reported in other reports in the literature [2–4, 6–8, 13–17, 19–23, 26, 28–32, 37–40].

Epidemiology and clinical features

This study provided the opportunity to calculate the approximate incidence of HFS within the geographic area of Lyon, France. By adding the 50 patients who underwent MVD within the past 12 years, and the 85 and 64 cases who were treated only with botulinic toxin over the same period of time, respectively by neurologists and ophthalmologists, the incidence of HFS was in the order of 6.6 for 100,000 population/12 years. These statistics on the incidence of HFS are not very different from those presented by Auger et al. [2] (7.4 for 100,000 males and 14.5 for 100,000 females).

In our series, females represented 61.5%, which is in the range of the percentages noted in various reports in the literature: 60.4% [7], 54% [14], 66.4% [18], and 77% [38].

The mean age at the time of surgery was 50 years in our series, which is close to the average ages noted in various publications: 53 years [14], 51 years [18], and 52 years [23].

As noted above, the left side was predominantly affected in our patients (61.5%). This is well in accordance with data noted in various reports in the literature: 54.2% [14], 58.5% [18], and 57 [38]. In our material, the left-sided predominance was more pronounced in males (72%) than in females (55%). This difference between the sexes regarding predominance, however, does not seem to have been addressed in other studies.

Our series of patients does not include cases of atypical HFS, as do those in other studies. In a study by Jannetta [18] 7.4% of the series of patients had atypical HFS.

It is interesting that of our 65 patients with (primary) HFS, there was only one case of symptomatic HFS, which revealed an eighth nerve schwannoma and disappeared after removal of the tumor.

Operative findings

A vascular compression was found in 95.4% of our patients. This is close to the percentages given in

Table 9. Postoperative EMG data in patients who did not have a pre-operative EMG

	Pre-op. clinical data	Post-op. clinical data		Post-op. EMG data	
1st Group: 8 cases	H.F.S.	No facial deficit:	7 cases	Normal: 6 cases Atrophy: 1 case	
(Total cure of HFS)	No facial deficit	Facial deficit:	1 case	Atrophy: 1 case	
2nd Group: 3 cases	H.F.S.	H.F.S. present No Facial deficit	2 cases	No Facial lesion Synkinesis Normal Blink ref.	2 cases
(Failure of HFS)	No Facial deficit	H.F.S. present Facial deficit	2 cases	Synkinesis Facial lesion Normal Blinked.	1 case

Table 10. Vascular compression series in patients with HFS with conflicts detailed, from literature reviews

Authors	NB Cases	Arteries AICA	PICA	VBA	Others	Veins	Others	No conflict seen
Loeser (1983)	21	9	5	4	–	1	–	–
Kaye (1984)	16	1	1	1	–	1	–	1
Auger (1986)	54	20	14	9	7	3	–	1
Huang (1992)	310	121	71	11	102	2	–	–
Sindou & Keravel	65	22	23	2	15	–	–	3
Total	466	173 (37,1%)	114 (24,5%)	27 (5,8%)	144 (30,9%)	7 (1,5%)	–	16 (3,4%)

Table 11. Vascular compression series in patients with HFS without conflicts detailed, from literature reviews

Authors	Nb cases	Arteries	Veins	Others (Tumor MAV, Anev)	No conclict seen
Neagoy (1974)	14	14	–	–	–
Jannetta (1980)	239	220	14	5	–
Wilson (1980)	22	22	–	–	–
Liu (1981)	16	16	–	–	–
Iwakuma (1982)	74	73	–	–	1
Authors with less than 10 cases	49	41		1	7
Total	414	386 (93.2%)	14 (3.4%)	6 (1.4%)	8 (1.9%)

various reports in the literature (see Tables 10 and 11): 98.1% [4], 100% [14], 98.6% [15], and 100% [17]. As noted in other studies [4, 14, 15, 17, 19, 21, 22, 28,39], the vascular compression in almost all our cases had an arterial origin (61 out of 62 patients, 93.8%).

Recently, thanks to special MRI procedures, it has become possible to reliably detect the existence of a vascular compression in the facial REZ and to accurately predict the type(s) of vascular compression (see reference 27 and the chapter by Froment and Ledelliou in this book). Froment and Ledelliou present evidence of a vascular loop in the REZ on the side of the face that is manifesting HFS in 19 of the 20 patients in their study. In these 19 patients there was no vascular loop present on the contralateral REZ. In the one remaining patient in their study, a vascular loop was visible on both sides, although the patient had the disease unilaterally. These facts are of prime importance, as the contralateral sides (together) to the disease contribute a kind of "control group."

Results of microvascular decompression to relieve HFS

A cure was obtained for 69.2% of our patients, and 30.8% were improved. This is in the range of the results published in other reports in the literature (see details in Table 12).

The reason(s) why surgery failed in some patients in our series—even in the patients who were more recently operated on (see Fig. 10)—is unclear, as it also is from other reports in the literature. Further analyses is necessary in this regard.

Some studies [14, 17, 21, 22, 39] report that re-operations in some patients improved the success rate, e.g., 88% to 93% in the report by Jannetta [17], 92% to 97% in the report by Huang et al. [14]. Both of these surgeons advocate re-operation as early as possible to avoid the technical difficulties of dissection related to adhesions due to fibrosis and arachnoiditis. The fact that in our series, 13.8% of the patients had a delayed relief of their HFS indicates to us that it would be appropriate to wait at least 12 months before considering re-operating in the case of failure.

Complications

In general, operative mortality involving HFS has been exceptional, as only 3 deaths have been reported [13, 39].

The rate of occurrence of transient neurological deficits after surgery is difficult to evaluate with accuracy because published reports rarely provide precise

Table 12. Results of MVD in patients with HFS, from literature reviews

Authors	Year	Nb	Nb of Oper.	Nb patients 1st operation	cured at 2nd operation	% Patients cured	% Partial remission	% Failure	Follow-up
Neagoy	1974	14	14	9 (64%)	–	64	–	–	5w–8y
Jannetta	1980	229	241	201 (88%)	12	93	5	2	1y–9y
Wilson	1980	22	24	16 (73%)	2	82	–	–	3m–y
Liu	1981	16	18	13 (81%)	2	94	6	0	6m–1y
Kaye	1981	16	16	10 (62%)	–	62	25	13	2m–5y
Iwakuma	1982	74	74	72 (97%)	–	97	1	2	1m–3y
Loeser	1983	20	21	11 (55%)	1	60	25	15	4m–7y
Piatt	1984	48	51	32 (67%)	–	67	25	13	42m
Auger	1986	54	54	38 (70%)	–	70	9	21	1y–10y
Huang	1992	310	326	286 (92%)	16	97	2	1	6m–8y
Sindou & Keravel	1994	65	65	45 (69%)	–	69	25	6	1m–12y
Authors with less than 10 cases		42	42	34 (81%)	–	81	9	10	

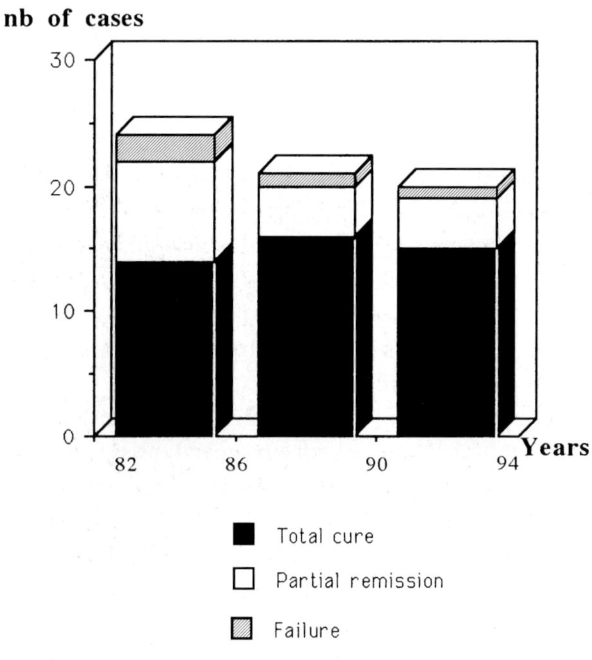

Fig. 10. Results of microvascular decompression in patients with HFS as noted over a period of years

information about such complications. The most frequent permanent neurological deficits observed were facial weakness and hearing loss. Data from the literature are summarized in Table 13.

Our rate of occurrence of permanent facial deficits (3.1%) is within the range of that reported in the literature (0% to 6.3%) [3, 4, 14, 17, 19, 22, 39]. A more precise evaluation would require systematic pre- and postoperative EMG and blink reflex recordings.

Our rate of permanent hearing loss (7.7%) is also within the range of that reported in the literature (1.5% to 20%) [3, 4, 14, 17, 19, 22, 39]. Systematic pre- and postoperative audiometric examinations and BAEP recordings are necessary to quantify this particular complication precisely.

The routine use of intraoperative BAEP monitoring has been reported to be of prime importance in reducing the risk of hearing loss, as pointed out by many investigators [4, 5, 12, 25, 29, 35, 38; for details, see the chapter by Fischer et al. in this book]. This is also our opinion, as derived from our experience with the present series of patients, in which 4 patients suffered a permanent hearing loss who were in the group of 25 patients operated on before the routine use of BAEP monitoring, versus only 1 patient who was in the group of 40 patients in whom BAEP were monitored. In addition, it is interesting to note that in our last 20 patients no decrease in hearing occurred, as shown in Fig. 8. The same is true in Jannetta's material: hearing loss reported in his earlier series of patients (1971–79) [17] was 7%, while in his later series of patients (1980–89) [18] it was reported to be 1.4%.

Mechanisms of HFS and causes of failure of MVD

Every neurosurgeon using microvascular decompression to relieve HFS is convinced that vascular compression is the main–if not the sole-origin of the disease [10, 11, 16]. All published surgical reports have noted the presence of an offending vessel in the facial REZ in more than 95% of the cases.

Table 13. Postoperative complications in patients with HFS, from literature reviews

Authors	Year	Nb Operations	Transient Facial Palsy	Hearing Loss	Permanent Facial Palsy	Hearing Loss	Mortality
Jannetta	1980	241		9		26	0
Wilson	1980	24		7		5	1
Kaye	1981	16	3	2	1	2	0
Iwakama	1982	74	0	0	0	12	0
Loeser	1983	21	1	0	1	4	0
Auger	1986	54	11	0	0	8	0
Huang	1992	326	15	2	0	5	0
Sindou & Keravel	1994	65	14	5	2	5	0

Although vascular contacts can be seen at the REZ of the facial nerve in autopsy studies on patients who did not have HFS (see the chapter by Mercier et al. in this book), MRI examinations in patients with HFS give clear evidence of a neurovascular contact. In fact, provided that an adequate technique be used, an MRI examination is able to show almost always, i.e., 95% of the time, an image of a neurovascular contact in the REZ on the ipsilateral side of the HFS; however, only occasionally (5% of the time) does an MRI examination show a neurovascular contact on the contralateral REZ (see the chapter by Froment and Ledelliou in this book).

Electrophysiological studies done both in humans and in laboratory animals by Møller and co-workers (see the chapter by Møller in this book) are very much in favor of the hypothesis that hyperactivity of the facial nucleus is generated by a vascular compression at the REZ of the nerve.

The reasons why a total and permanent cure of HFS is not always achieved after an MVD has been performed remain unclear. A variety of explanations for such a failure can be proposed. For examples:

1) As there may be several different vessels that are in contact with the facial nerve, the surgeon could well miss one of them, if not attentive enough.
2) Because the offending vessel (which in almost all cases is an artery) may be very rigid and/or have short stretched perforators to the brain stem, its transposition away from the REZ might well have been insufficient to completely decompress the nerve
3) The foreign material interposed between the REZ and the artery can be too soft (e.g., Teflon felt fibers) or too rigid (e.g., Dacron plaque) and, consequently, does not provide enough protection for or causes too much compression on the nerve, respectively.
4) Although the condition of the REZ is not usually described with precision in surgeons' reports, every neurosurgeon will remember the REZ of the seventh nerve as being grey and atrophic. This segmental atrophy, which is a sign of a significant neural degeneration, might explain why MVD may not have been effective in spite of the nerve being well decompressed.
5) Fibrosis and arachnoiditis, which might well occur postoperatively, could generate new "irritative" factors for the REZ of the seventh nerve and counterbalance the decompressive effect of the procedure.

If the reason for failure of MVD involves any of the explanations give in 1), 2), and 3) above, more careful surgical measures must be utlized. If the reason for failure of MVD is neural atrophy, such as that noted in example 4 above, the surgeon would be compelled to operate on patients with HFS as early as possible, to avoid the development of irreversible atrophy. If the reason for failure of MVD involves the postoperative development of fibrosis and/or arachnoiditis, as described in example 5 above, then attempts must be made to reduce the necessity to insert a foreign material (e.g., Teflon felt or Dacron plaque) between the artery and the REZ to maintain their separation, because such a foreign material might generate or increase "irritation" of the nerve and thus counterbalance the decompressive effect of MVD.

Finally, the problem of ascertaining whether or not MVD has been successful following a real decompressive or, rather, a neocompressive mechanism, is still not totally solved [1].

The results of all reports on surgical series, and the intraoperative EMG recordings as well as the laboratory studies by Møller [24] (also see chapter by Møller in this book) provide support for validity of the decompressive effect of the MVD procedure.

The comparative studies of the results of two series of patients with trigeminal neuralgia after treatment by MVD [33, 36]—the first study involving the interposition of foreign material between the nerve and the artery, and the second study involving the foreign material touching the nerve—give clear evidence of the decompressive effect of MVD on trigeminal neuralgia.

Much remains to be understood about the complex disease of HFS, and more long-term clinical studies as well as further laboratory work are needed.

References

1. Adams CBT (1989) Microvascular compression: An alternative view and hypothesis. J Neurosurg 70: 1–12
2. Auger RG, Whisnant JP (1990) Hemifacial spasm in Rochester and Olmsted County, Minnesota: 1960 to 1984. Arch Neurol 417: 1233–1234
3. Auger RG, Piepgras DG, Laws ER Jr, Miller RH (1981) Microvascular decompression of the facial nerve for hemifacial spasm: Clinical and electrophysiologic observations. Neurology 31: 346–350
4. Auger RG, Piepgras DG, Laws ER Jr (1986) Hemifacial spasm: Results of microvascular decompression of the facial nerve in 54 patients. Mayo Clin Proc 61: 640–644
5. Ciriano D, Sindou M, Fischer C (1991) Apport du monitorage per-opératoire des potentials évoqués auditifs précoces dans la décompression vasculaire microchirurgicale pour névralgie du trijumeau ou spasme hémifacial. Neurochirurgie 37: 323–329
6. Cook BR, Jannetta PJ (1984) Tic convulsif: Results in 11 cases treated with microvascular decompression of the fifth and seventh cranial nerves. J Neurosurg 61: 949–951
7. Ehni G, Woltman HW (1945) Hemifacial spasm: Review of 106 cases. Arch Neurol Psych 53: 205–211
8. Fabinyi GCA, Adams CBT (1978) Hemifacial spasm: Treatment by posterior fossa surgery. J Neurosurg Psychiatry 41: 829–833
9. Fischer C (1989) BAEP monitoring in posterior fossa surgery. In: Desmedt JE (ed) Neuromonitoring in surgery. Elsevier, Amsterdam, pp 191–207
10. Gardner WJ (1962) Concerning the mechanism of trigeminal neuralgia and hemifacial spasm. J Neurosurg 19: 947–958
11. Gardner WJ, Sava GA (1962) Hemifacial spasm: A reversible pathophysiologic state. J Neurosurg 19: 240–247
12. Grundy BL, Jannetta PJ, Procopio PT, Lina A, Boston JR, Doyle E (1982) Intraoperative monitoring of brainstem auditory evoked potentials. J Neurosurg 57: 674–682
13. Hanakita J, Kondo A (1988) Serious complications of microvascular decompression for trigeminal neuralgia and hemifacial spasm. Neurosurgery 22: 348–352
14. Huang C, Chen I, Lee LS (1982) Microvascular decompression for hemifacial spasm: Analyses of operative findings and results in 310 patients. Neurosurgery 30: 53–57
15. Iwakuma T, Matsumoto A, Nakamura N (1982) Hemifacial spasm. Comparison of three different operative procedures in 110 patients. J Neurosurg 57: 753–756
16. Jannetta PJ (1975) Trigeminal neuralgia and hemifacial spasm etiology and definitive treatment. Trans Am Neurol Assoc 100: 89–91
17. Jannetta PJ (1980) Neurovascular compression in cranial nerve and systemic disease. Ann Surg 192: 518–525
18. Jannetta PJ (1990) Cranial rhizopathies. In: Youmans JR (ed) Neurological surgery, 3rd edn. WB Saunders, Philadelphia, pp 4169–4182
19. Kaye AH, Adams CBT (1981) Hemifacial spasm: A long term follow up of patients treated by posterior fossa surgery and facial nerve wrapping. J Neurol Neurosurg Psychiatry 44: 1100–1103
20. Kelly DL (1977) Posterior fossa neuro-vascular decompression for tic douloureux and hemifacial spasm. N C Med J 38: 534–536
21. Liu KN, Wu JM, Fairholm D (1981) Hemifacial spasm treated by posterior fossa surgery. J Formosan Med Assoc 80: 1235–1239
22. Loeser JD, Chen J (1983) Hemifacial spasm treated by microsurgical facial nerve decompression. Neurosurgery 13: 141–146
23. Maroon JC (1978) Hemifacial spasm: A vascular cause. Arch Neurol 35: 481–483
24. Møller AR (1991) The cranial nerve vascular compression syndrome: A review of pathophysiology. Acta Neurochir (Wien) 113: 24–30
25. Møller AR, Jannetta PJ (1983) Monitoring Auditory Functions during cranial nerve microvascular decompression operations by direct recording from the eight nerve. J Neurosurg 59: 493–499
26. Naessens PJ, De Waele LF (1980) Microvascular decompression in the posterior fossa of the trigeminal nerve for tic douloureux and microvascular decompression of the facial nerve for hemifacial spasm. Acta Neurol Belg 80: 95–98
27. Nagaseki Y, Horikoshi T, Omata T, Ueno T, Ushida M (1992) Resonance imaging visualizing vascular compression of the trigeminal or facial nerve. J Neurosurg 77: 379–386
28. Neagoy DR, Dohn DF (1974) Hemifacial spasm secondary to vascular compression of the facial nerve. Cleveland Clin Q 41: 205–214
29. Piatt JH Jr, Wilkins RH (1984) Treatment of tic douloureux and hemifacial spasm by posterior fossa exploration: Therapeutic implications of various neurovascular relationships. Neurosurgery 14: 462–471
30. Rhoton AL (1978) Microsurgical neurovascular decompression for trigeminal neuralgia and hemifacial spasm. J Fla Med Assoc 65: 425–428
31. Rushworth RG, Smith SF (1982) Trigeminal neuralgia and hemifacial spasm. Med J Aust 1: 424–426
32. Saito H (1985) Neurovascular decompression for hemifacial spasm. Acta Otolaryngol [Suppl] 419: 149–154
33. Sindou M, Amrani F, Mertens P (1990) Decompression vasculaire microchirurgicale pour névralgie du trijumeau. Comparison de deux modalités techniques et déductions physiopathologiques. Neurochirurgie 36: 16–26
34. Sindou M, Fobe JL, Ciriano D, Fischer C (1990) Intraoperative Brain Stem Auditory Evoked Potentials in the microvascular decompression of the Vth and VIIth cranial nerves. Revue de laryngologie 111: 427–431
35. Sindou M, Ciriano D, Fischer C (1991) Lessons from brain stem auditory evoked potential monitoring during microvascular decompression for trigeminal neuralgia and hemifacial spasm. In: Schramm J, Møller AR (eds) Intraoperative neurophysiologic monitoring in neurosurgery. Springer, Heidelberg, pp 293–300

36. Sindou M, Mertens P, Amrani F (1991) Does microsurgical vascular decompression for trigeminal neuralgia work though a neocompressive mechanism? Anatomical–Surgical evidence for a decompressive effect. Acta Neurochir [Suppl] 52: 127–129
37. Wilberger J, Velo A (1981) Microneurosurgical treatment of trigeminal neuralgia and hemifacial spasm. South Med J 74: 1124–1126
38. Wilkins RH (1991) Hemifacial spasm: A review. Surg Neurol 36: 251–277
39. Wilson CB, Yorke C, Prioleau G (1980) Microsurgical vascular decompression for trigeminal neuralgia and hemifacial spasm. West J Med 132: 481–484
40. Witzmann A, Dieckmann G (1982) Intracranial facial nerve decompression in the management of hemifacial spasm. Appl Neurophysiol 45: 291–294

Correspondence: Marc Sindou, M.D., D.Sc. Department of Neurosurgery, Hôpital Neurologique Pierre Wertheimer, 59, Boulevard Pinel, F-69003 Lyon, France.

Monitoring of brainstem auditory evoked potentials during microvascular decompression for hemifacial spasm

C. Fischer[1], **M. Sindou**[2], **J. Bohorquez**[3], and **O. Bertrand**[3]

[1]Department of Clinical Neurophysiology, and [2]Department of Neurosurgery, Hopital Neurologique Pierre Wertheimer, Lyon, France
[3]Brain Signals and Processes Laboratory, Inserm 280, Lyon, France

Summary

Experience in the use of intraoperative monitoring of brainstem auditory evoked potentials (BAEPs) to relieve hemifacial spasm (HFS) in 42 patients is reported. No patient was deaf before surgery. Postoperatively, one patient (2.3%) was totally deaf. Mean preoperative pure tone average (PTA) was 12.5 ± 9.2 dB. Mean postoperative PTA was 20.5 ± 18 dB ($p < 0.001$). The wave I–V interval was elevated in 5 patients preoperatively and in 12 patients postoperatively. The postoperative BAEPs of the patient who became deaf were totally and definitely obliterated. During surgery changes in BAEPs were as follows: after anesthetic induction the mean I–V interval was significantly increased compared to the preoperative recordings ($p < 0.001$). In 5 patients retraction of the cerebellum led to either abolition of waves (transient in 4 cases, permanent in 1 case), which required removal or repositioning of the retractor, or to a significant delay of peak V (29 cases) or no change (8 cases). Microvascular decompression procedure led to transient abolition of all waves (4 cases) or to the abolition of all waves except peak I (4 cases) or to delays of peak V ranging from 0.5 ms to > 1 ms (18 cases). In 15 cases changes were negligible. The main concern in BAEP monitoring was to identify significant changes of the response waveform, latencies and amplitudes on-line, and to give functional warnings to the surgeon so that he or she could modify his or her maneuvers and thus prevent deterioration of the auditory pathway. It is concluded, as it has been in other studies, that intraoperative BAEP monitoring during microvascular decompression to relieve HFS reduces the risk of postoperative deafness.

Key words: Brainstem auditory evoked potentials, deafness, intraoperative monitoring, hemifacial spasm.

Introduction

Experience in the use of intraoperative monitoring of brainstem auditory evoked potentials (BAEPs) during surgical procedures to relieve hemifacial spasm (HFS) that have been performed at the Hopital Neurologique, in Lyon, France since 1985 is reported. It was found that BAEPs are helpful in evaluating the functional condition of peripheral and central auditory pathways during such surgical procedures [2, 11, 15]. Monitoring of BAEP is also widely used in clinical evaluations. BAEPs consist of 5 waves that are usually identified by Roman numerals. Waves I and II are probably generated at the level of the auditory nerve and waves III to V are generated in the brainstem.

Microvascular decompression (MVD) of the facial nerve is an effective method used to relieve HFS, despite a number of possible hazards such as postoperative unilateral deafness [1, 6, 9, 14, 15]. Wilkins [15] provided a detailed review of the medical literature, which included his own reports, that noted that according to several published series the rate of postoperative auditory nerve dysfunction ranged from 10 to 20% of all operated patients when intraoperative BAEP monitoring is not used. He added that in his own experience postoperative ipsilateral deafness could be avoided by using intraoperative monitoring of BAEPs [12, 15], as did Møller in previous reports [10, 11].

Patients and methods

Patients

Forty-two patients who presented with HFS were monitored intraoperatively using recordings of BAEP (see chapter by M. Sindou et al. in this book): 29 females (69%) and 13 males (31%) of mean age 52 ± 12 years (range 25–75 years); 15 of these patients (36%) had HFS on the right side and 27 (64%) had HFS on the left side.

Pure tone audiometry was performed in all patients sometime within the week before surgery and within ten days following surgery. Postoperative otoscopy and tympanometry were performed systematically in order to detect middle ear dysfunction, which is a common problem following this type of surgery. We calculated the pure tone average (PTA) to be within the speech frequency range (500, 1000, and 2000 Hz). We regarded all cases in which the postoperative PTA increased by more than 10 dB when compared to preoperative PTA as abnormal. Standard BAEP recordings were performed in all patients within the week before surgery and again within the first postoperative week in all patients except one. We calculated the peak latency of waves I, III and V, and the interpeak latencies (IPL) I–III and I–V, and the peak I/V amplitude ratio. Interpretation of the recordings was based on normative values (mean $\pm$ 2 standard deviation (SD)) that were established in our own clinical neurophysiology department in 20 subjects with mean age 33 years. The latencies (in milliseconds) of the peaks in this reference material were: peak I $= 1.71 \pm 0.12$; peak III $= 3.8 \pm 0.15$; peak V $= 5.74 \pm 0.23$; and peak I–V $= 3.97 \pm 0.21$. The amplitude ratio I/V < 1. Latencies longer than 2.5 SD of the normal mean values were considered abnormal. The conduction time of any IPL I–V that was equal to or greater than 4.5 ms was rated abnormal.

For statistical analysis of pre- and postoperative audiometric results and for pre-, intra-, and postoperative BAEP data we used the student's paired and unpaired t-Tests.

Intraoperative BAEP recording technique

BAEP were recorded throughout the surgical procedure between a positive electrode located in F_z and a reference electrode located at the earlobe ipsilateral to the stimulation site (A_1 or A_2). The ground electrode was placed on the shoulder. Sterile hypodermic needles placed after anaesthetic induction were used as electrodes. The electrode impedance was below 5000 ohms. Only in a few cases did we use a silverball electrode placed in contact with the cochlear nerve for direct recording of the nerve compound action potential (CAP), because inserting a direct recording electrode requires that the surgeon interrupt the procedure for some time. Our purpose was to develop a method of intraoperative monitoring that would neither interfere with the surgeon's work nor increase the duration of the operation. Between 1985 and 1989 we used a conventional, previously described, technique that did not employ digital filtering [7]. During that time it became clear that it was necessary to average 2000 response in order to obtain a reliable record, which took about 1.30 to 2 minutes, thus causing an unacceptable delay in making reliable neurophysiological data available. For this reason we developed and have used since 1989 a system using an adaptive digital filtering technique that produces new curves of BAEPs every 15 seconds without interfering with surgery [8].

The monitoring system used for this study has been described in detail elsewhere [4]. Briefly, it consists of a one-channel data acquisition system that makes use of a personal computer that also controls all operations. This system fulfills specific criteria for intraoperative monitoring, e.g., it is small in size and is easily portable on a small cart, and it has a high level of automation for on-line data processing and storage.

BAEPs obtained after 200 click stimulations are analog filtered with a filter having a bandwidth of 100-1500 Hz. A moving averaged response is then obtained from a set of 5 to 10 successive BAEPs. A time-frequency optimal digital filter, based on Wiener's filtering theory [3] and a wavelet decomposition of the signal [5], is automatically computed and adaptively updated for each new BAEP. With a stimulus rate of 20 clicks/sec, this provides a new filtered response every 15 sec, corresponding to the brain activity over the previous 2 minutes. Adaptive Wiener filter strategy based on successive sub-averages permits the implementation of algorithms to discard too highly artifacted evoked potentials. Thus, more reliable averaged BAEPs can be obtained within a shorter time.

Our main concern in BAEP monitoring is to be able to identify changes of the response waveform on-line, i.e., to continuously measure latency and amplitude of the waves of interest (waves I, III and V). Relative changes are in general more relevant in such monitoring than absolute comparisons to statistical norms. A computer algorithm that automatically tracks the peaks on successively filtered curves has been implemented [3]. Starting from an initial manual peak identification, local extrema are searched for within a time window centered around each peak. Latency values and peak-to-peak amplitudes are then computed and drawn on the video display as trend curves over a period of hours. Figure 1 illustrates this synthetic presentation of the processed data during a microvascular decompression procedure. Event markers can also be entered and used as indicators of the various surgical phases. Neuromonitoring relies on the fact that high-rate sequential recording increases the redundancy of the measured parameters and makes

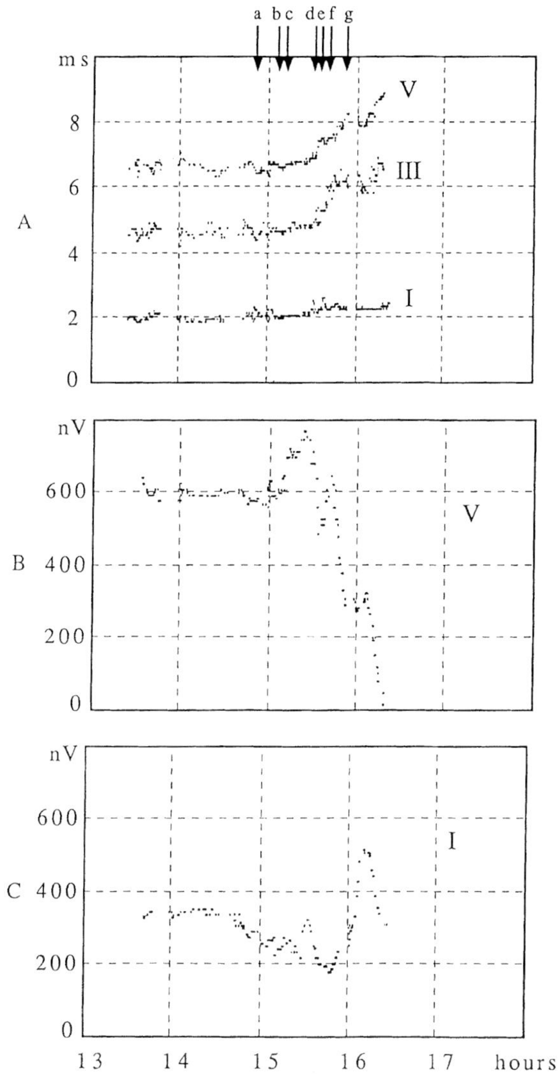

Fig. 1. Trend curves, with automatic detection of waves I, III, and V, of latencies and amplitudes during microvascular decompression to relieve hemifacial spasm and during which considerable changes in the BAEPs occurred. Abscissa: time from onset of the surgical procedure. Ordinate:
A: Latencies of waves I, III, and V in milliseconds. a/dura opening. b/retractor positioning followed by a slight delay of the waves. c/retractor adjusted; waves are stable for a while; d,e,f/warnings during microvascular decompression; g/retractor off; delay of waves is still increasing.
B: Amplitude of wave V in nanovolts. The amplitude of these peaks during the decompression, and at the end of the procedure wave V is seen to be drastically reduced.
C: Amplitude of wave I in nanovolts. Note the increase in the amplitude of wave I during decompression and the trend towards normalization after removing the retractor

the interpretation of response modifications more reliable.

An important additional capability of the monitoring system is to provide on-line data retrieval. Because all BAEP curves are stored, it is possible to recall and grand average previous responses at any time during the surgery. This facilitates global waveform comparison of the ongoing recordings of BAEP with previous responses, e.g., the reference BAEP recorded at the beginning of surgery, the BAEP recorded before retractor positioning, etc. This facility allows one to assess with more confidence a modification of the response. Functional warnings can be given to the surgeon, so that he or she may be able to modify his or her maneuvers, thus preventing the occurrence of strong and sometimes irreversible deterioration of the auditory nerve and the brainstem.

The monitoring equipment is placed in the operating room and the surgical procedure is displayed on a video screen coupled to a camera mounted on the operating microscope. This system enables us to observe the evoked potentials obtained by stimulation of the ear on the operated side and, occasionally, the potentials obtained by stimulation of the contralateral ear.

A reference grand average of BAEPs is obtained after anesthetic induction and prior to skin incision. Another reference BAEP is established after opening the dura mater but before placing the retractor on the flocculus. After placing the retractor, a 10-minute observation period (called the retractor test) is allowed. The surgeon will adjust the retractor if the monitor displays a peak delay of wave V greater than 0.5 ms, or if there are alterations affecting wave I or wave V, or if there are marked changes in the waveform of these waves. If any of these problems were to occur, the surgical procedure would only proceed when the BAEPs became stable. During microvascular decompression of the facial nerve, the occurrence of any alteration in the BAEPs may require a modification of the surgical procedure. Finally, after removing the retractor and during closure of the cutaneous planes, one last grand average of BAEPs is obtained in order to evaluate the patient's final neurophysiological condition.

Results

Pre- and postoperative audiometry

No patient in this study was deaf before surgery. Postoperatively one (female) patient (2.3%) was totally deaf.

Preoperatively, in 5 patients the PTA threshold was equal to or better than 15 dB, including the patient who became deaf postoperatively and whose preoperative PTA threshold (35 dB) was the highest in our series of 42 patients. Postoperatively, the PTA of 8 patients had worsened by 10 dB, as compared to their preoperative values.

Mean preoperative PTA: 12.5 ± 9.2 dB.
Mean postoperative PTA: 20.5 ± 18 dB ($p < 0.001$)

Pre- and postoperative BAEPs

The wave I–V interval was elevated in 5 patients preoperatively and in 12 patients postoperatively. The postoperative BAEPs of the patient who became deaf were totally obliterated. The mean values of IPL I–V and of wave V latency for all the cases ($n = 42$) were calculated and statistically compared (both before and after surgery). The results are as follows:

Mean I–V interval before surgery: 4.16 ± 0.25 ms
Mean I–V interval after surgery: 4.26 ± 0.34 ms ($p < 0.001$)
Mean wave V latency before surgery: 5.85 ± 0.29 ms
Mean wave V latency after surgery: 6.16 ± 0.36 ms ($p < 0.001$)

Changes in BAEP during surgery

The main intraoperative BAEP patterns are illustrated in Figs. 1, 2, 3, and 4.

After anesthetic induction, the mean ($n = 42$) I–V interval (4.57 ± 0.31 ms) was significantly increased compared to the preoperative recordings ($p < 0.001$). After opening the dura mater only minor BAEP changes were noted: I–V interval $= 4.67 \pm 0.4$ ms ($p < 0.04$).

The 10-minute retractor test was carried out for each patient. In 5 cases this test led either to totally abolished BAEPs (3 patients) or abolished waves III and V (2 patients), which required removal or repositioning of the retractor until BAEP components were restored. The patient who became deaf postoperatively had totally abolished BAEPs at this stage, while the 4 other patients had no hearing loss.

The intraoperative delays of peak V due to retraction were > 1 ms in 8 patients, between 0.5 and 1 ms in 10 patients, and equal to or < 0.5 ms in 11 patients. In 8 patients there was no change in BAEP values. The 19 patients with no change or who had a delay $\leqslant 0.5$ ms were operated on during the second half of our study.

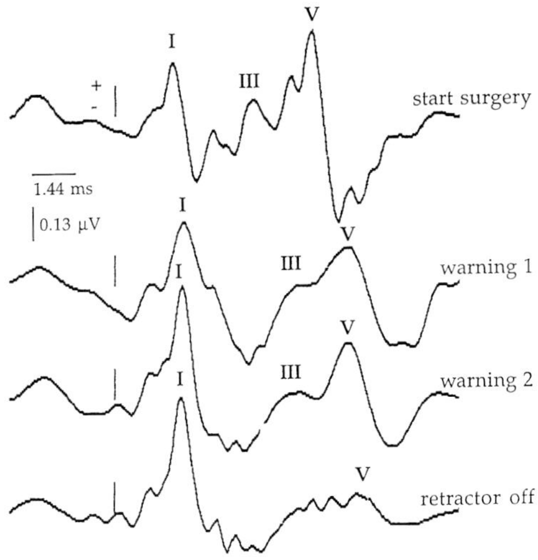

Fig. 2. Same patient as in Fig. 1. Off-line grand averages of 6000 responses. Before dura opening (start of surgery) all waves are present; I–V interval is 4.6 ms. Warning 1: wave V is delayed (+1.0 ms) from the reference grand average, and wave III is abnormal. Warning 2: the delay of wave V is greater (+1.5 ms), and wave I amplitude is increased. At the end of the operation (retractor off) wave V is so small as to be considered transiently absent

The mean duration of retraction required for decompression of the facial nerve was 44 ± 12 minutes. The mean number of warnings displayed on the monitor and of which the surgeon was notified was 1.45 ± 0.8. There was no warning in 5 cases.

The following *observations were made during the microvascular decompression procedures*:

- in 4 patients all BAEP components were abolished: 1 at the end of decompression, 1 very progressively, and 2 very abruptly, particularly in the patient who had not tolerated retraction of the cerebellum and became deaf.
- in 4 patients the structure of BAEPs was impaired, showing only wave I: 3 during dissection and 1 after the use of dacron (Figs. 1 and 2).
- in 6 patients wave V showed a peaking delay · 1 ms: 2 during dissection, 1 after the use of dacron, and 3 progressively; these 3 latter patients required increased retraction (Fig. 3).
- in 12 patients wave V showed a peaking delay in the range 0.6 to 1 ms: 5 after increased retraction, 7 progressively.
- in 15 patients there was a delay of peak V $\leqslant 0.5$ ms and the intraoperative changes were considered negligible (Fig. 4).

The last BAEP grand average was obtained about 30 minutes *after removing the retractor*. The following

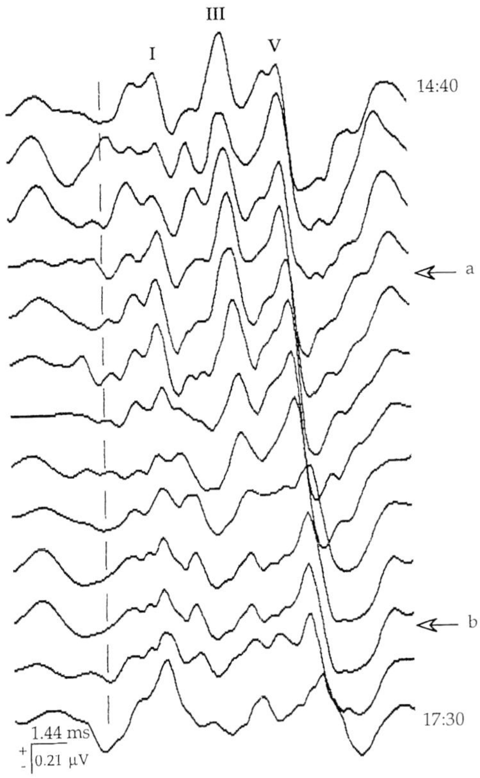

Fig. 3. Typical BAEP changes during microvascular decompression to relieve HFS. Off-line grand averages of 6000 responses. 14:40, start surgery. 17:30, end of monitoring. a/retractor on; b/retractor off. Note the transient decrease of wave I amplitude and the slowly progressive delay of waves III and V

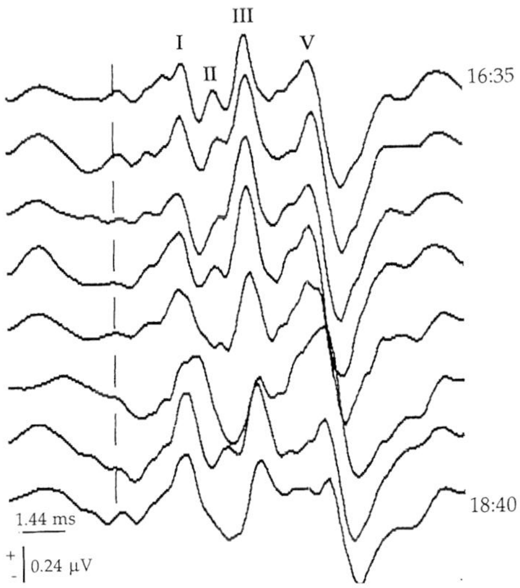

Fig. 4. Off-line grand averages of 8000 responses during BAEP monitoring. No significant modification of BAEPs occurred. At the end of the procedure, the delay in latency of wave V (+0.5 ms) as compared to the reference grand average was considered common

events were then observed: total BAEP obliteration (in 4 patients, including the patient with postoperative deafness), persistence of wave I alone with a latency that was abnormal—between 2.2 and 2.7 ms (in 5 patients), a persistent peak delay larger than 1 ms (in 6 patients), a persistent peak delay between 0.5 and 1 ms (in 12 patients), and a negligible delay of less than 0.5 ms in 15 patients.

Altogether, 42 patients were monitored intraoperatively. It was during the first half of our study that we noted that 4 patients had obliterated BAEPs at the end of surgery, and that in 3 patients only wave I was detectable at the end of surgery. In the second half of our study, BAEP changes were not so considerable.

Discussion

During the past 9 years, 42 patients operated on for HFS had intraoperative monitoring of BAEPs in our institution. Only 1 case of postoperative deafness occurred: the fifth patient, who was a 75 year-old woman and the oldest patient in our series, presented with arteriosclerosis and hearing loss prior to the operation (her PTA was 35 dB). None of the other 41 patients in this study who were treated for HFS complained of hearing loss during the weeks following their operation. The earliest postoperative PTA in 8 of these 41 patients showed an increase in threshold in the PTA in the range 15 to 35 dB.

The purpose of monitoring BAEP intraoperatively is to reduce, as much as possible, the risk of postoperative deafness [10, 11, 12, 14, 15]. In a study by Sindou, 4 of 25 non-monitored cases (i.e, 16%) resulted in postoperative deafness (see chapter by M. Sindou in this book). The results of this study can be compared with the results of the present study in which only 1 patient of 42 who were monitored intraoperatively acquired postoperative deafness. In a recent review of literature dealing with HFS, Wilkins [15] noted that the complication rate tended to diminish in direct correlation with the experience of the surgeon, with the exception of the incidence of significant ipsilateral postoperative hearing loss that did not improve until the institution of intraoperative monitoring of auditory evoked potentials. In Wilkins' own series of 48 patients operated on to relieve HFS, there were 2 cases of postoperative deafness (4%). Before the introduction of intraoperative monitoring of BAEP, 10 of 152 (6.6%) patients who underwent microvascular decompression to relieve HFS or trigeminal neuralgia (tic douloureux) were followed by profound hearing loss or deafness. A study by Barker et al. noted similar results: 2.6% of their patients presented with postoperative ipsilateral deafness. Based on 782 microvascular decompression procedures, they state that before routine monitoring 4.8% of such operations were complicated by ipsilateral hearing loss, whereas since the introduction of routine monitoring this rate has been reduced to 7.9% [2]. Without the use of intraoperative monitoring, a postoperative reduction in hearing may occur in as much as 15% [1] and 16% [9] of patients.

During microvascular decompression to relieve HFS, BAEPs may be altered at various stages. The reference traces that are plotted while the patient is under general anesthesia will be significantly different from the preoperative recordings. The mean delay of peak V may be as much as 0.4 ms, which could be an effect of the anesthetic drugs, the lowered central temperature, and/or the impairment of sound conduction in the middle ear due to artificial ventilation. It is therefore necessary to obtain reference data after anesthetic induction so that the BAEPs recorded continuously during surgery may be reliably interpreted. Positioning the retractor on the flocculus requires particular attention on the part of the neurophysiologist. The deleterious effect of an incorrect positioning of the retractor on the auditory nerve is well-known [13] and if not reversed, changes in the BAEP may increase and thus indicate injury to the auditory nerve that represents a risk of postoperative hearing impairment or postoperative deafness.

In the present study, during microvascular decompression of the facial nerve no noticeable BAEP changes were observed in only 12 of the 42 patients. In 4 patients there was complete BAEP obliteration without reversal before the monitoring ended. It was one of these 4 patients who experienced postoperative deafness. Two patients had transient BAEP obliteration and the others all had delays of the peaks of the BAEP intraoperatively, although in these latter patients the BAEP improved at the end of the operation. In 15 patients there was a delay of peak V of less than 0.5 ms at the end of the operation compared to that at the start of monitoring.

The IPL I–V was abnormal in 13 patients when tested postoperatively. Of these 13 patients, the IPL I–V was normal in 8 before the operation. The changes in IPL I–V noted intraoperatively may reflect a moderate retrocochlear dysfunction.

The technique of intraoperative BAEP monitoring requires training of personnel and, like that of surgery, should improve as the operator's experience increases. This assumption is supported by the fact that in our study the 4 patients with totally obliterated BAEPs were among the first 10 patients who were monitored. There was no sustained obliteration of BAEPs in the 32 remaining patients in our study who were monitored.

Since 1989 we have been using a system that allows us to visualize immediately any modifications affecting the function of the auditory pathways. Little use has been made of the recording of the auditory nerve action potential, as this technique may interfere with the progress of an operation, and we have therefore preferred to optimize the recording of farfield potentials [8]. These plotted curves provide an overall picture of all the data made available by monitoring BAEPs and enable us to check the functional condition of auditory pathways more efficiently during microvascular decompression to relieve HFS. Although the surgeon's skill usually improves with each operation, it is indisputable that BAEP monitoring helps the surgeon to improve the quality of his operative technique.

References

1. Auger RG, Piepgras DG, Laws ER Jr (1986) Hemifacial spasm: results of microvascular decompression of the facial nerve in 54 patients. Mayo Clin Proc 61: 640–644
2. Barker FG, Jannetta PJ, Bissonette DJ, Shields PT, Larkins MV, Jho HD (1995) Microvascular decompression for hemifacial spasm. J Neurosurg 82: 201–210
3. Bertrand O, Garcia-Larrea L, Artru F, Mauguiere F, Pernier J (1987) Brainstem monitoring. I. A system for high-rate BAEP recording and feature extraction. Electroenceph Clin Neurophysiol 68: 433–445
4. Bertrand O, Bohorquez J, Pernier J (1990) Technical requirements for evoked potential monitoring in the intensive care unit. In: Rossini PM, Mauguiere F (eds) New trends and advanced techniques in clinical neurophysiology. Electroenceph Clin Neurophysiol [Suppl] 41: 51–70
5. Bertrand O, Bohorquez J, Pernier J (1994) Time-frequency digital filtering based on an invertible wavelet transform: an application to evoked potentials. IEEE Trans BME 41: 77–88
6. Ciriano D, Sindou M, Fischer C (1991) Apport du monitorage peropératoire des potentiels auditifs précoces dans la décompression vasculaire microchirurgicale pour névralgie du trijumeau ou spasme hémifacial. Neurochirurgie 37: 323–329
7. Fischer C (1989) BAEP monitoring in posterior fossa surgery. In: Desmedt JE (ed) Neuromonitoring in surgery. Elsevier, Amsterdam, pp 191–207
8. Fischer C, Bertrand O (1993) Evoked potentials in posterior fossa surgical lesions. Basic principles and intraoperative monitoring. In: Raimondi A et al (eds) Posterior fossa tumors. Springer, New York, pp 158–168

9. Iwakuma T, Matsumoto A, Nakamura N (1982) Hemifacial spasm. Comparison of three different operative procedures in 110 patients. J Neurosurg 57: 753–756
10. Møller AR, Jannetta PJ (1983) Monitoring auditory functions during cranial nerve microvascular decompression operations by direct recording from the eigth nerve. J Neurosurg 59: 493–499
11. Møller AR, Møller MB (1989) Does intraoperative monitoring of auditory evoked potentials reduce incidence of hearing loss as a complication of microvascular decompression of cranial nerves? Neurosurgery 24: 257–263
12. Radtke RA, Erwin W, Wilkins RH (1989) Intraoperative brainstem auditory evoked potentials: significant decrease in postoperative morbidity. Neurology 39: 187–191
13. Sekiya T, Iwabuchi T, Kamata S, Ishida T (1985) Deterioration of auditory evoked potentials during cerebellopontine angle manipulations. J Neurosurg 63: 598–607
14. Sindou M, Ciriano D, Fischer C (1991) Lessons from brain stem auditory evoked potential monitoring during microvascular decompression for trigeminal neuralgia and hemifacial spasm. In: Schramm J et al (eds) Intraoperative neurophysiologic monitoring in neurosurgery. Springer, Heidelberg, pp 427–431
15. Wilkins RH (1991) Hemifacial spasm: a review. Surg Neurol 36: 251–277

Correspondence: Catherine Fischer, M.D., Lab Neurophysiologie Clinique, Hopital Neurologique, 59 Blvd Pinel, F-69003 Lyon, France.

ENT Surgical treatments of hemifacial spasm

J. Soudant[1], **J. Willer**[2], and **G. Lamas**[1]

[1]Service Otorhinolaryngology, and [2]Neurophysiology and Electrophysiology Research Departments, Groupe Hospitalier Pitie-Salpetriere, Paris, France

Summary

The technique of microvascular decompression in the cerebellopontine angle that was initially described by Jannetta has initiated many questions and has precipitated new work concerning the facial nerve.

Many authors have noted spectacular improvement in patients' HFS following microvascular decompression, but how this technique works is still unclear.

It is known that HFS may have several causes, some of which may be unsuspected. Many methods of treatment, mainly surgical, have had long-lasting results. Thus a single mechanism, which was advocated by Jannetta, is not certain. The peroperative experience of Møller is decisive. Møller demonstrated that HFS disappears as soon as the compressing blood vessel is moved off the nerve, but that the HFS reappears when the vessel is allowed to again touch the nerve. However, this does not prove that HFS is a direct consequence of a conflict, as other techniques are also effective.

The present paper reports on several personal cases of HFS. An attempt is made to list the different causes and the different treatments are described.

Electrophysiologic studies, especially the blink reflex, are combined with a conditioning double stimulation, which led the authors to conclude, in accord with Møller, that probably several factors are involved in the generation of HFS, but that hyperexcitability of the motor nucleus of the facial nerve is always essential. On a strict scientific level, the authors have not declared microvascular decompression to be the single treatment for HFS, because a satisfactory treatment does not necessarily demonstrate a physiopathologic hypothesis and thus validate the theory of a vascular neural conflict.

Key words: Hemifacial spasm, etiology, electrophysiology, treatments, surgery.

1. Introduction

There is no univocal treatment for hemifacial spasm (HFS). Jannetta [1] and Fukushima [2] have shown that microvascular decompression (MVD) of the facial nerve is very effective in alleviating the symptoms of HFS, as have others. However, HFS could probably be caused by many factors, and the best treatment for this condition is still controversial [3].

The results of treating HFS by MVD, as described by Jannetta [1], Fukushima [2], and others have been so successful that the good results achieved using surgical techniques other than MVD may have been overlooked. Such results have included complete recovery from HFS as well as long-lasting improvements, as shown in many cases of long-term follow-up. This is the reason why we must be very skeptical about the unique mechanism of HFS. Thus it is important that we consider surgical techniques other than MVD for treating HFS.

It is not in accordance with a scientific approach to assume that good results with a certain therapy demonstrates the absolute value of a theory that supports this therapy. In fact, we agree with Møller and Jannetta [4], who hypothesized that many factors are probably combined to initiate HFS and to make the condition become prominent at a certain time following a long, asymptomatic period.

We agree with Møller and Jannetta's [4] theory, based on electrophysiological data, that hyperactivity of the motonucleus of the seventh cranial nerve (CN VII) is involved in generating the signs of HFS. In our department, jointly with J.C. Willer, we have studied 7 patients who had typical HFS of confirmed peripheral origin. Of the 7 patients in whom a distal origin was confirmed, 6 underwent decompression of the peripheral portion of the facial nerve, which led to a complete recovery in 4 patients with no recurrence noted at follow-up more than 2 years postoperative;

the other 2 patients were improved at more than 2 years postoperative follow-up, but they still had some degree of spasm (50% improvement). These results are similar to those described by Pulec [5] and demonstrate that true HFS can be caused by a lesion on the facial nerve along its course through petrous bone.

2. Pathophysiology

2.1. Three theories of pathophysiology of HFS

2.1.1. Ephaptic transmission

Ephaptic transmission is assumed to occur directly between nerve fibers because of a contact zone or a close relationship between two active functional areas. It has been assumed that two nerve fibers actually do not need to be in a direct contact for ephaptic transmission to occur. Ephaptic transmission is not mediated through a neurotransmitter, as is synaptic transmission, but rather as an electric transmission. In an experimental procedure, Granit et al. [6] demonstrated how an artificial synapse can be created between afferent and efferent fibers in a peripheral nerve by placing a suture on the sciatic nerve "so gently that impulses were still available." After removing the sutures and irrigating with Ringer's solution these authors noted that the experimentally created synapse completely reversed. Ephaptic transmission is assumed to always occur in one direction, from slow- to fast-conducting fibers. Gardner [7] and Gardner and Sava [8] gave credibility to the ephaptic transmission theory of HFS. The ephaptic hypothesis has also been supported by Nielsen [9], who studied the delayed muscle response elicited by stimulation of the zygomatic branch of the facial nerve and recorded from the mentalis muscle on the HFS side [9–12]. This response has a smaller amplitude than the maximal amplitude obtained in response to direct stimulation of the mentalis branch itself. Nielsen also found the latency of the R_1 response of the blink reflex to be longer on the HFS side than on the normal side. Nielsen [9] noted that hyperventilation causes HFS patients to have tonic and clonic contractions of the lower eyelid and of the submental area, which cease after a short period of apnea. He took this as support for the hypothesis that ectopic excitation in the facial nerve causes HFS.

2.1.2. Hyperexcitability of the facial motonucleus

Ferguson [13] presented the hypothesis that hyperexcitability of the facial motonucleus is the cause of HFS, and he assumed that somehow vascular compression causes that hyperexcitability. This nucleus hypothesis has been supported by intraoperative electrophysiologic studies done by Møller and Jannetta [1] and Møller [14, 15]. These investigators proposed that the damaged area of the facial nerve initiates electric impulses that are transmitted both to the distal portion of the nerve and to its nucleus. The impulses traveling proximally will activate the motoneurons, and over a period of time will make the motonucleus hyperactive and create self-sustained activity in the motonucleus. This supports the hypothesis that it is the neural activity in the facial motonucleus that creates the spasm of HFS (16). This has been described by Møller and co-workers as being similar to the "kindling effect" that is caused by novel input to a nucleus. The kindling effect was first described by Goddard [17] for the amygdala, and it was later found to be a more general principle in that it caused different nuclei to become hyperactive [18]. Digre et al. [19], however, were skeptical of the nucleus hypothesis, because medications that stabilize the nerve cell membrane do not have a noticeable effect on HFS.

2.1.3. Abnormal regeneration of the facial nerve

This theory assumes that it is a lesion on the facial nerve that causes the manifestation of HFS. This hypothesis has not been easily accepted, particularly because most patients with HFS never manifest signs of facial palsy. However, Frueh et al. [20] provided proof of an aberrant regeneration of the facial nerve in 25 of the 60 (42%) patients they studied. Frueh believed that such a condition probably occurs in more patients than expected. Frueh et al. [20] states that "a chronic pressure on the seventh nerve produced by an adjacent pulsating artery, the most common cause of hemifacial spasm, might reasonably be expected to damage the nerve as well as stimulate its firing. Seventh nerve damage is common in HFS, which substantiates the hypothesis that there would be evidence of ipsilateral damage to some or all branches of the facial nerve in most patients with HFS."

2.2. Electrophysiologic signs of HFS

The delayed muscle response has been described as a typical sign of HFS [9]. It is often followed by after-discharges.

The amplitude of the R_1 component of the blink reflex response on the affected side is larger (up to twice the value) than the amplitude of this response on the normal side. This indicates that the number of activated fibers on the affected side is greater. Ninety-seven percent of patients with HFS have a synkinetic response in muscles of the lower face (orbicularis oculi and mentalis muscles) [9].

After facial nerve decompression the abnormal muscle response is no longer present [12, 21–23]. In a study of 60 patients with HFS who underwent MVD in the cerebellopontine angle using Jannetta's technique, it was shown:

- that the abnormal muscle response was present in only 27% of the cases and that after-discharges disappeared in 90% of the cases after the operation.
- that the amplitude of the blink reflex was normal in 100% of the cases, and that postoperatively the R_1 latency was significantly shorter than preoperatively.
- that synkinesis was only present in 13% of the patients, as evidenced from an examination of the blink reflex.

2.3. Is the trigeminal nerve (CN V) involved in HFS?

The trigeminal nerve is generally assumed to provide proprioceptive information from the face, but its role in HFS has not yet been clearly defined. It seems that both CN V and CN VII would participate in the development of HFS, because there are many interconnections between these two nerves. This could be an explanation as to why some treatments that act to block the trigeminal nerve are used to treat a HFS [19, 24].

2.4. New evidence in favor of facial motonucleus hyperexcitation in HFS

Subjects without HFS and patients with HFS have been studied using electrophysiological techniques in order to obtain a better understanding of the pathophysiology of HFS [21, 25–28].

2.4.1. Electrophysiologic technique

Each of the 7 patients in the Poignonec et al. [27] study was comfortably seated in an armchair with his/her upper body tilted backwards at approximately 45 degrees, with the head resting on a pillow to provide good muscular relaxation. The patient was asked to stay still and not speak.

In one patient adequate relaxation could not be achieved because of unrelated major lumbar pain, and the experimental session was thus discontinued. Electromyograms of the facial muscles with measurements of threshold, latency, and conduction velocity were previously obtained in all of the patients with HFS. During a second session, trigeminal-facial reflexes (blink reflexes) were successively studied on the normal side and on the side of the spasm according to the method previously described by Willer and Lamour [25].

In short, we stimulated the supraorbital nerve electrically with bipolar electrodes after identifying the supraorbital notch by means of touch. The stimuli were 0.2-ms square impulses generated by a constant-current stimulator and presented at a rate of 17 pulses per second (pps). The reflex responses were recorded from the right and the left orbicularis oculi muscles and orbicularis oris muscles by surface electrodes placed on the overlying cleansed skin. The responses were monitored on an oscilloscope, from which photographs were taken and processed by a computer in real-time. The recorded potentials were stored on magnetic tape for later processing.

The characteristics of the recorded responses (threshold, latency, and amplitude) were studied in this way following stimulation of the right and the left supraorbital nerves while the patients were relaxed. In the individuals without HFS, the R_1 component of the response is entirely ipsilateral to the stimulation during the first set of experiments. During the second set of experiments [29], the excitability of the early blink response (R_1) was studied using methods described previously. The R_1 response evoked by the stimulation of the ipsilateral supraorbital nerve (stimulation-test) was conditioned by a preceding stimulation of the contralateral supraorbital nerve, the intensity of which was below threshold.

After a period of control (4 to 5 minutes), during which only the stimulus test was carried out, the conditioning stimulation was applied together with the test stimulation to create an interstimulus that varied between 0 and 600 ms.

The response to 10 successive stimulations were obtained at each value of the delay to minimize variability. The same procedure was used on both the normal side and the affected side of the patients with HFS as well as on 5 voluntary subjects from our medical team.

2.4.2. Data analysis

For each subject the numeral values of latencies and thresholds of the R_1 and R_2 responses are expressed in percentage of the average value of the last 40 control responses (100%). (Four normal subjects were tested, and this group was used as a control group—2 males and 2 females. Then the seven patients were tested using the same procedure first on the HFS side and then on the normal side. For each electric stimulation a double choc was used with an interstimulus interval going from 0 to 600 ms. The last 40 responses for each subject and for each double choc (normal and with HFS) were expressed by calculating the average value. This value was said, for each of them, as being the 100% value.) In this way an inter-individual study was made possible.

For each parameter, the mean value with the standard deviation was calculated. The significance, if there were variations using these mean values, were assessed by a factorial ANOVA analysis.

2.4.3. Results

Basic characteristics of the facial trigeminal reflex responses

In normal cases, electrical stimulation of the supraorbital nerve produces a response with two components (R_1 and R_2) in the ipsilateral orbicularis oculi muscle and only the R_2 component in the contralateral orbicularis oculi muscle. The latency of the R_1 component was 10.8 ± 0.16 mse and its threshold was 1.84 ± 0.08 mA. The R_2 component was bilateral, with a mean latency 33.88 ± 1.04 ms and its threshold was slightly lower than that of the R_1 component (1.69 ± 0.9 mA). These reflex responses were generated in the orbicularis oculi muscle only when a subject was in a state of muscular relaxation, and no response could be detected in the orbicularis oris muscle or in the mentalis muscles in response to stimulation of the supraorbital nerve. When a subject initiated selective and moderate voluntary contractions, either of the orbicularis oris muscle or of the mentalis muscles, a blink reflex response appeared in the muscle that was activated (synkinesis). The blink reflex response was similar (in latency, shape, and duration) to the R_1–R_2 complex that was recorded from the orbicularis oculi muscles.

In patients with HFS the general organization of the blink reflex is different from normal subjects.

Indeed, stimulation of the supraorbital nerve on the affected side evoked blink reflex responses with an R_1–R_2 complex in all of the muscles of that side of the face—the orbicularis oculi, orbicularis oris, and mentalis muscles, and these responses in all three muscles had a similar threshold (1.45 ± 0.08 mA). The latency of the R_1 response, which is the more stable of the two components, was 11.5 ± 0.5 ms, 13.8 ± 0.4 ms, and 14.4 ± 0.4 ms in the orbicularis oculi, orbicularis oris, and mentalis muscles, respectively.

The R_1 component of the blink reflex is seen to follow stimulation at even high rates (up to 0.5 Hz), as is typical of an oligosynaptic reflex response. On the other hand, the R_2 component has the characteristics of a polysynaptic reflex with variable shape, long and variable latencies, and signs of habituation when the stimulus rate is increased to 0.25 Hz.

Excitability cycle of the R_1 component

The excitability of the R_1 response was studied using a conditioning technique with double shocks, with the delay between the conditioning stimulus applied to the contralateral supraorbital nerve and the stimulus being varied between 0 and 600 ms. We have used this technique on both the normal and the affected sides of patients with HFS. In subjects without HFS we used this technique during a complete relaxed state and during voluntary and prolonged moderate contractions. The EMG activity could be monitored by all subjects through a loudspeaker so that the subject could maintain his/her voluntary contraction.

When the results obtained in patients with HFS were compared with the results from subjects who did not have HFS, it appears that the excitability of the R_1 component of the blink reflex on the normal side of the patients with HFS was not different from that obtained in the subjects who did not have HFS. The conditioning stimulus produced a facilitation of the R_1 component (50%) that was significant ($t = 6.95$, $P < 0.001$, $N = 7$) at 30 ms interstimulus delay, and the facilitation reached 140% at 50 ms interstimulus delay. The facilitation progressively decreased with increasing interstimulus delay, but it remained significant up to an interstimulus delay of 80 ms (+25% of facilitation) ($t = 3.11$, $P < 0.05$, $N = 7$). There was no noticeable effect from contralateral stimulation for longer intervals between the conditioning stimulus and the stimulus (from 90 to 600 ms). On the HFS side, there was a facilitating effect of the conditioning stimulus within a larger range of delays, and it reached significance ($t=4.29$, $P<0.01$, $N=7$) at no delay between conditioning stimulus and the stimulus (simultaneous stimulations), at which level it increased the amplitude of the R_1 component by 38%. The facilitation reached a higher peak (+220%) than what was obtained on the normal side at a delay of 60 ms. The facilitation progressively decreased with increasing delays, but remained significant for longer delays than what was the case for the normal side. At a delay of 80 ms the facilitation was approximately 80%. The facilitation was not significant beyond 300 ms ($t=2.15$, not significant, $N=7$) where it was 18%.

Thus the change in the excitability of the R_1 component of the blink reflex response as a function of delay between a contralaterally-applied conditioning stimulus is similar to what it is on the normal side. However, this change tends to be identical to the one recorded on the HFS side during a sustained moderate voluntary contraction of the orbicularis oculi muscles.

This study, using contralateral conditioning of the blink reflex, has thus demonstrated that the change in the excitability of R_1 component of the blink reflex response, as a function of the delay between the (ipsilateral) stimulus and the (contralateral) conditioning stimulus, is similar in both the involved orbicularis oculi muscle and the orbicularis oris muscle. This shows indications of a hyperexcitability of the entire population of motoneurons of the facial nerve. On the other hand, on the normal side and in normal subjects at rest, we recorded no spontaneous ectopic reflex response, neither did we find any response to be enhanced by double shock stimulations.

2.4.4. Discussion

The results of this study indicate that facial motoneurons in the entire motonucleus of the facial nerve are hyperexcitable in patients with HFS, and there is evidence of an abnormal crossing of the R_1 component of the blink reflex in the orbicularis oculi muscle on the HFS side when stimulating the contralateral supraorbital nerve. The presence of synkinesis of the blink reflex responses, including both the R_1 and the R_2 components in the orbicularis oris and mentalis muscles on the HFS side but not on the normal side or in a normal individual at rest, is in agreement with earlier results Frueh et al., 1990. However, we interpret the underlying mechanisms for the synkinesis differently from Nielsen [11], who assumed that the synkinesis was caused by ephaptic transmission in the facial nerve at the site of compression by a vascular loop that would result in a cross-transmission of the blink reflex response to all of the branches of the facial nerve. Although the ephaptic transmission hypothesis may be probable, our qualitative results suggest that synkinesis that causes the blink reflex response to occur in all facial muscles is more likely a result of a diffuse hyperexcitability of the entire motonucleus of the facial nerve. The finding that there is a crossed R_1 component in the response demonstrates that the motoneurons of the orbicularis oculi muscles are hyperexcitable.

Another factor in favor of the hypothesis that the synkinesis in HFS is a result of hyperexcitability of the facial motonucleus is the fact that a blink reflex response (with an R_1 and R_2 component) can be recorded in the orbicularis oris and the mentalis muscles during voluntary contractions of individuals who do not have HFS. This finding makes it unlikely that ephaptic transmission is the cause of the synkinesis of the blink reflex that has been observed in patients with HFS, and that such synkinesis can be physiologically present under certain experimental conditions in individuals who do not have HFS.

There is also quantitative evidence that supports the hypothesis that the signs of HFS are caused by a central hyperexcitability of the motonucleus of the facial nerve. Thus the larger increase in excitability of the R_1 component of the blink reflex produced by a contralateral conditioning stimulus on the HFS side is an indication of hyperexcitability of the motonucleus of the facial nerve [29]. The fact that this hyperexcitability occurs on the HFS side over a larger range of delays (up to 200 ms) compared to the normal side indicates that the facial motonucleus on the affected side is more excitable than it is on the normal side. This was demonstrated in the orbicularis oculi muscle as well as in the other muscles on the affected side of patients with HFS. The early facilitation of the R_1 response on the affected side suggests that the motoneurons of the facial nerve that generate the R_2 component receive facilatatory input from similar oligosynaptic channels that originates from both ipsi- and contralateral pathways.

The finding that a moderate voluntary contraction of the orbicularis oculi muscle in a subject who does not have HFS increases the excitability of the R_1 response in a way similar to that seen on the affected side of a patient with HFS demonstrates that a neural circuitry that can cause such central hyperexcitability of the entire facial motonucleus is present in all individuals, but it is activated at rest only on the side of the lesion in patients with HFS.

Since this hyperexcitability is also physiologically recorded in a normal individual during voluntary contractions, it seems to be directly related to an increase in the basal tones of these motoneurons.

In patients with HFS, this central hyperexcitability and the increase in the basal tones of the motoneurons of the facial nerve may have been brought about by the "irritation" of the facial nerve at the site of vascular contract, thus continuously stimulating the motoneurons with an antidromal influx initiated in this focus.

3. Etiology

In accordance with common methods, we will classify HFS in patients with symptomatic HFS and in those with essential HFS (with postparalytic HFS being considered a particular case). Several studies of the etiology of HFS have been published. Digre et al. [19], after reviewing the literature, reported on the etiology of HFS in 1688 reported cases as follows:

Vascular causes	509
Tumors	19
Bony abnormalities	7
Others	4
Unspecified	986
Unknown-essential	163

(all confirmed by imaging techniques, surgery, or autopsy)

Sprick and Wirtschafter [30] studied patients with HFS who were treated with botulinum toxin, and after reviewing the literature, reported that of 1676 patients with HFS the number of tumors recorded was only 9. However, only 52% of the patients with HFS who were treated with botulinum toxin had a radiologic investigation using computer tomograph (CT-scan) or magnetic resonance imagery (MRI).

3.1. Vascular etiology

Jannetta (see Chapter by Jannetta in this volume) reported a compressing vessel in 98% of the operated patients. The vascular conflict was caused either by an artery (loop, mega-dolicho- artery, malformation, etc), a vein, or both. The authors of the present paper [as well as the others] found that a vessel at the root exit zone of the facial nerve was involved in every case.

3.2. Bony abnormalities

Many bony abnormalities, such as the following, have been described as possibly causing HFS:

Paget's disease, osteogenesis imperfecta, abnormalities of the cranio-facial junction, occipital bone hyperplasia, stenosis of the internal auditory canal [5]. Systemic diseases such as multiple sclerosis [31, 32]. Cholesteatomas [5, 19, 32].

3.3. Distal traumatisms of the facial nerve [20, 33–35]

3.4. Inflammatory diseases [5]

Cerebellopontine angle arachnoiditis [36].

Inflammation of the sheath of the facial nerve in the petrous bone. This type of inflammation has been described by Pulec [5] as a possible cause of HFS, and we have also seen 7 cases of HFS related to a lesion in the petrous bone. Five of these 7 cases were obvious, but in 2 cases we found no significant lesion. A histologic examination of the inflammatory portion of the nerve sheath that was observed during facial nerve decompression noted an "unspecified inflammation of the sheath".

3.5. Familial HFS

There are indications that HFS can have a genetic disposition. Friedman et al. [38] reported on five members of the same family within three generations who were suffering from typical HFS on the left side.

4. Treatment for HFS

Alt-hough Micro-Vascular Decompression (MVD) seems to be the best treatment for HFS (39), it is important to know that many different treatments have been used with more or less of success.

4.1. An injection of botulinum toxin seems to give HFS patients some relief for a period of 3 to 4 months and, therefore, should be repeated as needed. However, complications with this treatment have been described and many patients do not elect to continue such injections after three or four years. Møller (personal communication) has expressed worries about the long-term risks related to the accumulation of botulinum toxin in the body.

4.2. *Non-selective symptomatic treatments, such as facial nerve blocks with morphine* [19, 40], may provide improvement for 1 to 2 months, but have side-effects such as pain and transitory facial paralysis. *Alcohol* is also a symptomatic treatment that was used in the past for peripheral neurologic disorders. A solution of 60-80% alcohol was injected in front of the mastoid at the stylomastoid foramen until the face was paralyzed. The paresis characteristically persisted for months and the spasm would have been absent for 1–2 years [41].

Other methods have been used in order to perform a facial nerve block while preventing post-treatment fibrosis. *Pricking (needling)* the nerve with a needle without any injection [5, 42] has been reported to give 10 months relief from HFS. This method of needling has also been combined with thermotherapy by heating the needle at a temperature of 55 degrees Celsius, with some temporary results.

4.3. *Sectioning of the facial nerve and anastomosis* of the facial nerve with CN XII have been tried. Surprisingly, recurrences of HFS have been seen after such operations [43].

4.4. Fan [44], in his study of 33 patients with HFS in whom *longitudinal incisions of the facial nerve in the cerebellopontine angle* were made via a retrosigmoid approach, reported excellent results in 26 of the 33 patients (78%), 6 of them having a very mild HFS postoperatively that disappeared completely between 3 and 13 days after the operation. Twenty of these 33 patients who were followed postoperatively were free of spasm for more than 1 year, with only 1 patient experiencing a recurrence.

4.5. Youngs et al. [45] *decompressed the facial nerve in the mastoid segment* to create damage to the nerve in its peripheral course to the geniculate ganglion. Nine patients in this study had initially good results with clinical resolution of HFS for at least 1 month following surgery. Four of the patients experienced later recurrence of HFS to varying degrees. Two patients, both undergoing revision procedures, received no subjective benefits from surgery. Paulsen and Neveling, whose technique is described in a report by Pfaltz and Podvinec [quoted in 46], performed a microcoagulation of the facial nerve via a spiral pathway. But the selectivity is, at least, hazardous. In 1974, Castillo [46], using the same spiral pathway approach, severed through half the diameter of the nerve and prevented a "regrowth" of the nerve by interpositioning a piece of silicone. Scoville [46], performed a partial resection of the nerve, but extended it down to the stylomastoid foramen. No definite facial palsy was reported after any of these operations, but there was a recurrence of the HFS that was less pronounced than before the operation. Stieda and co-workers [46], and then Nosik and Weill [46], partially sectioned the terminal branches of the facial nerve in the parotid gland and obtained similar results. Miehlke [47] performed a resection that was more than 5 millimeters long in order to avoid a regeneration. After a short period of paresis in the area of this part of the facial nerve, recovery of facial function occurred shortly after 5 weeks, but 9 of the 28 patients in this series had recurrence of HFS within 2 years postoperatively.

4.6. *Selective neurectomy* of the facial nerve was introduced by Fisch and Esslen [48]. The principle is to resect all involved extratemporal branches of the facial nerve and none of the others. After dissection of the facial nerve in the parotid area, each of the extratemporal branches are stimulated electrically with a bipolar electrode in order to identify the branches. The branches of the facial nerve that are producing the hyperkinetic facial movements are divided and coagulated, and a clip is applied on each of them (Fisch [46], found that revision surgery was easier and took less time than a primary operation). All of the branches for the orbicularis oculi muscles and all of the superior branches for the orbicularis oris muscles are divided. In a study of 191 patients having any kind of hyperkinesia, 94 of them had HFS. Of these 191 patients, 90 were operated on to relieve HFS or blepharospasm. Sixty-nine had follow-up examinations between 1 and 12 years (39 HFS and 30 blepharospasm patients). Twenty-six percent of the patients who underwent operation to relieve HFS had no postoperative HFS, 26% had a 75% improvement in their HFS, 28% had a 50% improvement in their HFS, and the remaining 20% were poorly or not improved at all [47]. Of the 8 patients who had unsatisfactory results, 6 of them had been reoperated on using the same technique with good results. On 7-year follow-up, 80% of the patients were satisfied, but Fisch noted his belief that the greater experience of the surgeon, the better the results.

The success rate of this operation differs among different investigators. Marinello and Sade [46], reported an 80% success rate, Sade [46] reported a 100% recurrent rate, Diamond and Frew [49] noted that it was impossible to reoperate on a patient, and Fisch [46] expressed no difficulty at all.

4.7. Pfaltz and Podvinec [46] described *selective funicular neurectomy* as a treatment for HFS. This technique is related to the organization of the fibers in a nerve. These investigators decompressed the facial nerve in its mastoid segment, opened the nerve sheath, and stimulated the fibers electrically, after which they separated the nerve in very small bundles; 30 to 50% of the nerve fibers that are involved in the abnormal facial movements of the patient are resected as long as 5 mm. Following this procedure there is always a facial palsy which takes 6 weeks to recover. Three patients in Pflatz and Podvinec's report had been operated on using this method. One patient had been nonsymptomatic for more than 8 years, and the other two had a partial recurrence after one and five years postoperatively, respectively.

4.8. Selective thermocoagulation was described by Chauveau [50]. This method for treating HFS is based on a stimulation- coagulation of the terminal branches of the facial nerve performed transcutaneously. These investigators describe the main difficulty to be in detecting the correct branches and then to coagulate them by using the coagulator. This procedure is performed under local anesthesia. Chauveau reported that 50% of his patients had very good results, with improvement of the HFS that lasted for several years. He also noted three incomplete remissions and one failure. One patient suffered a paralysis of the orbicularis oculi muscle.

Conclusions

HFS is a rare disease and therefore only a few surgeons have extensive experience in its treatment. The pathophysiology of HFS is still controversial, as is its etiology. A peripheral lesion of the facial nerve in the petrous bone should be considered to be a cause of HFS.

In cases where no lesion is diagnosed, a vascular exploration of the root entry zone has to be done, but this must be performed by a team of very specialized surgeons.

References

1. Jannetta PJ (1986) Microvascular decompression for hemifacial spasm. In: May M (ed) The facial nerve. Thieme, New York, pp 499–508
2. Fukushima T (1984) Results of posterior fossa microvascular decompression in the management of hemifacial spasm. Facial N Res Jpn 4: 9–14
3. Adams CBT (1989) Microvascular compression: an alternative view and hypothesis. J Neurosurg 57: 1–12
4. Møller AR, Jannetta PJ (1986) Physiological abnormalities in hemifacial spasm studied during microvascular decompression operations. Exp Neurol 93: 584–600
5. Pulec JL (1972) Idiopathic hemifacial spasm: Pathogenesis and surgical treatment. Ann Otol 81: 664–676
6. Granit R, Leksel L, Skoglund CR (1944) Fibre interaction in injured or compressed region of nerve. Brain 67: 125–140
7. Gardner WJ (1966) Crosstalk, the paradoxal transmission of a nerve impulse. Arch Neurol 14: 149–156
8. Gardner WJ, Sava G (1962) Hemifacial spasm. A reversible pathophysiologic state. J Neurosurg 19: 240–247
9. Nielsen VK (1988) Electrophysiology of hemifacial spasm. In: May M (ed) The facial nerve. Thieme, New York, pp 487–497
10. Esslen E (1957) Der Spasmus facialis eine Parabiosserscheinung: Elektrophysiologische Untersuchungen zum Entstehungsmechanismus des Facialisspasmus. Dtsch Z Nervenheil 176: 149–172
11. Nielsen VK (1984) Pathophysiological aspects of hemifacial spasm. Part I. Evidence of ectopic excitation and ephaptic transmission. Neurology 34: 418–426
12. Nielsen VK, Jannetta PJ (1984) Pathophysiological aspects of hemifacial spasm. Part III. Effects of facial nerve decompression. Neurology 36: 891–897
13. Ferguson JH (1978) Hemifacial spasm and the facial nucleus. Ann Neurol 4: 97–103
14. Møller AR (1987) Hemifacial spasm: Ephaptic transmission or hyperexcitability of the facial motor nucleus? Exp Neurol 98: 110–119
15. Møller AR (1993) Cranial nerve dysfunction syndromes: Pathophysiology of microvascular compression. In: Barrow DL (ed) Neurosurgical Topics Book 13. Surgery of Cranial Nerves of the Posterior Fossa, Chapter 2. American Association of Neurological Surgeons, Park Ridge, Illinois, pp 105–129
16. Fligny I, Lamas G, Soudant J, Azerad J, Willer JC (1993) Etude electrophysiologique du reflexe de clignement chez le rat Wistar. An electrophysiological investigation into the rat's blink reflex. CR Acad Sci Paris, Life Sci 316: 598–602
17. Goddard GV (1964) Amygdaloid stimulation and learning in the rat. J Comp Physiol Psychol 58: 23–30
18. Wada JA (1981) Kindling 2. Raven Press, New York
19. Digre KB, Corbett JJ, Smoker WR, McKuskers S (1988) CT and hemifacial spasm. Neurology 38: 1111–1113
20. Frueh BR, Preston RA, Musch DC (1990) Facial nerve injury and hemifacial spasm. Am J Ophthalmol 110: 421–423
21. Auger RG (1979) Hemifacial spasm: Clinical and electrophysiological observations. Neurology (NY) 29: 1261–1272
22. Auger RG, Piepgras DG (1989) Hemifacial spasm associated with epidermoid tumor of the cerebellopontine angle. Neurology 39: 577–580
23. Auger RG, Whisnant JP (1990) Hemifacial spasm in Rochester and Olmsted County, Minnesota, 1960 to 1984. Arch Neurol 47: 1233–1234
24. Kitahara M, Saito H (1984) Hemifacial spasm, the role of the trigeminal nerve. In: Portmann M (ed) The facial nerve. Proceedings of the Fifth International Symposium on the Facial Nerve (held in Bordeaux, France, September 3–6, 1984). Masson, New York Paris, pp 49–53
25. Willer JC, Lamour Y (1977) Electrophysiological evidence for a facio-facial reflex in the facial muscles in man. Brain Res 119: 459–464
26. Willer JC, Lamas G, Fligny I, Soundant J (1993) Hypoglosso-facial anastomosis alters excitability of hypoglossal motoneurons in man. Neurosci Lett 155: 212–215

27. Poignonec S, Vidailhet M, Lamas G, Fligny I, Soudant J, Jedynak P, Willer JC (1994) Electrophysiological evidence for central hyperexcitability of facial motoneurons in hemifacial spasm. Eur Arch Otorhinolaryngol [Suppl] 216–217
28. Kugelberg E (1952) Facial reflexes. Brain 75: 385-396
29. Willer JC, Roby A, Boulu P, Boureau F (1982) Comparative effects of electroacupuncture and transcutaneous nerve stimulation on the human blink reflex. Pain 14: 267–278
30. Sprick C, Wirtschafter JD (1988) Hemifacial spasm due to intracranial tumor. An international survey of botulinum toxin investigators. Ophthalmology 95: 1042–1045
31. Telischi FF, Grobman LR, Sheremata WA, Apple M, Ayyar R (1991) Hemifacial spasm: Occurrence in multiple sclerosis. Arch Otolaryngol Head Neck Surg 117: 554–556
32. Biezenbos van de JBM, Horstink MWIM, Vlasakker van de CJW, Engelen van BGM, Eikema Hommes OR, Barkhof F (1992) A case of bilateral alternating hemifacial spasm. A brief report. Mov Disord 7: 68–70
33. Martinelli P, Gabellini AS, Lugaresi E (1983) Facial nucleus involvement in post-paralytic hemifacial spasm. J Neurol Neurosurg Psychiatry 46: 586–587
34. Martinelli P, Giuliani S, et al (1992) Hemifacial spasm due to peripheral injury of facial nerve: A nuclear syndrome? Mov Disord 7: 181–184
35. Parisi L, Ferrante L, et al (1990) On a case of early onset post-traumatic HFS. Zentralbl Neurochir 51: 223–224
36. Laine E, Graux P, Fontan M (1951) A propos de 2 nouvelles observations d'hemispasme facial gueri par une intervention sur une arachnoidite de l'angle ponto-cerebelleux. Rev Neurol (Paris) 84: 38–40
37. Adler CH, Zimmerman RA, Savino PJ, Bernardi B, Bosley TH, Sergott RC (1992) Hemifacial spasm. Evaluation by magnetic resonance imaging and magnetic resonance tomographic angiography. Ann Neurol 32: 502–506
38. Friedman A, Jamrozik Z, Bojakowski J (1989) Familial hemifacial spasm. Mov Disord 4: 213–218
39. Loeser JD, Chen J (1983) Hemifacial spasm: Treatment by microsurgical facial nerve decompression. Neurosurgery 13: 141–146
40. Gowers WR (1897) A manual of diseases of the nervous system, 2nd edn. Blakiston Publishing, Philadelphia
41. Russel JSR (1910) Facial spasm. In: Allbut C, Rolleston HD (eds) A System of Medicine, Volume 8. Macmillan, London, pp 638–649
42. Wakasugi B (1972) Facial nerve block in the treatment of facial spasm. Arch Otolaryngol 95: 356–358
43. Stennert E, Limberg R, Laskawi R, Haubrich J (1984) Recurrence of hemifacial spasm after hypoglossal-facial nerve anastomosis. In: Portmann M (ed) The facial nerve. Proceedings of the Fifth International Symposium on the Facial Nerve (held in Bordeaux, France, September 3–6, 1984). Masson, New York Paris, pp 48
44. Fan Z (1993) Intracranial longitudinal splitting of facial nerve: A new approach for hemifacial spasm. Ann Otol Rhinol Laryngol 102: 108–109
45. Youngs R, Ludman H, Smith S (1988) Transtympanic surgery for hemifacial spasm. An electrophysiological study. Clin Otolaryngol 13: 331–333
46. Portmann M (1984) The facial nerve. Proceedings of the Fifth International Symposium on the Facial Nerve (held in Bordeaux, France, September 3–6, 1984). Masson, New York Paris, p 56
47. Miehlke A (1981) Management of hemifacial spasm. In: Samii M, Jannetta PJ (eds) The cranial nerves. Springer, Berlin, pp 478–483
48. Fisch U, Esslen E (1972) The surgical treatment of facial hyperkinesia. Arch Otolaryngol 95: 400–405
49. Diamond C, Frew I (1979) The facial nerve. Oxford University Press, Oxford
50. Chauveau JM (1990) L'hemispasme facial essentiel, nouvelle technique therapeutique par la stimulation-coagulation transcutanee des branches de terminaison du nerf facial au niveau de la face. Medical Thesis, Faculty of Medecine, Paris, France. (French Faculties will supply anyone with any thesis upon request)

Correspondence: Prof. Jacques Soudant, Service ORL, Groupe Hospitalier Pitie-Salpetriere, 47 —83, bd de l'Hopital, F-75013 Paris, France.

Pharmacology of hemifacial spasm

H. Ollat

Association pour la Neuro Psycho Pharmacologie (A.N.P.P.), Paris, France

Summary

For many years carbamazepine and baclofen have been the only pharmacological treatments for hemifacial spasm (HFS), but their efficacy is low and they have noticeable side-effects.

Local injections of botulinum toxin (Bo-Tx) is now the reference treatment for HFS. This toxin binds selectively to cholinergic presynaptic endings of the peripheral nervous system (motor endplates and postganglionic parasympathetic fibers), translocates into presynaptic cytosol, and inhibits vesicular release of acetylcholine, resulting in muscular paralysis. Bo-Tx is very effective in treating HFS but is not truly appropriated to its pathophysiology. In addition, it may have adverse side-effects due to spreading beyond its target, and it may induce plastic changes in the peripheral nervous system.

Key words: Hemifacial spasm, anticonvulsants, botulinum toxin, motor endplate, acetylcholine release.

Introduction

Carbamazepine and baclofen were the first two pharmacological treatments considered to be efficacious in the treatment of hemifacial spasm (HFS) [15], although controlled studies on their use have never been performed. However, their efficacy has been proven to be rather low; according to some investigators carbamazepine (600-1200 mg/day) provides only 20% complete resolution of the spasm and only 30-35% good and durable improvement, and baclofen (40-60 mg/day) is even less efficacious [2, 3, 21].

Carbamazepine and baclofen have pharmacokinetic properties that hamper their utilization. Thus carbamazepine (CBZ) is nearly totally metabolized, mainly by epoxydation. Among the metabolites, CBZ-E is very active. The reason for differences in sensitivity to treatment with CBZ may be that the quantities of CBZ that are transformed into CBZ-E vary among individuals [4]. Because CBZ is an enzymatic inductor that is able to increase its own metabolism, which results in its plasmatic half-life being noticeably reduced during prolonged administrations, it is often recommended to control plasmatic levels of CBZ when starting the treatment and after 3–4 weeks of administration. CBZ can also increase the metabolism of numerous other drugs and thereby reduce their efficacy. Baclofen also has important individual variations in its absorption and its elimination during prolonged administrations. In addition, it is important to note that both CBZ and baclofen have numerous adverse side effects (see Table 1) [16]. Some of the side effects of CBZ are due to too high plasmatic levels but they disappear when the daily dose is reduced. The most frequent side effect of treatment with CBZ is of a sedative nature, which occurs slowly over a period of time as a result of chronic CBZ intoxication, and the risk is that it goes unnoticed or that when noticed may be attributed to other causes such as brain aging for example. Other side effects of CBZ are of the idiosyncratic type, which necessitate immediate cessation of the treatment. Such side effects are often severe but fortunately they are also very rare. The main undesirable side effects of treatment with baclofen are also sedative in nature, and which, like those of CBZ, cease when the daily dosage is reduced.

The low efficacy of treatment with these drugs and their noticeable side effects can explain why CBZ and baclofen have been supplanted by botulinum toxin for treating HFS when the latter became available. Nevertheless, knowledge acquired from using these drugs CBZ and baclofen to treat HFS and analyses of their mechanisms of action on HFS have helped to clarify the pathophysiology of HFS. Compared with these two drugs, the effectiveness of botulinum toxin (Bo-Tx) in reducing the symptoms of HFS is high and its mechanism of action is well known, although the latter

Table 1. Adverse side-effects of carbamazepine and baclofen (from 16)

Carbamazepine Related to plasmatic levels	Idiosyncrasic type	Baclofen
Sedation		Sedation
Cronic intoxication	Exanthemes	
	Hypersensibility syndrome	Cardiorespiratory depression
Digestive symptoms	Anemia, agranulocytosis	Hypotension
Extrapyramidal signs	Lyell's epidermolysis	Confusional state
Biological endocrine effects	Stevens-Johnson's syndrome	Ataxia
Decrease of seric folates	Acute hepatitis	Digestive symptomes
Induction of hepatic enzymes		Vertigo

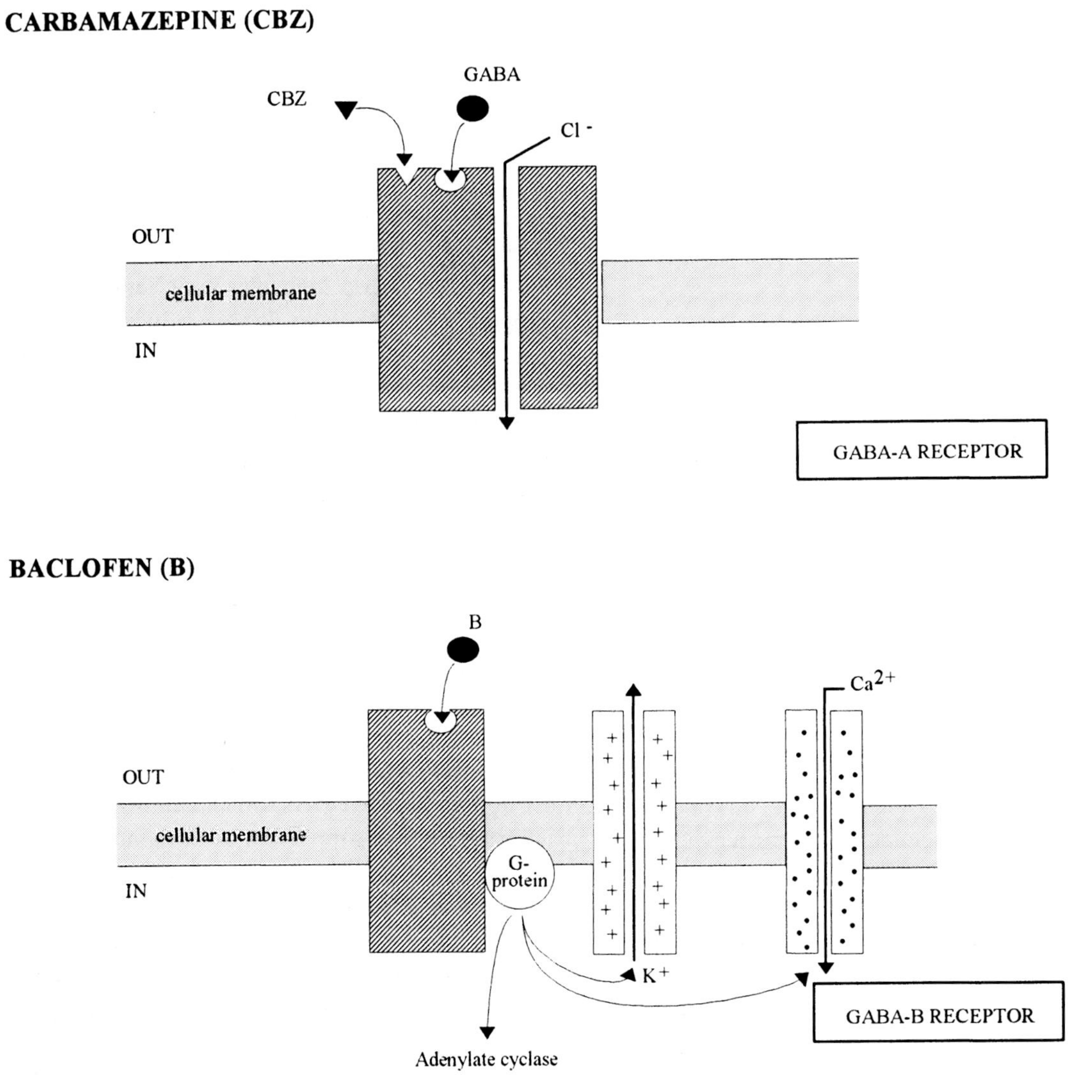

Fig. 1. Schematic drawing of the neurobiochemical effects of the drugs carbamazepine and baclofen

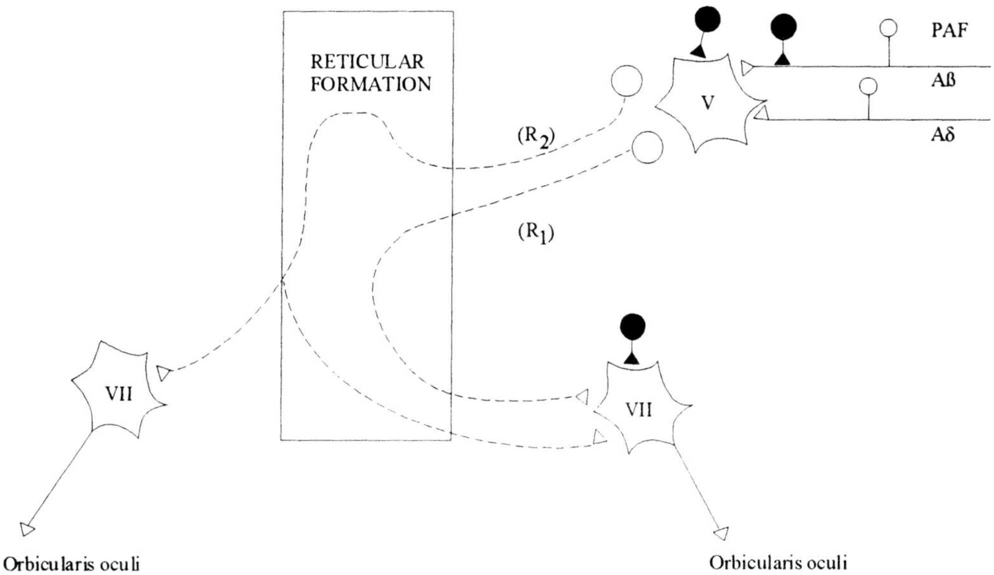

Fig. 2. Schematic drawing of the blink reflex and its control by GABAergic interneurons. Primary afferent fibers (*PAF*) of the blink reflex are A type (those of the corneal reflex are A type); they make synapses on trigeminal nucleus neurons (*V*). A polysynaptic chain of interneurons (dashed lines) links the trigeminal nucleus and the facial motor nucleus (*VII*) innervating the orbicularis oculi muscle (ipsilaterally for R_1 and bilaterally for R_2). GABAergic interneurons (black) make synapses on motor neurons, sensitive neurons, and presynaptic endings of PAF

does not affect the functional disturbances that cause HFS (or other abnormal movements).

Mechanisms of action of carbamazepine and baclofen

Although there have been no specific studies of the mechanisms of action of CBZ and baclofen on HFS, other studies have provided enough information in this regard to allow the presentation of three hypotheses on these mechanisms:

a) baclofen and CBZ may reduce transmission between primary afferent fibers and trigeminal neurons
b) baclofen affects excitability in motor neurons (as suggested in studies of patients with spastic disorders), and
c) baclofen and CBZ affect nociceptive transmission (as suggested in studies in animals).

CBZ and baclofen are GABAergic agonists (Fig. 1). CBZ is a benzodiazepine; it binds to specific receptors associated with GABA-A receptors and increases the chloride influx induced by their stimulation.

Baclofen is a direct agonist; it binds to GABA-B receptors and stimulates them, which results in an increase in potassium efflux or a decrease in calcium influx.

An increase in chloride influx or potassium efflux induces a hyperpolarization of the cellular membrane, thereby causing the cell to be less excitable.

A decrease in calcium influx into axonal endings reduces the presynaptic release of neurotransmitters and thus, theoretically, CBZ and baclofen would be able to act directly as well as indirectly on facial motor neurons, as suggested by the organization of the blink reflex (Fig. 2): GABAergic interneurons make synapses with facial motor neurons, trigeminal nucleus neurons, and primary afferent fibers; GABAergic agonists, such as CBZ and baclofen, could therefore reduce the excitability of facial and trigeminal neurons and thereby decrease neural transmission between primary afferent fibers and trigeminal neurons. Some of these effects have been confirmed by clinical and experimental studies [21].

Electrophysiological studies in patients with spastic disorders showed that baclofen:

a) reduces the excitability of spinal alpha motor neurons,
b) reduces the activity of intrinsic spinal circuits that have excitatory effects on alpha motor neurons (such as the circuits involved in the flexor reflexes), and
c) facilitates presynaptic inhibition of primary afferent fibers [5, 17].

Table 2. GABAergic agonists and neuronal transmission in the trigeminal spinal nucleus (pars oralis) (from 9)

	Ethosuximide	Valproate	CBZ Phenytoine	Baclofen
Segmental excitation	no effect	no effect	depression	depression
Segmental inhibition	depression	depression	facilitation	facilitation
Descending inhibition	depression	depression	depression	facilitation
Descending excitation	no effect	depression	depression	no effect

Fromm and colleagues showed that baclofen and CBZ reduce the efficacy of excitatory influx afferent to the trigeminal spinal nucleus. These investigators recorded the neuronal responses of the trigeminal spinal nucleus to stimulation of the maxillar nerve in anesthetized cats both without a conditioning stimulus (simple segmental excitation) and with a conditioning stimulus that induced either a segmental inhibition, a descending inhibition, or a descending excitation. These studies showed that CBZ and baclofen share two properties that pure anticonvulsive drugs do not have (see Table 2): a) they depress segmental excitatory transmission and b) they facilitate the mechanisms of segmental inhibition. In addition, baclofen facilitates the mechanisms of descending inhibition and CBZ depresses the mechanisms of descending excitation (for a review see 9).

It is thus possible that the effects of baclofen on HFS result from its actions on several types of neurons and neuronal circuitries: for example, it may cause a reduction in the excitability of facial motor neurons and reduce the efficacy of excitatory influx reaching them. The effects of CBZ on HFS may mainly be due to a potentiation of the efficacy of circuits inhibiting facial motor neurons. It thus seems that these two drugs may act to reduce an abnormal activity of facial motor neurons, but it seems unlikely that either drug would have any effect on the ephaptic transmission between fibers of the facial nerve. Thus, the low clinical effectiveness of these two drugs may be taken as an indication that the pathophysiology of HFS can be ephaptic transmission just as well as hyperactivity of the facial motor nucleus.

Botulinum toxins

Botulinum toxins are synthesized by Clostridium botulinum, a strictly anaerobic bacterium, and they are probably the most powerful of the biological and chemical toxins.

Botulinum toxins specifically inhibit the release of acetylcholine by cholinergic endings of the peripheral nervous system, such as the motor endplates of skeletal muscles and postganglionic parasympathetic fibers. Clostridium botulinum synthesizes seven kinds of toxins (A, B, C1, D, E, F and G) in this way. These substances all have the same structure but they are coded by different genes that were recently cloned. The pharmacological properties of these different substances and their powers as toxins are different. Type A botulin toxin, used in patients, is most powerful (see reviews by Simpson: 25, 26). It should be noted that Clostridium botulinum produces toxins other than those noted above, such as C2 and C3, which have different effects but the same mechanism of action [1, 12, 27].

After that thousands of people who ate domestic tinned foods have been poisoned by botulinum toxins, the A type of the botulinum toxin came into use as a treatment for muscle hyperactivity of various kinds beginning at the end of the seventies, thanks to A.B. Scott, an ophthalmologist from San Francisco who was the first to use them to treat strabismus [22, 23]. Later its indications were quickly expanded to treat abnormal movements of the face as well as of the limbs (see Table 3).

Table 3. Current clinical indications for botulic toxin injections

Blepharospasm
Hemifacial spasm
Spasmodic torticollis
Oromandibular dystonia
Laryngeal dystonia (adductor type)
Occupational dystonias
Laryngeal dystonia (abductor type)
Spasticity
Tremor
Detrusor-sphincter dyssynergia
Rectal sphincter spasm

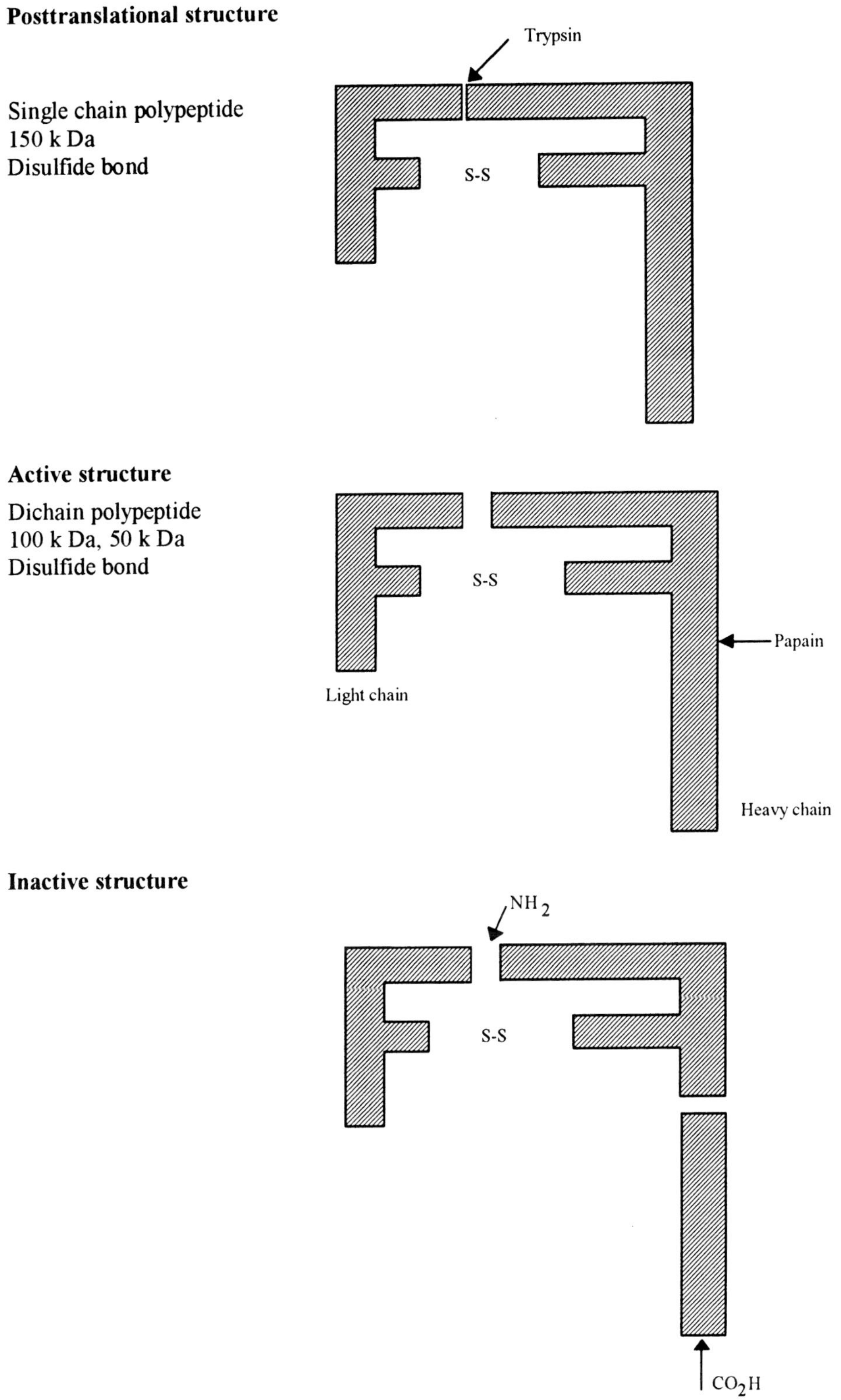

Fig. 3. Diagram of post-translational, active, and inactive structures of botulinum toxins (from 25)

Synthetic botulinum toxins, known as Bo-Txs, are synthesized as relatively inactive single chain polypeptides that contain at least one disulfide bond (Fig. 3). Their cleavage by trypsin produces an active and bicatenary molecule with a heavy chain (100 kDa) and a light chain (50 kDa) linked by a disulfide bond. A supplementary cleavage provided by papain cuts the heavy chain into two segments of equivalent molecular

Table 4. Structure of Botulinum toxin (Bo Tx), Tetanus toxin (Te Tx) and Diphteria toxin (Di Tx) (modified from 25)

	Bo Tx	Te Tx	Di Tx
Origin	Clostridium botulinum	Clostridium tetanus	Corynebacterium diphteria
Post translational structure	Single chain polypeptide	Single chain polypeptide	Single chain polypeptide
Active structure	Dichain polypeptide	Dichain polypeptide	Dichain polypeptide
Molecular weight			
Heavy chain	100 kDa	100 kDa	40 kDa
Light chain	50 kDa	50 kDa	20 kDa
Ratio	2:1	2:1	2:1
Binding domain	Carboxyterminus of heavy chain	Carboxyterminus of heavy chain	Carboxyterminus of heavy chain
Channel forming domain	Aminoterminus of heavy chain	Aminoterminus of heavy chain	Aminoterminus of heavy chain
Enzyme domain	C_2, D:light chain	?	Light chain
Site of action	Peripheral cholinergic terminals	Central inhibitory synapses	Systemic protein synthesis

weight. None of the three segments of Bo-Tx has toxic effects by itself; only holotoxin blocks the release of acetylcholine and a breaking of the disulfide bond inactivates Bo-Tx as well [24].

It should be noted that the structure of Bo-Txs is comparable to those of toxins synthesized by Clostridium tetani or by Coryne bacterium diphtheria (see Table 4). Type C2 botulinum toxin is synthesized as two polypeptide chains (100 and 50 kDa), which are not linked but which must act together to induce toxic effects [24].

Neurotoxic effects of Bo-Txs result from a three-step process that was described by Simpson [28]: 1) the toxin binds in a specific way to presynaptic membranes of peripheral cholinergic nerve endings; 2) the toxin then translocates into the presynaptic cytosol; 3) the release of acetylcholine then becomes inhibited.

The presynaptic binding has been proven, and its characteristics have been precisely determined by the use of iodine-labeled toxin : it is very fast and important (150-500 sites/μm^2 of membrane), saturable, and poorly reversible. This presynaptic binding also has a low dependence on both temperature and the activity of the cholinergic nerve endings. Above all, the binding of Bo-Txs is very specific to cholinergic nerve endings (for example Bo-Txs can bind to noradrenergic nerve endings but the necessary concentrations are one hundred times higher than those which are sufficient to block cholinergic transmission) [25].

The binding of Bo-Txs is probably made possible by the carboxyterminus of its heavy chain. It should be stressed that the binding site is different from the antigenic site and that, consequently, antibodies can still neutralize the toxin at this step. The presynaptic receptors are unknown. Membrane gangliosides or other proteins containing sialic acid are probably involved but their functions would more likely be to concentrate toxin molecules next to their receptors and/or to facilitate their cytosolic translocation [6, 7, 8].

The cytosolic translocation of Bo-Txs has also been studied using labeled toxin, and the results show that the mechanisms are probably the same as those of the Diphtheria toxin (see Fig. 4); namely, that a Bo-Tx is internalized after binding in vesicles formed by an invagination of the presynaptic membrane during endocytosis, and then endosomes migrate to combine with lysosomes and that during this migration intraendosomial pH decreases and the conformation of the toxin changes. At the same time, an aminoterminal of the heavy chain enters the vesicular membrane, after which its light chain finally gets through the formed channel.

This mechanism explains that an activation of cholinergic fibers shortens the delay of paralysis, because the nervous activity induces an exocytosis and then a compensatory endocytosis. It also explains that chloroquine, a drug raising the intraendosomial pH, can antagonize the effects of Bo-Tx [26].

It should be stressed that the translocational process is specific to peripheral cholinergic nerve endings ; Bo-Tx can bind to central cholinergic nerve endings, but very high concentrations are needed to inhibit their release of acetylcholine [11].

The paralytic phase is the last phase of the neurotoxic process. Bo-Tx inhibits the vesicular (quantic)

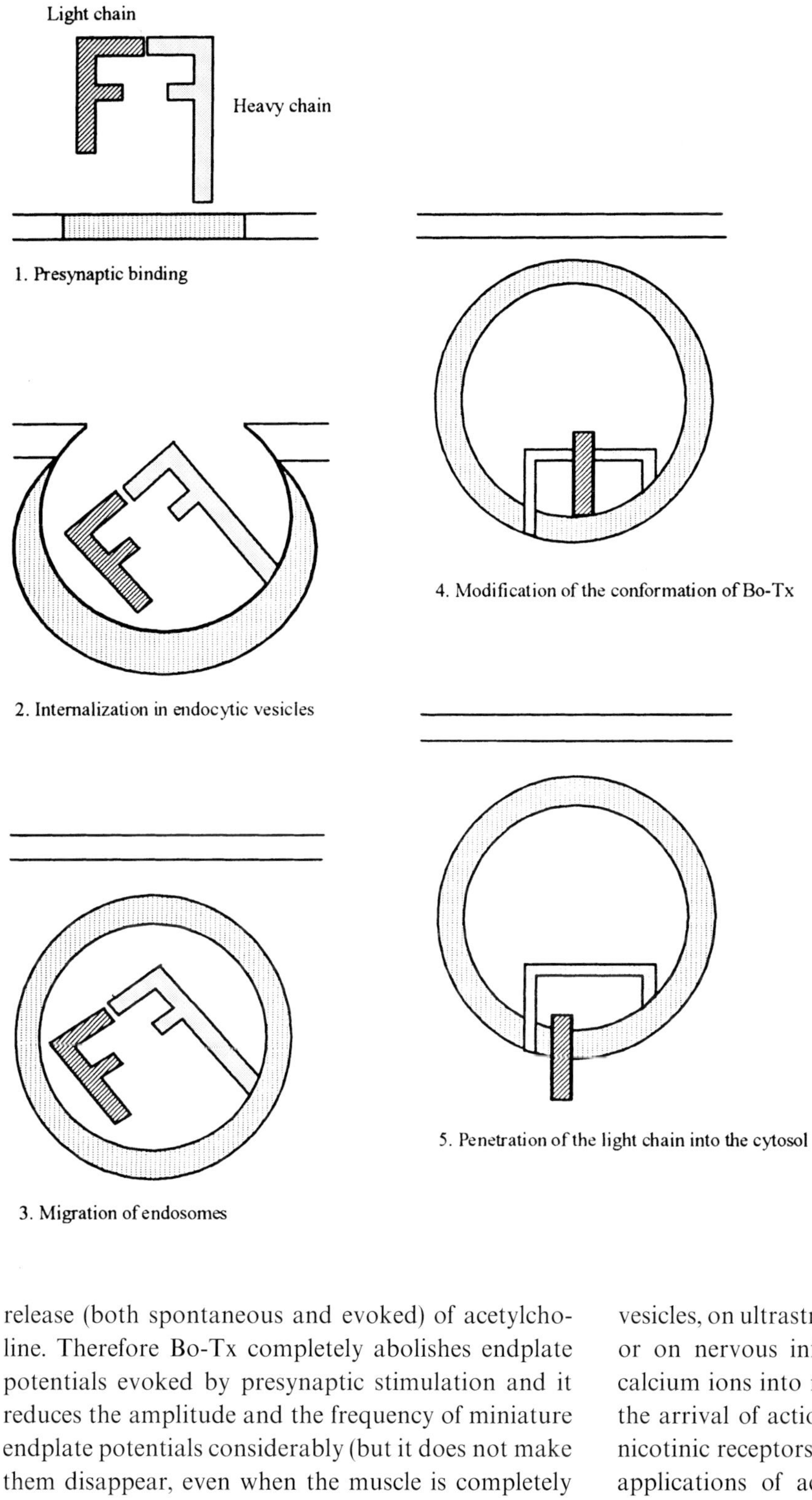

Fig. 4. Diagram of the mechanism of the cytosolic translocation of botulinum toxin (from 25)

release (both spontaneous and evoked) of acetylcholine. Therefore Bo-Tx completely abolishes endplate potentials evoked by presynaptic stimulation and it reduces the amplitude and the frequency of miniature endplate potentials considerably (but it does not make them disappear, even when the muscle is completely paralyzed).

Bo-Txs' effects on the molecular release of acetylcholine have been discussed by several investigators [19, 30]. Bo-Txs have no effect on synthesis or vesicular storage of acetylcholine, on the number of synaptic vesicles, on ultrastructure of cholinergic nerve endings, or on nervous influx transmission and entrance of calcium ions into nerve endings that are triggered by the arrival of action potentials. Bo-Txs do not block nicotinic receptors, because they still respond to local applications of acetylcholine (or nicotine) even in a paralyzed muscle [8]. It thus seems that Bo-Txs disturb the exocytic process itself, and the most likely hypothesis for this is that it reduces the effects of Ca^{2+}, but the exact mechanisms of this action are not precisely understood [28].

Table 5. ADP-ribosylating activity of bacterial toxins (modified from 1)

Toxin	Substrate	Consequences
Diphteria Pseudomonas	Elongation Factor 2	Inhibition of protein synthesis
Cholera	Gs protein	Permanent activation of Gs
Pertussis Anthrax	Gi protein	Permanent inhibition of Gi
Clostridium ● perfringens ● spinoform ● difficile ● botulinum (C_2)*	Actin (monomeric form)	Inhibition of actin polymerization Disorganization of cytoskeleton
Clostridium botulinum ● C_3 ● C_1, D	Protein "ras-like"	Disorganization of exocytosis (?)

*C_2 acts only on actin of smooth muscles and not on actin of skeletal muscles

Several bacterial toxins, and particularly some toxins synthesized by Clostridium botulinum, have an ADP-ribosyl transferase activity that catalyzes the transfer of an adenosine-diphosphate-ribose on an amino acid of a proteic substrate. Their substrates, and then their effects, vary (see Table 5). The C2 type of the toxin, which is not strictly speaking a Bo-Tx, inhibits actin polymerization and disorganizes the cytoskeleton. The C3 type of the toxin and the true Bo-Tx types C1 and D act on "ras-like" proteins, which are GTP-binding proteins of low molecular weight, probably involved in the guidance of synaptic vesicles to the presynaptic active zones. Other Bo-Txs are devoid of ADP-ribosyl transferase activity, but they likely have another enzymatic activity that allows them to inhibit the phosphorylation of synapsin I (dephosphorylated synapsin I stows synaptic vesicles in the cytoskeleton, and its phosphorylation releases them and enables them to migrate to the active zone) [24].

In conclusion, although botulinum toxin is very effective in treating HFS and its mechanism of action is well known, it is not truly appropriate for serving the pathophysiology of HFS because its effectiveness is achieved by its ability to block normal neuromuscular transmission, which is not disturbed in patients with HFS.

The side effects of botulinum toxin injection is another negative aspect. The usual opinion is that these injections only induce a little cumbersome local and transitory side-effects due to the spreading of the botulinum toxin beyond its target. In patients with HFS (or blepharospasm) such spreading of the toxin produces mainly ptosis, diplopia, and/or eversion of the lower eyelid (10–30% of the cases); more serious side effects such as facial paralysis, dysphagia, or modifications in lachrymal secretion are rarely observed. However, when the side effects become too severe and/or are too cumbersome we can control them by administering 3,4-diaminopyridine; this substance, which is also used in the treatment of Lambert-Eaton Syndrome, acts by extending the opening of the presynaptic voltage-dependent calcic channels and then increasing the release of dependent-calcium acetylcholine.

Systemic effects from botulinum toxin injections are very rare, which is amazing because the botulinum toxin can enter the blood system and block cholinergic transmission at the level of the autonomic nervous system and because vegetative disorders are quite ordinary in cases of botulism. Actually, the amount of botulinum toxin that can spread to and through the circulatory system are probably too weak to have effects that can be easily detected in the clinic; however, paraclinical investigations have detected some effects of botulinum toxin that were a distance from the injection site and that involved the skeletal musculature and cardiovascular reflexes [10].

Single fibre electromyography recorded from muscles distant to the site of botulinum toxin injection in response to stimulation of the motor nerve gave responses that indicated a neuromuscular transmission disorder similar to that noted in patients with botulism. Such an indication did not exist before the treatment with botulinum toxin, it appeared precociously, and it increased over a period of several weeks: the time between the action potential that was recorded at the level of the motor nerve and that which was recorded at the level of the muscle fibre was abnormally long and very fluctuable; this "jitter" was reduced by increasing the frequency of the nerve stimulations. These anomalies can be explained by two non-exclusive mechanisms: a reduction in the release of acetylcholine or a terminal sprouting of the motor axons responsible for the creation of neuromuscular junctions in excess. In support of the former hypothesis, it is noteworthy that the "jitter" may depend on the frequency of the nerve stimulations, but this has not been confirmed by all investigators [18]. In support of the latter hypothesis, there were two observations made in this study when the muscles intoxicated by the injection of botulinum toxin were recuperating : a) sprouting and collateralisation of the terminals of the motor axons, which develop a few days after the presynaptic blockage and that are made in excess, so that a unique muscular fibre is often innervated by several neurons; b) synthesis and membrane incorporation of new nicotinic receptors by inactivated muscular fibres [13, 32]. This axonal sprouting process, which is likely initiated by a tropic factor synthesized by the inactivated muscle, could explain the reduction in the effect of the botulinum toxin that occurs in some patients.

Moreover, systematic studies of cardiovascular reflexes point out anomalies in 80% of patients treated with botulinum toxin. These anomalies consisted of variations in the R–R interval, modifications in pulse and blood pressure due to hyperpnea or orthostatism, and disorders of adaptation to effort [10].

Some investigators have reported side effects of the botulinum toxin other than those noted above, but these have not yet been confirmed. For example, the development of antitoxin antibodies when treatment with botulinum toxin is prolonged has been reported, which could explain the decrease in the therapeutic effects of such treatment as well [14, 31].

In the future we should continue to study the pathophysiology of HFS and develop experimental models, such as the one developed by Saito and Møller [20] in order to develop pharmacological treatments for this disorder that are better suited to its pathophysiology. Such treatments would be expected to be effective but devoid of the adverse side effects that we presently see in botulinum toxin treatments.

References

1. Aktories K, Hall A (1989) Botulinum ADP-ribosyltransferase C3: A new tool to study low molecular weight GTP-binding proteins. Tips 10: 415–418
2. Arthurs B, Flanders M, Codere F, Gauthier S, Dresner S, Stone L (1987) Treatment of blepharospasm with medication, surgery and type A botulinum toxin. Can J Ophthalmol 22: 24–28
3. Auger RG, Litchy WJ, Casano TL, Ahlskog JE (1992) Hemimasticatory spasm: Clinical and electrophysiologic observations. Neurology 42: 2263–2266
4. Bertilsson LF, Tomson T (1986) Clinical pharmacokinetics and pharmacological effects of carbamazepine and carbamazepine-10,11-epoxide. An update. Clin Pharmacokin 11: 177–198
5. Delwaide PJ (1985) Electrophysiological analysis of the mode of action of muscle relaxants in spasticity. Ann Neurol 17: 90–95
6. Dolly JO, Halliwell JV, Black JD, Williams RS, Pelchen-Matthews A, Breeze AL, Mehraban F, Othman IB, Black AR (1984) Botulinum neurotoxin and dendrotoxin as probes for studies on transmitter release. J Physiol 79: 280–303
7. Dolly JO, Black J, Williams RS, Melling J (1984) Acceptors for botulinum neurotoxin reside on motor nerve terminals and mediate its internalization. Nature 307: 457–460
8. Dolly JO, Ashton AC, Evans D, Richardson PJ, Black JD, Melling J (1987) Molecular action of botulinum neurotoxins: role of acceptors in targeting to cholinergic nerves and in the inhibition of the release of several transmitters. In: Dowdall MJ, Hawthorne J (eds) Cellular and molecular basis of cholinergic function. Ellis Horwood, Chichester, United Kingdom, pp 517–535
9. Fromm GH (1985) Effects of different classes of antiepilectic drugs on brainstem pathways. Fed Proc 44: 2432–2435
10. Girlanda P, Vita G, Nicolosi C, Milone S, Messina C (1992) Botulinum toxin therapy: Distant effects on neuromuscular transmission and autonomic nervous system. J Neurol Neurosurg Psychiatry 55: 844–845
11. Gundersen CB (1980) The effects of botulinum toxin on the synthetis, storage and release of acetylcholine. Prog Neurobiol 14: 99–119
12. Habermann E, Dreyer F (1986) Clostridial neurotoxins: Handling and action at the cellular and molecular level. Curr Top Microbiol Immunol 129: 93–179
13. Holland RL, Brown MC (1981) Nerve growth in botulinum toxin poisoned muscles. Neuroscience 6: 1167–1179
14. Jankovic J, Brin MT (1991) Therapeutic uses of botulinum toxin. N Engl J Med 324: 1186–1194
15. Jesel MM, Isch-Treussard C (1964) Essai de traitement de l'hémispasme facial primitif par le tegretol (Geigi). Rev Otoneuro-ophthal 39: 130–135
16. Loiseau P, Larousse C, Bourin M (1984) Antiepileptiques. Sem Hop Paris 60: 2741–2764
17. Milanov IG (1992) Mechanisms of baclofen action on spasticity. Acta Neurol Scand 85: 305–310
18. Olney RK, Aminoff MJ, Gelb DJ, Lowenstein DH (1988) Neuromuscular effects distant from the site of botulinum neurotoxin injection. Neurology 38: 1780–1783
19. Polak RL, Sellin LC, Thesleff S (1981) Acetylcholine content and release in denervated or botulinum poisoned rat skeletal muscle. J Physiol 319: 253–259
20. Saito S, Møller AR (1993) Chronic electrical stimulation of the facial nerve causes signs of facial nucleus hyperactivity. Neurol Res 15: 225–231
21. Sandyk R, Gillman MA (1987) Baclofen in hemifacial spasm. Int J Neurosci 33: 3–4
22. Scott AB (1980) Botulinum toxin injections into extraocular muscles as an alternative to strabismus surgery. Ophthalmology 87: 1044–1049
23. Scott AB (1981) Botulinum toxin injection of eye muscles to correct strabismus. Trans Am Ophthalmol Soc 79: 734–770
24. Sellin LC (1985) The pharmacological mechanism of botulism. Tips 6: 80–82
25. Simpson LL (1981) The origin, structure and pharmacological activity of botulinum toxin. Pharmacol Rev 33: 155–188
26. Simpson LL (1982) The interaction between aminoquinolines and presynaptically acting neurotoxins. J Pharmacol Exp Ther 222: 43–48
27. Simpson LL (1984) Molecular basis for the pharmacological actions of clostridium botulinum type C2 toxin. J Pharmacol Exp Ther 230: 665–669
28. Simpson LL (1986) Molecular pharmacology of botulinum toxin and tetanus toxin. Ann Rev Pharmacol Toxicol 26: 427–453

29. Spitzer N (1972) Miniature endplate potentials at mamalian neuromuscular junctions poisoned by botulinum toxin. Nature 237: 26–27
30. Stanley EF, Drachman DB (1983) Botulinum toxin blocks quantal but non non-quantal release of Ach at the neuromuscular junction. Brain Res 261: 172–175
31. Tsui JK, Wong NLM, Wong E, Calne DB (1988) Production of circulating antibodies to botulinum A toxin in patients receiving repeated injections for dystonia. Ann Neurol 23: 181 (Abstract)
32. Yee WC, Pestronk A (1987) Mechanisms of postsynaptic plasticity: Remodeling of the junctional acetylcholine receptor cluster induced by motor nerve terminal outgrowth. J Neurosci 7: 2019–2024

Correspondence: Hélène Ollat, M.D., Association pour la Neuro Psycho, Pharmacologie (A.N.P.P.), 25 rue de la Plaine, F-75020 Paris, France.

Hemifacial spasm: treatment with botulinum toxin (a report of 50 patients)

C. Vial and **A. Vighetto**

EMG Laboratory, Botulinum Toxin Clinic, Hôpital Neurologique, Lyon, France

Summary

In this study the effectiveness of botulinum toxin injection in a group of 50 consecutive patients with hemifacial spasm was investigated. Two hundred and thirty injections were performed over a period of 46 months. Each patient received 2 to 12 injections (mean = 4.5). Mean delay of reinjection was 17.4 weeks. Mean duration of effective relief from spasms following all injections was 15 weeks. Ninety percent of patients improved more than 70%. Efficacy is maintained for up to 12 injections. Complications were noted in one-third of the injections: blurred vision (7.4%), excessive upper facial weakness (5.2%) or excessive lower facial weakness (5.6%), ptosis (4.3%), tearing (3.5%), and dry eye (1.7%). Any systemic effects were registered. Some questions related to botulinum toxin treatment are addressed.

Key words: Hemifacial spasm, botulinum toxin, treatment.

Introduction

The clinical application of the known potent muscle paralytic effect of botulinum toxin (BT) was pioneered by Scott [21] in the pharmacologic treatment of strabismus. Use of BT in treating blepharospasm and hemifacial spasm (HFS) was investigated in 1985 [8, 20, 22]. Assessment was given in 1989 by the American Academy of Ophthalmology [2] and in 1990 by the American Academy of Neurology [17]: "Local injections of BT into facial muscles are accepted as a safe and efficacious modality in treating the hyperkinesis of HFS." Herein we report our own experience in a series of 50 patients.

Material and methods

Population

Fifty patients with primary HFS (36 women and 14 men) were selected for the present study. All were patients referred to our outpatient Botulinum Toxin Clinic between June 1990 and March 1994 for treatment of HFS, and all had at least two sessions of BT injections. This present population was a part of the series of 61 patients who were presented in another chapter of these Proceedings (see Vighetto and Vial in this book). The average age of the patients was 60 years, ranging between 22 and 82 years. There were 17 patients (13 women and 4 men) with right-sided HFS and 33 patients (23 women and 10 men) with left-sided HFS (66%). The average duration of the symptoms prior to treatment was 7.5 years, ranging between 8 months and 37.5 years. All patients initially underwent a complete neurologic examination. Computer tomography (CT-scan) or magnetic resonance imagery (MRI) was performed on all patients to rule out symptomatic HFS.

Prior to this study, 19 of the patients were treated with carbamazepine without satisfactory effect (no effect in 10, side effects in 4, and insufficient effect in 5 patients). Two patients underwent a microvascular decompression (MVD) operation previously, with only a transient efficacy.

Initial visit

A severity score (0–4) was determined on the first visit to evaluate the intensity of each patient's HFS: 0 = no spasm (0 patients); 1 = mild, barely noticeable spasm (2 patients); 2 = mild spasm without functional impairment (17 patients); 3 = moderate functional impairment (26 patients); 4 = severe muscle involvement and synkinesis (5 patients).

BT Treatment

Botulinum toxin-A, supplied by Porton (United Kingdom), was prepared in two dilutions: first concentration of 20 units/0.1 ml for upper facial muscles, and second concentration of 5 units/0.1 ml for lower facial muscles. Intradermic or subcutaneous injections were administered with a 30-gauge needle on a 1-ml syringe. After informed consent was obtained from the patient, injections were given at 3 to 5 sites in the upper facial territory, including the medial and lateral pretarsal upper lid, the lateral pretarsal lower lid, the lateral canthal angle, and the medial brow. Injections in the upper lid were administered slowly to prevent the intradermic diffusion of liquid away from the injection site and to avoid levator weakness and ptosis. Injections were never given in the lower facial territory during the first time injections were given but only on subsequent visits, if necessary. The sites of injection in the lower facial territory were: the zygomatus, the levator labii, and the lateral part of the orbicularis oris muscle. After accruing one year of experience, we changed the latter sites of injections to more external sites (Fig. 1) to avoid drooping of the corner of the mouth.

The dose of BT was modified, if necessary, at each session: it was increased if the expected effects were insufficient in quality or duration, and decreased if complications were reported. When indicated, the modification was about 25% of the previous dose. The goal of these adjustments was to obtain for each patient an appropriate dose that would lead to the cessation of HFS within at least 3 months or, if there was any weakness in the usual movements of the face movements, it should not be easily detected.

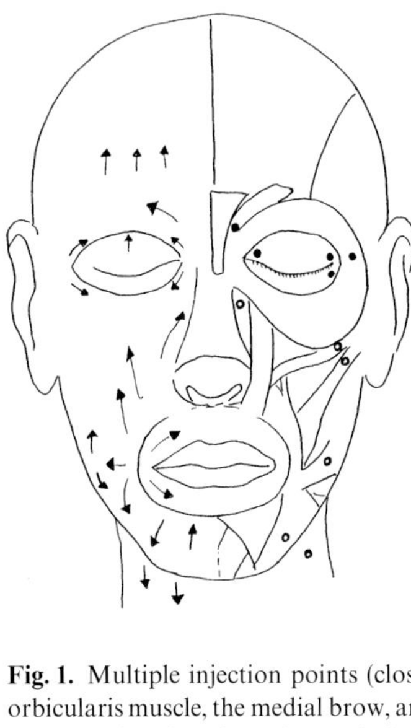

Fig. 1. Multiple injection points (closed circles ●) in the pretarsal orbicularis muscle, the medial brow, and the lateral canthal angle. In the lower facial territory (open circles ○), injection points must be distant from the corner of the mouth (levator labii superioris, zygomatus, risorius, depressor anguli oris, platysma). Arrows indicate the action of the muscles

Clinical assessment

To comprehend the overall benefits of treatment, the patients were systematically asked on each visit to estimate the percentage of improvement in their condition as compared to the initial status. Each patient was informed that the estimated percentage had to take into account both the duration and the quality of improvement, as well as any side effects. Patients were also asked to record when their improvement began and how long was the total duration of their spasm-free period. The duration of the effect of each injection session was considered not to be the time of relief before the patient's condition returned to its baseline condition, but more often as the time between the last injection session and when their symptoms and discomfort reappeared. For this purpose, each patient was given a questionnaire and was asked to write down their assessment of the severity (mild or severe) and duration (more or less than 15 days) of any side effects. At examination muscle weakness was considered to be a side effect when it was excessive (e.g., Charles Bell's sign or drooping of the corner of the mouth). Patient evaluation was performed one month after the first injection and at each reinjection session.

The injections were repeated every 3 months, but in case of sustained improvement they were delayed until the reappearance of HFS.

Results

A total of 230 injections were given to the 50 patients over a period of 46 months. Each patient received 2 to 12 injections, with a mean value of 4.5 injections. Mean delay of reinjection was 17.4 weeks (range of 4 to 52 weeks). For upper facial muscles mean doses of BT were 50 ± 16 units (range of 20 to 160 units), and for lower facial territory mean doses of BT were 10 ± 5.5 units (range of 1.5 to 40 units). In the lower facial territory, only 102 injections were performed. The results are summarized in Fig. 2.

Following the first injection, 80% of the patients experienced a beneficial effect of at least 75% improvement in HFS (Fig. 2A) and only 2 patients had no improvement. An analysis of global results for 230

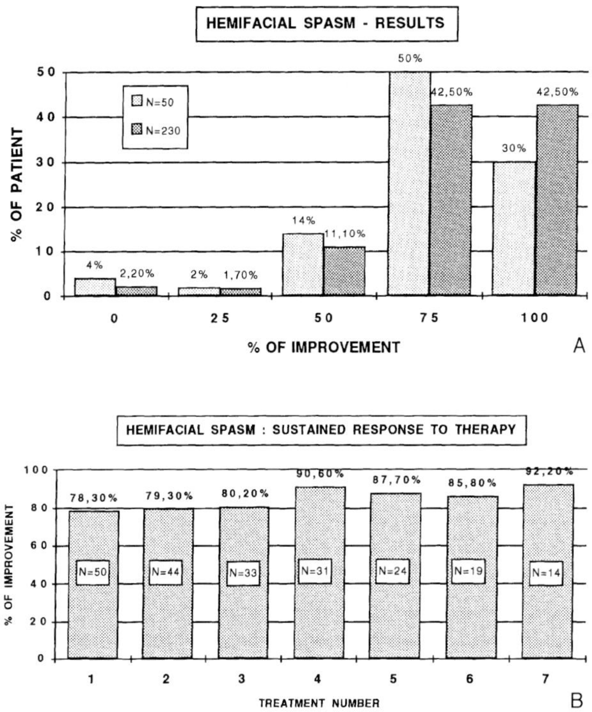

Fig. 2. **A** Precentage of improvement after the first injection (N = 50) and after all of the injections (N%230). More than 80% of the patients report a beneficial effect of 75% improvement or more. **B** There is a sustained improvement after each therapy session

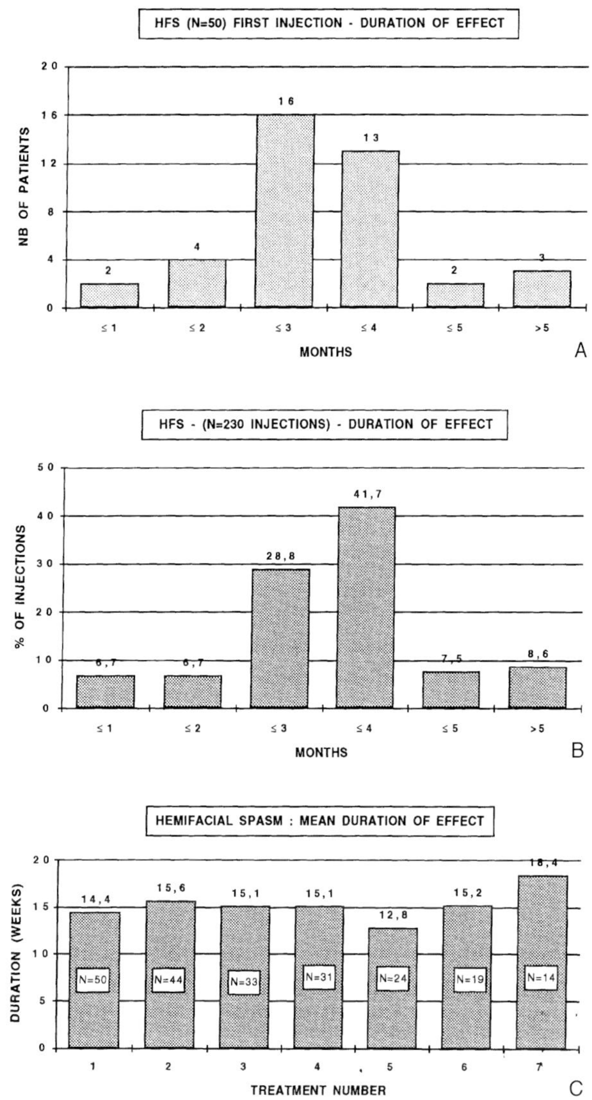

Fig. 3. Duration of improvement after the first injection (**A**) and after all of the injections (**B**). There is a sustained duration of effect after each therapy session (**C**)

injections revealed similar results, with the number of totally satisified patients being greater than those who had no improvement. Long-term follow-up of improvement (Fig. 2B) after each injection (1 to 7 sets) revealed a sustained response to BT and even a slight increase in effectiveness following latter injections (mean value of improvement was 78% for the first injection in 50 patients, and 92% for a smaller group of patients following the seventh set of injections). With repeated injections all of the patients experienced some beneficial effects.

An improvement in HFS occurred within the first week of the first session. The mean delay of improvement was 5.2 days (median 2 days, range of 0 to 15 days). The mean duration of effect was 14.7 weeks after the first injection (Fig. 3A), and 15 weeks with a maximal value of 77 weeks (Fig. 3B) after all of the injections. Long-term follow-up revealed sustained results in mean duration of improvement (Fig. 3C).

There were no systemic complications. All side effects were transitory and abated within 2 to 3 weeks. The incidence of side effects was not rare, as they occurred in one third of the injections and in 30 of the 50 patients (see Table 1).

Discussion

The effectiveness of BT injections in treating HFS is well established by a placebo-controlled blind study [26] and by numerous open trials [1, 4, 7, 9, 10, 14, 15, 18, 20, 22, 24, 27] that are summarized in Table 2. A beneficial effect is reported in more than 90% of BT-treated patients. Our results are consistent with these findings.

Table 1. Complications after BT injections related to the number of patients (N = 50) and to the number of injections (N = 230)

Complications (%)	N = 50	N = 230
% of Patients	60	74
% of Injections	60	34
Blurred vision	14	7,4
Burning	12	5,6
Weakness		
– upper	12	5,2
– lower	8	5,6
Ptosis	6	4,3
Tearing	10	3,5
Dry eye	4	1,7
Diplopia	4	1,3
Hematomas	4	1,3
Keratitis	0	0,4

How BT improves HFS

The straightforward explanation of BT efficacy in treating HFS is its peripheral action on the neuromuscular junction. However, several uncertainties remain concerning both the pathophysiology of HFS and the possible other neurological targets of BT action.

With regard to the pathophysiology of HFS, the site of the generation of the spasms remains controversial. Twitches can be due either to abnormal discharges peripheral to the facial nucleus (ectopic excitation, ephaptic transmission, and lateral spread of impulses), or to hyperexcitability of the facial nucleus. In the latter case, a central action of BT may be indicated. Indeed, botulinum toxin, like tetanus toxin, can be carried by retrograde intraaxonal transport to motoneurones [25]. In this line one could expect that BT could modify the reactions of brainstem interneurons. However, Geller et al. [11] demonstrated that after BT injection, whenever spasms disappear clinically, there persists abnormal electromyographic responses such as spontaneous bursts, after activity following stimulation of distal branches of the facial nerve, blink reflex, and synkinesis. In addition, only the amplitude of the muscle responses to stimulation decreases due to a reduction in the number of muscle fibers. Thus it is readily understandable that local denervation of the periocular muscles is sufficient to reduce the intensity of facial spasms. Another possible mechanism has been suggested by Hallett et al. [12]. BT apparently acts by preferentially blocking the neuromuscular junctions of the muscle fibers that are involved in the involuntary movements of HFS while leaving other muscle fibers relatively spared. The beneficial effects on spasms of the muscles of the lower face [16] following BT injections that are limited to the periocular muscles can include the BT spreading or the synkinetic decrease.

What are the main side effects after BT injection?

The main side effects of BT injections result from excessive dosages or excessive spreading. In fact, most of the side effects are well tolerated by the patients, and they rarely renounce reinjection because of the side effects. Most patients stated that the improvement in their HFS outweighed the inconvenience of any side effects that occurred. Moreover, all complications have been transient.

Ptosis is one of the most frequent complications following BT injections and clinically it is the most relevant one. Ptosis seems to be dose-dependent [6], and the risk of developing ptosis increases with the number of reinjections. Ptosis results from weakness of the levator palpebrae superioris muscle due to BT spreading. This muscle is more sensitive to the effects of the toxin than are the extraocular muscles, and injection near the mid-portion of the upper eyelid must be avoided.

Excessive weakness of the orbicularis oculi muscles produces Souques' sign in its minor form, which is clinically well tolerated, or Charles Bell's sign in its major form. Excessive lower facial weakness can be the result of excessive amounts of BT injected into the lower territory of the face or of local spreading of BT to the zygomatic muscles from a more inferior and external injection site in the orbicularis oculi muscles. Electromyographic abnormalities detected before BT injection could indicate a risk factor for excessive facial palsy following BT injection [3]. In our experience, the incidence of these side effects was greater following first injection as compared to subsequent injections. Dose modifications were sufficient to avoid recurrence of the side effects.

Which muscle should be injected?

To avoid BT spreading some investigators have injected the toxin as close to the motor endpoint as possible, after identifying it by percutaneous electrical stimulation. In fact, the response is better when BT is injected in different sites in the muscle [6]. Our own experience in the few patients in this study is in accord with indications that multiple injection sites are su-

Table 2. Some American and European reports using the two different presentations of BT-A. (*) indicates the percentage of patients with more than 75% improvement. Units are different for Oculinum (*U*) and Dysport (*u*), with a 1 to 4 ratio. In some reports, the side effects are mixed (*mx*) and concern blepharospasms and hemifacial spasms

Series	Savino	Biglan	Dutton	Jankovic	Adenis	Flanders	Yu	Soulayrol	Elston	Jedynak	Ruban	Vial
Date	1985	1988	1988	1990	1990	1993	1992	1992	1992	1993	1993	1994
N° of patients	15	24	60	13	35	51	12	46	73	54	72	50
N° of injections	20	70	148	29	–	241	76	–	–	—	280	230
Inject/patients	1	2,9	–	2,2	–	4,7	6,3	–	–	3,9	–	4,5
Duration (w)	12,2	–	14,4	15,1	13	17,4	10,8	–	15	9	10	15
Response rate(%)	100	100	96,9	92	92	100	94,7	91	75*	83	83*	83*
BT	Oculinum	Oculinum	Oculinum	Oculinum	Oculinum	Oculinum	Dysport	Dysport	Dysport	Dysport	Ocul. + Dysp.	Dysport
Mean dose	17,5U	37,9U	12,5-25U	17,5U	25U	34U	(?)	88u	120u	104u	–	60u
Complications(%)	35	18,6	(mx) 22,6	–	(ms) 13,4	–	–	17	19*33	–	16	34
Ptosis	–	20%	7,30%	–	–	8%	16,6%	–	–	16%	–	6%
Weakness	20%	5,70%	1,10%	21%	–	–	75%p	–	–	–	–	10,80%
Tearing	20%	–	1,10%	–	–	–	–	–	–	–	–	3,50%
Dry eyes	–	–	7,50%	–	–	–	–	–	–	–	–	1,70%

perior to a single motor point [14]. This can probably be explained by the diffuse innervation zone for the upper orbicularis muscle [5]. On the other hand, the number of complications can be correlated with the number of injection points [9].

The choice of injection sites is critical. The major symptoms of HFS are due to spasmodic eye closure, and abolishing this alone is often sufficient to relieve the patient's discomfort. We prefer to inject BT botulinum in the lower facial muscles only on the second or third injection session, if the patient's condition requires and, if so, only after the risks of lower facial weakness are fully explained to the patient.

Which optimal dose of BT should be administered to the patient?

Two different preparations of BT-A are available (Botox^R and Dysport^R), but the units are different with a ratio of 1 to 4. For each of these manufactured BT, the range of mean doses is large (see Table 2). In fact, doses of BT depend on age, severity of spasm, and the patient's susceptibility. We prefer to use a low dose for the first injection to test susceptibility of the patient and, if necessary, we increase the dose for the second injection. Our BT doses are lower than those used in other series [9, 15, 18, 24, 27]. Usually, 40 to 50 units (Dysport^R) are sufficient for the first injection into the orbicularis oculi muscle and 10 units are sufficient for injection into the lower facial muscles using a different dilution).

Long-term efficacy and safety

A sustained effect of BT after each injection was observed in our series that had a follow-up of 46 months. These results are in accordance with other series that had a longer follow-up of 7 years [9, 10].

What is the "curative" effect of BT? The therapeutic effect of BT on HFS is largely symptomatic. However, a more lasting effect may be expected over a long time. After repetitive injections, successive denervation may overstep the sprouting process and induce a sustained relief of spasm via a muscle weakness. However, as yet such a phenomenon has not been demonstrated.

Can there be an acquired immunization to BT? The development of a resistance to BT after repeated injections is largely debated [13]. Such an acquired immunization seems possible when treating spasmodic torticollis, but it has not been demonstrated in patients treated for HFS. The risk of sensitization is probably less in patients with HFS, because the dose requirement for treating HFS is lower. Moreover, antibody production to BT-A appears to have no direct effect on the patient's clinical response to treatment [23].

Are there systemic effects of BT? Single fiber electromyographic abnormalities have been demonstrated in distant muscles after BT injection to treat HFS (19). These abnormalities remain in all cases subclinical. However, future studies will have to precise if these distant effects may be cumulative.

Place of BT injections in hemifacial spasm therapy

The effectiveness of microvascular facial nerve decompression has been demonstrated (see other chapters in this book), but definite complications to this procedure such as hearing loss and facial weakness have been reported. Transitory effectiveness constitutes the great advantage of treatment with BT, but it is also its main disadvantage. BT therapy can be considered an effective and safe therapy for controlling HFS. The use of BT in treating HFS is particularly advised in three situations: 1) in the beginning stages of HFS, when the spasms are mild; 2) when the patient is a poor operative candidate or simply refuses to undergo neurosurgical decompression; and 3) if the patient develops recurrent muscle spasms following neurosurgical decompression. In fact, it is our experience that most HFS patients would prefer having BT injections as the initial therapy for their disorder.

References

1. Adenis JP, Smolik I, Maes S (1990) Traitement des spasmes faciaux par la toxine botulinique A. J Fr Ophthalmol 13/5: 259–264
2. American Academy of Ophthalmology (1989) Botulinum toxin therapy of eye muscle disorders. Safety and effectiveness. Ophthalmology (Instrument and Book Issue) 37–41
3. Angibaud G, Simonetta-Moreau M, Rascol O, Clanet M (1995) Treatment of hemifacial spasm with botulinum toxin. Eur Neurol 35: 43–45
4. Biglan AW, May M, Bowes RA (1988) Management of facial spasm with clostridium botulinum toxin, Type A (Oculinum). Arch Otolaryngol 114: 1407–1412
5. Borodic GE, Cozzolino D, Ferrante R, Wieger AW, Young RR (1991) Innervation zone of orbicularis oculi muscle and implications for botulinum A toxin therapy. Ophthalmic Plast Reconstr Surg 7/1: 54–50
6. Borodic GE (1994) Hemifacial spasm: evaluation and management with emphasis on botulinum toxin therapy. In: Jankovic J, Hallett M (eds) Therapy with botulinum toxin. Marcel Dekker, New York, pp 331–351
7. Dutton JJ, Buckley EG (1988) Long term results and complications of botulinum toxin in the treatment of blepharospasm. Ophthalmology 95: 1529–1534
8. Elston JS, Russell RW (1985) Effect of treatment with Botulinum toxin on neurogenic blepharospasm. Br Med J 290: 1857–1859
9. Elston JS (1992) The management of blepharospasm and hemifacial spasm. J Neurol 1: 5–8
10. Flanders M, Chin D, Boghen D (1993) Botulinum toxin: preferred treatment for hemifacial spasm. Eur Neurol 33: 316–319
11. Geller B, Hallett M, Ravits J (1989) Botulinum toxin therapy in hemifacial spasm: clinical and electrophysiologic studies. Muscle and Nerve 12: 716–722
12. Hallett M, Glocker FX, Deuschl G (1994) Mechanism of action of Botulinum toxin. Ann Neurol 36: 449–450
13. Hambleton P, Cohen HE, Palmer BJ, Melling J (1992) Antitoxins and botulinum toxin treatment. Br Med J 304: 959–960
14. Jankovic J, Schwartz K, Donovan DT (1990) Botulinum toxin treatment of cranial cervical dystonia, spasmodic dysphonia, other focal dystonias and hemifacial spasm. JNNP 53: 633–639
15. Jedynak CP, Palfi S, Vidailhet M, Kullmann B (1993) Traitement du spasme hémifacial par la toxine botulique. Rev Neurol 149/3: 202–206
16. Mauriello JA, Coniaris H, Haupt EJ (1987) Use of botulinum toxin in the treatment of one hundred patients with facial dyskinesia. Ophthalmology 94: 976–979
17. Report on the Therapeutics and Technology Assessment Subcommittee of the American Academy of Neurology (1990) Assessment: The clinical usefulness of botulinum toxin-A in treating neurologic disorders. Neurology 40: 1332–1336
18. Ruban JM, Pelissier de Feligonde O, Benillouche P (1993) Analyse de l'éfficacite de la toxine botulique A dans le traitement du blépharospasme et de l'hémispasme facial. A propos de 160 cas. Ophtalmologie 7/6: 481–482
19. Sanders DB, Massey EW, Buckley EC (1986) Botulinum toxin for blepharospasm: single fiber EMG studies. Neurology 36: 545–547
20. Savino PJ, Sergott RC, Bosley TM, Schatz NJ (1985) Hemispasm facial treated with botulinum A toxin injection. Arch Ophthalmol 103: 1305–1306
21. Scott AB (1981) Botulinum toxin injections to eye muscles to correct strabismus. J Am Ophthalmol 79: 734–770
22. Scott AB, Kennedy RA, Stubbs HA (1985) Botulinum A toxin injections as a treatment for blepharospasm. Arch Ophthalmol 103: 347–350
23. Siatkowski RM, Tytyunikov A, Biglan AW, Scalise D, Genovese C, Raikow RB, Kenerdell JS, Feuer WJ (1993) Serum antibody production to botulinum A toxin. Ophthalmology 100: 1861–1866
24. Soulayrol S, Caperan A, Penot-Ragon C, Beaulieu JP, Gastaut JL (1993) Traitements par injections locales de toxine botulique en neurologie. Presse Med 22: 957–963
25. Wiegand H, Erdmann G, Wellhoner HH (1976) I125-labeled botulinum A neurotoxin: pharmacokinetics in cats after intramuscular injection. Naunyn-Schmiedebergs Arch Pharmacol 292: 161–165
26. Yoshimura DM, Aminoff MJ, Tami TA, Scott AB (1992) Treatment of hemifacial spasm with botulinum toxin. Muscle and Nerve 15: 1045–1049
27. Yu YL, Fong KY, Chang CM (1992) Treatment of idiopathic hemifacial spasm with botulinum toxin. Acta Neurol Scand 85: 55–57

Correspondence: Christophe Vial, M.D., EMG Laboratory, Botulinum Toxin Clinic, Hôpital Neurologique, 59 boulevard Pinel, F-69003 Lyon, France.

Hemifacial spasm: treatment with botulinum toxin (long-term results)

M.-H. Marion

Summary

The first report of the beneficial effects of botulinum toxin in treating hemifacial spasm appeared ten years ago; subsequent reports have confirmed these benefits, and these reports are reviewed here. The results of long-term (5 year) follow are also presented and details on the injection technique are discussed.

Key words: Long-term results, botulinum toxin, hemifacial spasm.

Introduction

There have been many reports [1–11] on the treatment of hemifacial spasm (HFS) with botulinum toxin (Botox). These articles as well as the pharmacology of this toxin are reviewed in the present paper, and the technical aspects of injection technique are discussed. The long-term results of a personal series of patients (author's private practice) with a 5-year follow-up are presented and discussed.

Pharmacology of botulinum toxin

Botulinum toxin is the most powerful neurotoxin known to man. There are eight distinct botulinum toxins labelled A, B, C1, C2, D, E, F and G, that are produced by the bacterium, Clostridium botuli [12]. Type A is used for human therapy. Botulism is an acute symmetrical descending paralytic illness that follows the ingestion of food (most often imperfectly sterilized canned food) that contains the botulinum toxin A, B and E produced under anaerobic conditions by Clostridium botuli. The structure of botulinum toxin is now well established; it has a heavy chain (molecular weight of 1,000,000) and a light chain (molecular weight of 50,000), joined together by a disulfide bridge [13]. The paralytic effect of botulinum toxin is explained by a peripheral action of the toxin on the neuromuscular junction. Botulinum toxin blocks the release of acetylcholine from nerve terminals. The action of botulinum toxin on the neuromuscular junction is based on three steps [13]; 1) a specific and saturable binding to presynaptic nerve membranes, 2) an active internalization, and 3) an intracellular activity. The exact process by which the toxin prevents the release of acetylcholine from the presynaptic vesicles has recently been elucidated. Botulinum toxin A is a zinc protein [14] with an enzymatic activity that selectively cleaves the synaptic protein SNAP-25 [15]. However, the paralysis is transient because of the apparition of new neuromuscular junctions sprouting from presynaptic axons [16].

There are two preparation of botulinum toxin available. The American botulinum toxin, now commercialized by Allergan Co., was first named Oculinum and then Botox. The English botulinum toxin, commercialized by Speywood, is named Dysport. There is no dose standardization between the two preparations [17]. Laboratories [18] and clinical data [19] suggest the ratio 1:3. One unit of Botox is equivalent to 3 units of Dysport.

Review of the literature

Savino et al. [6] reported the successful treatment of 15 patients with hemifacial spasm (HFS) with botulinum toxin. They injected 2.5 units of Oculinum (Allergan) in each of 5 sites in the orbicularis oculi and 2 sites in the zygomatic major. Two patients were injected on more than one occasion. All patients reported relief from their spasms for approximately 12.2 weeks after treatment began. Complications included excessive tear production in 4 patients, corneal exposure in 1 patient, ectropion in 1 patient, and some facial weakness that lasted no more than 2 weeks. Some investigators [1–5, 9–10] reported results with Oculinum (Allergan) using a similar protocol for injection sites and dosages that confirmed the beneficial effects of botulinum toxin in treating patients with HFS.

Elston [7, 8] published two reports on 6 and 73 patients, respectively, using Dysport (Speywood). In these reports Elston compared the long-term results of these patients in which he used two different protocols of injection with the same initial standard dose of 120 units (Dysport) in the orbicularis oculi muscle. The first protocol involved 4 injection sites (40 units lateral and 20 units medially at the junction of the orbital and preseptal orbicularis oculi muscle) resulted in 15 weeks improvement and a 33% incidence of side effects (lid oedema, partial ptosis, entropion, and lid droop). The second protocol, which omitted the lower medial site and for which the injections were given farther from the lid margin in the orbital orbicularis oculi muscle, resulted in a slightly shorter period of improvement (12 weeks) but fewer side effects (19% incidence rate). In both treatment groups, the spasms were reduced by 75% and Elston concluded that botulinum toxin is the simplest and safest treatment for HFS.

Jedynak et al. [11] published the results of their series of 54 patients with HFS; final results were available on 42 of the 54 patients, with 57% of the 42 patients reporting an overall improvement of more than 50%. However, when Jedynak adjusted his injection protocol, a final benefit of more than 50% in 24 of 27 patients was achieved. The final average effective dose was 104 units (using Dysport). Jedynak's initial protocol that involved 3 injection sites in the orbicularis oculi muscle and 1 injection site in the levator labii superior muscle was abandoned because of side effects; instead these investigators opted for a protocol that involved 2 injection sites in the orbicularis oculi muscle and 1 injection site in the zygomatic major muscle. The mean interval between injections was 9 weeks (injections were given at all 3 sites every 9 weeks). The most frequent side effect was ptosis, which was observed in 1 out of 6 injections.

All these reports are open studies, with variations in the toxin chosen for treatment, in the sites of injection, in the initial standard dose, and in the criteria for benefit evaluation and need for re-injection. However, these reports mentioned above (from America, England, and France) are representative of the beneficial effects of Botox in treating HFS.

Long term follow-up in this personal series of HFS patients treated with botulinum toxin

Patients and methods

The present author looked in more detail at the long-term results of 68 patients with HFS who were treated with botulinum toxin. Of these 68 patients, 28 had been followed for 3.5 to 7.2 years (4.75 years average). Forty of these 68 patients had dropped out of our follow-up study for various reasons (see Table 1).

Initial doses and injection sites depended very much on a clinical assessment of each patient, particularly with regard to the frequency and severity of the spasms and the patient's age. At each follow up visit, the dosage and the site of injection were adjusted, depending on the initial improvement in the spasms, duration of benefit, and any side effects.

Results

The patients were followed for 3.5 to 7.2 years (mean 4.75 years) and the number of injections was between 4 and 29 (average 13.4). The average initial effective dose (in practice, usually the second injection) was 84 units (Dysport) for the orbicularis oculi muscle and 12 units (Dysport) for the muscles of the lower face, with the average duration of improvement being 16 weeks (see Table 2).

The average dose for the last injection was 72 units (Dysport) for the eyes and 20 units (Dysport) for the

Table 1. 1988–1994: 256 patients

HFS Patients seen before 1990: 68	
Follow up:	28
Surgery:	5
Other center:	15
Lost:	20

Table 2. Long term result

	Eye	Lower Face	Benefit Duration
Initial dose (units)	84	12	16 weeks
Final dose (units)	72	20	13 weeks

mouth (risorius muscle). For 25 patients, the average duration of improvement of the spasm was 13 weeks; 3 patients had been in remission for more than 18 months and did not require further injection.

Side effects of these treatments included partial ptosis, vertical diplopia, blurred vision, excessive tearing, exposure keratitis, lower facial weakness, and a lop-sided smile. The incidence of side effects was 15% at the beginning of treatment and 4% following adjustment of the injection site and dose. In particular, diplopia and lower facial weakness were no longer seen in any of the patients at the last follow-up visit.

Discussion

All of the studies mentioned above confirm the beneficial effects of botulinum toxin in treating HFS. Three points need to be considered:

1) Site of injections

The American studies [6, 10, 20] traditionally used 5 periocular sites and didn't indicate any change in their injection strategy. The English study [8] started with 4 periocular sites but the lower medial site was omitted and, in general, the injection sites were moved farther from the lid margin to minimize any side effects.

The present author also adjusted the subsequent sites of injection, depending on the exact location and severity of the spasms. For example, with a predominant upper lid spasm, pretarsal injections were performed. If the spasm was predominant in the orbital part, the injection site was moved farther from the lid margin. Additional injections above the middle of the eyebrow at the junction between the frontalis and the orbicularis oculi muscles were helpful when the forehead was markedly involved in spasm. When the mouth was involved in the spasms, injections into the levator labii superior muscle or the zygomatic major muscle often resulted in a disfiguring droop of the upper lip and a lop-sided smile. Spasms of the lower part of the face can be predominant in patients with HFS, and they can produce a severe cosmetic disability. For the last 4 years, we have injected the risorius muscle with up to 40 units (Dysport) without noticing any side effects. This muscle should be injected in the line of the smile, just lateral to the nasolabial fold. Additional injections of the platysma are indicated when this muscle is involved in the HFS.

2) Dosage

It is our experience that the average effective dose of Dysport is 72 units per eye. However, there is a large range of 20 to 130 units (Dysport) that is acceptable for treatment of HFS; low dosages are used for elderly patients with mild HFS-higher dosages are used for patients with severe facial spasms. Hence, it's important to adjust the dosage according to clinical circumstances. It is also important to remember that 1 unit of Dysport (Speywood) is not the same as 1 unit of Botox (Allergan); the approximate clinical equivalence is 3:1 (i.e., 3 units Dysport = 1 unit Botox).

The present study also shows that there is little difference between the average dosage of 84 units (Dysport) at the beginning of treatment and 72 units (Dysport) after 5 years. Hence this study has shown no evidence of toxin resistance. The slight reduction from 84 to 72 units (Dysport) is probably due to attempts to minimize side effects; this may explain also the slightly shorter average duration of improvement in the spasm (4 to 3 months). It is also interesting to note that 3 patients appeared to be in remission since their last injection and they have not required further injections since that time. Whether this result is spontaneous or is related to treatment remains to be judged.

The earlier injection site for the lower face (in the levator labii superior muscle or in the zygomatic major muscle) was often associated with side effects that necessitated lowering the dose; if the injection is made in the risorius muscle, a more effective dose (20 units Dysport) can be given that will result in an improvement without side effects.

3) Side effects

Side effects are related to both the site of injection and the dosage, and they are probably due to local diffusion. We believe that our low incidence of side effects is due to the individual assessment of each patient; we do not employ identical doses and sites for each case. Rather, the treatment is carefully adjusted to each patient, taking into consideration the patient's age, the severity and extent of the spasms, and the response to previous injections.

Conclusions

Many trials have shown that botulinum toxin is effective in the treatment of HFS, and this is confirmed by our long-term follow-up study. Dose and injection sites around the eye must be adjusted for each patient and the lower face should be injected in the risorius muscle to preserve facial symmetry. Repeated injections at 3–4 month intervals continue to be as effective, without evidence of toxin resistance or other new side effects.

References

1. Frueh BR, Felt DP, Wojno TH, Musch DC (1984) Treatment of blepharospasm with botulinum toxin A: A preliminary report. Arch Ophthalmol 102: 1464–1468
2. Shorr N, Seiff SR, Jopelman J (1985) The use of botulinum toxin in blepharospasm. Am J Ophthalmol 99: 542–546
3. Lingua RW (1985) Sequelae of botulinum toxin injection. Am J Ophthalmol 100: 305–307
4. Mauriello JA (1985) Blepharospasm. Meige syndrome and hemifacial spasm: treatment with botulinum toxin. Neurology 35: 1499–1500
5. Dutton JJ, Buckley EG (1986) Botulinum toxin in the management of blepharospasm. Arch Neurol 43: 380–382
6. Savino PJ, Sergott RC, Bosley TM, Schatz NJ (1985) Hemifacial spasm treated with botulinum toxin A injection. Arch Ophthalmol 103: 1305–1306
7. Elston JS (1986) Botulinum toxin treatment of hemifacial spasm. J Neurol Neurosurg Psychiatry 49: 827–829
8. Elston JS (1992) The management of blepharospasm and hemifacial spasm. J Neurol 239: 5–8
9. Tolosa E, Marti MJ, Kulisevsky J (1988) Botulinum toxin injection therapy for hemifacial spasm. In: Jankovic J, Tolosa E (eds) Advances in neurology, vol. 49. Raven Press, New York, pp 479–491
10. Jankovic J, Schwartz K, Donovan DT (1990) Botulinum toxin treatment of cranial-cervical dystonia, spasmodic dysphonia, other focal dystonias and hemifacial spasm. J Neurol Neurosurg Psychiatry 53: 633–639
11. Jedynak CP, Palfi S, Vidailhet M, Kullmann B (1993) Traitement du spasme hemifacial par la toxine botulique. Rev Neurol (Paris) 149: 202–206
12. Simpson LL (1981) The origin, structure and pharmacological activity of botulinum toxin. Pharmacol Rev 33: 155–188
13. Melling J, Hambleton P, Shone CC (1988) Clostridium botulinum toxins: nature and preparation for clinical use. Eye 2: 16–23
14. Schiavo G, Rossetto A, Santucci A, Das Gupta BR, Montecucco C (1992) Botulinum neurotoxins are zinc proteins. J Biol Chem 267: 23479–23483
15. Blasi J, Chapman ER, Link E, Binz T, Yamasaki S, Camilli P, Sudhoff TC, Niemann H, Jahn R (1993) Botulinum neurotoxin A selectively cleaves the synaptic protein SNAP-25. Nature 365: 160–163
16. Duchen LOW (1971) An electron microscope study of the changes induced by botulinum toxin in the motor end plates of slow and fast skeletal muscles fibers of the mouse. J Neurol Sci 14: 47–60
17. Quinn N, Hallet M (1989) Dose standardization of botulinum toxin. Lancet i: 964
18. Pickett AM, Hambleton P (1994) Dose standardisation of Botulinum toxin. Lancet 344: 474–475
19. Marion MH, Sheehy M, Sangla S, Soulayrol S (1995) Dose standardisation of Botulinum toxin. J Neurol Neurosurg Psychiatry 58: 102–103
20. Jankovic J, Brin MF (1991) Therapeutic uses of botulinum toxin. N Engl J Med 324: 1186–1194

Correspondence: Marie-Helene Marion, M.D., 4 rue Leon Delhomme, F-75015 Paris, France.

Conclusions

Hemifacial spasm (HFS) consists of unilateral paroxysmal involuntary tonic-clonic spasms occurring in the muscles innervated by the facial nerve.

In almost every case operated on an arterial compression of the facial nerve at its root exit zone from the brain stem could be found. In a majority of cases it was an arterial loop originating from the posterior-inferior cerebellar artery, in most of the other cases it belonged to the anterior-inferior cerebellar artery. The neuro-vascular conflict (i.e., a cross-compression of the inferior aspect of the root exit zone) can almost always be seen on MRI combined with AngioMR.

Botulinum toxin is able to alleviate the symptoms, most often transiently. The definitive conservative treatment is microvascular decompression. In experts' hands and under intraoperative electrophysiological monitoring (BEAP recordings for hearing) and EMG recordings (for checking the good quality of the decompression), the MVD procedure is generally effective, and with minimal morbidity and rare mortality.

Springer-Verlag and the Environment

WE AT SPRINGER-VERLAG FIRMLY BELIEVE THAT AN international science publisher has a special obligation to the environment, and our corporate policies consistently reflect this conviction.

WE ALSO EXPECT OUR BUSINESS PARTNERS – PRINTERS, paper mills, packaging manufacturers, etc. – to commit themselves to using environmentally friendly materials and production processes.

THE PAPER IN THIS BOOK IS MADE FROM NO-CHLORINE pulp and is acid free, in conformance with international standards for paper permanency.